Nurses as Health Teachers

A Practical Guide

JUDITH WARING RORDEN, RN, MS, BSEd

Program Director, KOALA Associates
San Jose, California

W. B. SAUNDERS COMPANY

Harcourt Brace Jovanovich, Inc.
Philadelphia, London, Toronto, Montreal, Sydney, Tokyo

W. B. Saunders Company: The Curtis Center
                          Independence Square West
                          Philadelphia, PA 19106

Library of Congress Cataloging-in-Publication Data

Rorden, Judith Waring.

Nurses as health teachers.

Bibliography: p.

1. Patient education.   2. Nurse and patient.
   I. Title.   [DNLM: 1. Nurse-Patient Relations.
   2. Patient Education—nurses' instruction.
   WY 87 R7878n]

RT90.3.R67   1987   610'.7   86–27913

ISBN 0–7216–1804–9

Acquisition Editor: Dudley Kay
Production Manager: Frank Polizzano
Manuscript Editor: Barbara Hodgson
Indexer: Judith Waring Rorden

NURSES AS HEALTH TEACHERS—*A Practical Guide*   ISBN 0–7216–1804–9

Last digit is the print number: 9   8   7   6   5   4   3

ACKNOWLEDGMENTS

I would like to express my thanks to those who participated in special ways in the completion of *Nurses as Health Teachers*. I am especially indebted to James P. McLennan for his significant contribution to Chapters 3 and 8. As a long-time colleague, good friend, and former coauthor (Waring and McLennan, 1979), he has positively influenced my thinking on many of the issues discussed in this book. I would also like to thank those who reviewed the manuscript, giving me helpful guidance for its improvement, especially Edwina McConnell and Susan Berg-Levy. The efforts of Dudley Kay, publisher, and the production staff of W.B. Saunders Company, especially those of Donna Walker and Al Beringer, are greatly appreciated. I would also like to thank my husband, Bud, for his continued encouragement, loving support, and technical assistance in the preparation of the manuscript.

JUDITH WARING RORDEN

CONTENTS

FIGURES, TABLES, EXAMPLES viii

INTRODUCTION xi

1

PATIENT TEACHING AND THE NURSE 1

1.1 Nurse-Patient Interaction and Teaching............................ 3
1.2 Nursing Process and Patient Teaching 6
1.3 Issues That Influence Patient Teaching 10
1.4 A Historical Perspective on Patient Teaching..................... 18

Summary.. 23
Study Questions and Exercises 23

2

THE PATIENT AND THE LEARNING PROCESS.. 25

2.1 An Overview of the Learning Process 27
2.2 Experience as a Factor in Learning 32
2.3 Perception of Need as a Factor in Learning 38
2.4 The Social and Cultural Context of Learning..................... 46
2.5 Stress and Its Effects on Learning 52

Summary.. 61
Study Questions and Exercises 62

3

THE NURSE-PATIENT RELATIONSHIP AND TEACHING 64

3.1 How to Encourage Trust... 66
3.2 How to Use Nonverbal Communication Skills 70
3.3 How to Use Questions Effectively................................. 75
3.4 How Personalities Interact 77

Summary.. 83
Study Questions and Exercises 84

v

4

HOW TO PREPARE FOR TEACHING 88

4.1   How to Assess a Patient's Health Balance 90
4.2   How to Gather Assessment Data 94
4.3   How to Identify Learning Goals and State Objectives............. 101
4.4   How to Plan Teaching Intervention 108

Summary... *112*
Study Questions and Exercises *112*

5

HOW TO CHOOSE AND USE TEACHING STRATEGIES 114

5.1   What to Consider When Choosing a Teaching Strategy 116
5.2   Using Explanation or Lecture as a Teaching Strategy 123
5.3   Using Discussion as a Teaching Strategy 127
5.4   Using Demonstration-Coaching as a Teaching Strategy.......... 131
5.5   Using Experimental Strategies: Role Play, Behavioral Rehearsal, and Exercises.. 134

Summary... *141*
Study Questions and Exercises *141*

6

HOW TO CHOOSE AND USE TEACHING MATERIALS 143

6.1   Choosing Effective Teaching Materials 146
6.2   Using Written Materials... 150
6.3   Using Pictures and Diagrams 157
6.4   Using Audiovisual Programs....................................... 160
6.5   Using Self-Paced Learning Programs 164

Summary... *165*
Study Questions and Exercises *166*

7

HOW TO USE SPONTANEOUS TEACHING OPPORTUNITIES........................ 168

7.1   Handling Requests for Advice and Information................... 171
7.2   Responding to Requests for Diagnosis............................ 176
7.3   Handling Complaints and Complex Problems 179
7.4   Teaching Without Preparation 184

Summary... *189*
Study Questions and Exercises *190*

8

WHEN AND HOW TO USE LEARNING GROUPS..................................... 192

    8.1   How Groups Promote Learning...................................... 195
    8.2   Planning and Organizing a Learning Group...................... 200
    8.3   Leading Group Learning 208
    8.4   Making Referrals to Community Groups........................... 213

    Summary.. 217
    Study Questions and Exercises 217

9

HOW TO EVALUATE LEARNING...................................... 219

    9.1   Making Use of Feedback During Teaching 221
    9.2   Evaluating Learning by Observing Behavior...................... 226
    9.3   Using Verbal Methods of Evaluation 231
    9.4   Avoiding Evaluation Errors.. 234

    Summary.. 237
    Study Questions and Exercises 238

10

HOW TO DEVELOP A PATIENT EDUCATION PROGRAM 239

    10.1   The Assessment Phase of Program Development 241
    10.2   The Planning Phase of Program Development.................. 245
    10.3   The Organizational Phase of Program Development 249
    10.4   The Implementation Phase of Program Development.......... 253
    10.5   A Checklist for Program Development.......................... 257

    Summary.. 265
    Study Questions and Exercises 265

Appendix A   APPROACHES TO COMMON PATIENT-TEACHING SITUATIONS 267

    App 1.   Admission Teaching 267
    App 2.   Properative or Pretreatment Teaching......................... 272
    App 3.   Teaching Patient Care Procedures............................. 277
    App 4.   Discharge Teaching 284

    Summary.. 288

Appendix B   SOURCES OF EDUCATIONAL MATERIALS INFORMATION.......... 289

REFERENCES AND BIBLIOGRAPHY 293

INDEX 299

FIGURES, TABLES, EXAMPLES

LIST OF FIGURES AND TABLES

FIGURE 1–1   Influences on the teaching role of nurses 3
FIGURE 1–2   Phases of the nursing process 8
TABLE 1–1   Ethical Questions Related to Informed Consent 13
TABLE 1–2   Preparing for Discussion of Patient Teaching Role 17

FIGURE 2–1   Factors influencing the learning process 28
FIGURE 2–2   An apparent lack of relevant experience......................... 29
FIGURE 2–3   Help with recognizing a need to learn 30
TABLE 2–1   Learning Principles and Factors That Influence Learning 31
TABLE 2–2   Piaget's Stages of Cognitive Development....................... 36
TABLE 2–3   Levels of Learning 37
FIGURE 2–4   Maslow's Hierarchy of Needs 39
TABLE 2–4   Helping to Meet Patients' Basic Needs 42
TABLE 2–5   Beliefs About Control Over Health............................... 44
TABLE 2–6   Elements of the Health Belief Model............................. 45
FIGURE 2–5   Components of a patient's social world.......................... 47
FIGURE 2–6   Stress gauge... 55

FIGURE 3–1   The expressive and instrumental roles of the nurse 66
TABLE 3–1   Attitudes Toward Helping Others 70
TABLE 3–2   Summary of Jung's Personality Dimensions.................... 83

FIGURE 4–1   The health balance model 91
TABLE 4–1   Sources of patient data.. 96
FIGURE 4–2   Steps in the "CONE" interview.................................. 98
TABLE 4–2   Notes for Health Balance Assessment Interview 100
TABLE 4–3   Comparison of Goals of Care Terminology.................... 104
TABLE 4–4   The Care Planning Process....................................... 107
TABLE 4–5   Levels of Learning 109
TABLE 4–6   A Teaching Outline 112

TABLE 5–1   Sequence of Steps in a Lesson................................... 119

FIGURE 6–1   Pamphlet on breast self-examination 154

FIGURE   6–2   Graphs showing risks to smokers 159
FIGURE   6–3   Prompts for learner responses 165

FIGURE   7–1   Goals of personal problem solving............................. 172

TABLE   8–1   Behaviors That Promote Group Process 208
TABLE   8–2   Summary of Group Leadership Strategies 214

FIGURE   9–1   Feedback and the Nursing Process "system"................. 221
TABLE   9–1   Sources of Feedback 222
TABLE   9–2   Steps in Analyzing a Problem Behavior 226
TABLE   9–3   A CPR Checklist Used in Evaluations 229
TABLE   9–4   A Rating Scale for Two Learning Objectives 230

TABLE   10–1   Phases of Educational Program Development 240
FIGURE   10–1   The "PRECEDE" model for health education planning 242
TABLE   10–2   Elements of Marketing and Their Application to
                  Education 250

TABLE   A–1   Sample Plan for Admission Teaching 269
TABLE   A–2   Sample Plan for Preoperative or Pretreatment Teaching..... 275
TABLE   A–3   Sample Objectives and Content for Teaching Patient Care .. 281
TABLE   A–4   Sample Plan for Discharge Teaching........................... 286

LIST OF CASE EXAMPLES

EXAMPLE 1.1   An overheard conversation....................................... 5
EXAMPLE 1.2   Observation of a procedure 6
EXAMPLE 1.3   An emergency hospital admission................................. 9
EXAMPLE 1.4   Glaucoma treated with laser surgery............................ 14

EXAMPLE 2.1   An apparent lack of relevant experience....................... 29
EXAMPLE 2.2   Help with recognizing a need to learn 30
EXAMPLE 2.3   Two patients with hypertension................................ 35
EXAMPLE 2.4   A mother's motivation to learn................................ 40
EXAMPLE 2.5   Beliefs about AIDS... 45
EXAMPLE 2.6   Family acceptance of new behavior 50
EXAMPLE 2.7   Stress influences attitudes toward learning................... 53
EXAMPLE 2.8   A crisis of accumulated stress 57

EXAMPLE 3.1   Admission for exploratory surgery 73
EXAMPLE 3.2   A distressing diagnosis....................................... 73
EXAMPLE 3.3   Community care for a patient with Alzheimer's Disease...... 75

EXAMPLE 4.1   The health balance of a postpartum patient................... 92

EXAMPLE 5.1   Patient preparation for a cardiac procedure.................. 117
EXAMPLE 5.2   Use of an organizer in teaching.............................. 120
EXAMPLE 5.3   An uncommunicative learner................................... 126

EXAMPLE 5.4   Statements suggesting experiential strategies 136
EXAMPLE 5.5   Appreciating another's feelings 137

EXAMPLE 6.1   Appointment cards as a teaching material 146
EXAMPLE 6.2   Preparation for surgery on videotape 163

EXAMPLE 7.1   Getting help with a hidden problem.......................... 170
EXAMPLE 7.2   Some consequences of advice................................. 174
EXAMPLE 7.3   A problem of both mind and body 177
EXAMPLE 7.4   A problem of medical communication........................ 178
EXAMPLE 7.5   Upsetting event masks long-term problem................... 182
EXAMPLE 7.6   Asking directions to the lab................................. 186

EXAMPLE 8.1   A group tackles the problem of fear.......................... 198
EXAMPLE 8.2   Poor preparation for an activity group....................... 205

EXAMPLE 9.1   Evaluating resuscitation competence.......................... 228
EXAMPLE 9.2   Self-fulfilling prophecy in a classroom....................... 236

EXAMPLE 10.1   An educational program for family members 243
EXAMPLE 10.2   Program philosophies 248
EXAMPLE 10.3   Solving procedural problems 252

INTRODUCTION

Nursing practice combines scientific knowledge with technical, human relations, and communication skills in unique ways. It is the constantly changing combinations of these elements and the opportunity to solve problems in many areas which make nursing a challenging and exciting profession. Patient teaching presents special kinds of challenges and opportunities. It demands that the nurse combine a wide range of knowledge and skills. It demands that she relate effectively to the patient and his needs, and that she adjust her communication to his concerns, interests, and level of understanding. Her success in helping the patient learn has a continuing positive impact on his life, health, and future well-being. This book is intended as a practical guide for the nurse who recognizes the importance of patient teaching in nursing practice and who wishes to develop her ability to teach effectively.

A well-planned educational program begins with a statement of philosophy and purpose or goal (see Chapter 10). The program is then designed to reflect this philosophy and accomplish this purpose or goal. This text also began with a philosophy about the purpose of patient teaching and its place in nursing practice.

> The purpose of patient teaching, as described in these pages, is to help people acquire the tools with which they can take greater responsibility for their own well-being.

This philosophy is reflected in three principles that have been chosen for emphasis:

Principle 1—Effective teaching results in learning.

Principle 2—Patient teaching is concerned with helping people acquire the knowledge, attitudes, skills, and behaviors that will not only allow them to regain and maintain their health, but to attain even higher levels of wellness.

Principle 3—The identification of learning needs and patient teaching based on these needs are integral parts of the Nursing Process and of excellent nursing care for every patient.

The first of these principles appears to be self-evident. Upon reflection, however, it is clear that teaching does not always result in learning, in spite of the good intentions of the teacher. This text is devoted to helping the reader develop the practical understanding and teaching skills that will lead to patient learning.

Patient teaching has both short-term and long-term goals. By helping the patient learn, the nurse contributes to his ability to understand and participate in his own care. The nurse's concerns go beyond the treatment of ill health, however.

The teaching-learning process is the means for helping the patient improve his level of wellness in the longer term.

Patient teaching is not a process which is separate from other aspects of excellent patient care. As the nurse uses the Nursing Process to assess patient needs and plan and implement care, her broad concern for his well-being will lead her to identify learning needs. Teaching is one of the ways the nurse intervenes to meet patient needs. It is an important part of the comprehensive care of all patients.

With this philosophy as a framework, and a goal of offering practical guidance for nurse teachers, we will begin with an exploration of some of the basic principles affecting the teaching-learning process. Special emphasis is given to the interactive nature of that process in the first three chapters. With these as background, the remainder of the book is organized in a "how to" format, reflecting the kinds and sequence of decisions that the nurse makes in determining how best to help the patient learn.

In order to increase the book's practical usefulness, a large number of examples have been included that demonstrate how the ideas presented can be applied to practical situations. Study questions and exercises at the end of each chapter, appropriate for either individual or group learning, encourage the development of teaching skills. Their use will help the reader bridge the gap between theory and practice. Important points, such as the statement of philosophy above, are in special type so that the text can serve as a continuing reference for the reader.

Most of the teaching that nurses have the opportunity to do concerns individuals in a one-to-one relationship or very small groups of two to four. For that reason, the majority of this book focuses on this kind of setting for the teaching-learning process. The immediacy of this process has led to the use of the phrase "patient teaching" rather than "patient education." The latter has been reserved for formal, planned, less individualized approaches to helping with learning.

A number of other terms used in these pages need to be clarified. The word "patient" has been chosen as the most frequent alternative to "person," "client," or "learner." Although certainly not all of the people whom the nurse helps with learning are ill and hospitalized, use of this term lends clarity to the discussions. For the same reason, the "patient" is generally referred to with the male pronoun while the nurse is referred to as female. The author readily acknowledges that not all nurses are female, just as not all patients are male. One other short-hand term has been used throughout the book: reference to "family members" is intended to signify those people who are concerned about and have especially significant relationships with the "patient" and is not limited to those within his biological family.

The author is strongly committed to the belief that people have a right to learn about their bodies, their care, how to protect and improve their future health, and how to guard the well-being of their families. Nurses increasingly have opportunities to help with this learning. This book is offered as a guide for learning the effective teaching skills which will make possible this important contribution to the health of our patients and our communities.

1

PATIENT
TEACHING AND
THE NURSE

This chapter introduces the reader to the general context within which the teaching-learning process occurs in nursing. As part of this introduction, some of the major influences acting on patient teaching are explored. The main points contained in this chapter, including in the introduction, are as follows:

- Recent changes in health care delivery and attitudes toward health have increased nurses' opportunities to help with learning. (Introduction)
- Factors which have special impact on the nature of patient teaching include nurse-patient interaction, the Nursing Process, legal, medical care and administrative issues and historical precedent. (Introduction)
- Because patient teaching is basically a communicative process, nurse-patient interaction is at its core. (Section 1.1)
- Nurses teach constantly as they interact with others helping people to learn not only through prepared teaching but also spontaneously and indirectly. (Section 1.1)
- Teaching is an integral part of the Nursing Process. It is one of a number of actions that might be taken by the nurse in an effort to help the patient reach his health goals. (Section 1.2)
- In order to plan effective teaching, learning goals should be identified as part of the nurse's assessment of patient needs. (Section 1.2)
- Nurses have a professional obligation and legal responsibility to help with learning. (Section 1.3)
- Increased specialization and the use of technology in the delivery of medical care have resulted in new teaching challenges for nurses. (Section 1.3)
- Economic issues are of growing concern to administrators, who must be helped by nurses to appreciate the value of patient teaching. (Section 1.3)
- The teaching role of nurses has been an integral part of nursing practice throughout nursing history. (Section 1.4)

- Traditional values, which are the foundation of quality patient care, continue to motivate and direct the nurse's approach to patient teaching. (Section 1.4)

Helping patients learn how to care for themselves has been part of nursing care since the beginning of our professional history. In recent years, however, changes in medical and health care delivery and in social attitudes toward health have led to increased opportunities for patient teaching. Three of the changes that have focused new attention on self-care, illness prevention, and wellness are as follows:

1. Nurses and others in the health professions have become increasingly alert to the patient's right to share in decision making and actively participate in his care. In order for the patient to exercise this right, he must become knowledgeable enough to ask pertinent questions, accept responsibility for his own well-being by adjusting his behavior appropriately, and be able to articulate health needs in response to physical signals of distress or dysfunction. Learning enables patients to do these things.

2. Increasing costs and extremely rapid advances in medical care have led to distinct changes in being a patient. No longer do patients stay in the hospital until they are nearly well and able to care for themselves with ease. Instead, they are discharged sooner, often with complex care regimens. People who, a few years ago would have died, now live, although sometimes with chronic health problems and ongoing medical needs. Learning enables patients to take responsibility for their continuing care outside hospital walls.

3. Recent years have seen a surge of public interest in wellness. People have become increasingly aware that they can choose actions and life-styles that lessen their chances of ill health, promote their general well-being, and help them to attain positive good health. Although general principles of healthy living are widely publicized, individuals need help in applying those principles to their own lives. Learning that is focused on their individual needs enables them to do this successfully.

The interactive nature of nursing care gives the nurse unique opportunities to assess individual health goals. Her medical knowledge and expertise are excellent sources of information and skills to those with learning needs. Unfortunately, neither one's good intentions nor previous experience as a student necessarily makes one an effective teacher.

This book is devoted to helping nurses develop the teaching skills that will allow them to take full advantage of opportunities to help with patient learning. The starting point in this endeavor will be to examine some of the factors that influence the roles of the two persons primarily involved in the teaching-learning process: the nurse as teacher and the patient as learner. We will begin with the nurse's role and proceed to the patient's role in Chapter 2. Four general factors have been identified as being especially important to the nurse as health teacher.

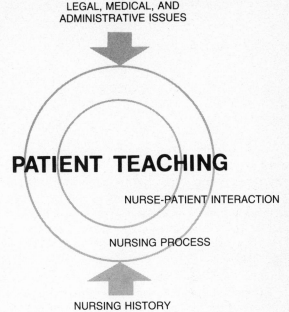

LEGAL, MEDICAL, AND
ADMINISTRATIVE ISSUES

Figure 1–1. Influences on the teaching
role of nurses.

PATIENT TEACHING

NURSE-PATIENT INTERACTION

NURSING PROCESS

NURSING HISTORY

Effective patient teaching

— occurs within the context of nurse-patient interaction,

— is surrounded by the skills and methods of the Nursing Process,

— is influenced by a variety of legal, medical care, and administrative issues,
   and

— is supported by a long and distinguished history of nurses as teachers.

These four general factors in combination have a major impact on the specific
nature of any given instance of patient teaching. They influence the relative
priority the nurse places on teaching, her choice of content, and her approach to
the learning needs of the patient and his family. The relationship of these four
factors to patient teaching is summarized in Figure 1–1.

In the four sections of this chapter we will look at each of these factors,
beginning with the core of patient teaching, the interpersonal relationship within
which it occurs.

1.1 NURSE-PATIENT INTERACTION AND TEACHING

Nursing is, by nature, a process based on communication and interpersonal
relationships. Even the most technical of nursing activities is surrounded by verbal
and nonverbal communication as the nurse assesses needs, plans care, notes
patient responses, coordinates care with colleagues, and records her observations
and interventions.

Within the context of giving care, the nurse often explains what she or others are doing and what the patient can expect or shows the patient or his family members a procedure or piece of equipment. These activities may be done without prior planning, or even without awareness by the nurse that she is teaching. At other times the nurse carefully selects teaching as a nursing intervention, planning exactly how to approach a topic so that the patient's learning needs will be met. In still other instances, the person who sees the nurse as a representative of an organization or as an "expert" learns simply by observing her behavior. In all of these situations involving nurse-patient interaction, the nurse is actually teaching. She may deliberately plan a lesson, help others learn spontaneously and without prior planning, or teach indirectly and inadvertently.

Prepared Teaching

Because of their own classroom experiences, people often think of teaching as a more or less formal activity in which the teacher decides in advance what will be taught and how the subject will be presented. This is the kind of teaching most often discussed in textbooks on patient education because it is the most easily dissected, examined, and interpreted. In order to be effective, this kind of teaching requires time: time to assess patient needs carefully, time to develop the interpersonal communication on which learning depends, and time to plan and prepare teaching strategies and materials. In many ways it is the most rewarding kind of teaching for the nurse teacher because the subject matter is often so very important to the person's well-being. With learning goals well defined, the nurse is able to see progress toward goals as positive reinforcement for her efforts. Because prepared teaching is approached deliberately, it is the kind of teaching in which the nurse can hone her skills in helping others learn.

The nurse has many opportunities for prepared teaching. Whenever patients and their family members need to acquire complex knowledge, perform new skills, or practice new patterns of behavior or attitudes, a prepared teaching approach is most likely to be successful because preplanning allows material to be presented logically and in depth. Prepared teaching may be conducted either in groups or on a one-to-one basis. It may be part of a formal patient education program, or it may be a nurse's individual response to meeting a patient's unique learning needs. It may consist of a formally structured lesson, or it may be a series of informal discussions on planned topics.

Spontaneous Teaching

In the course of a working day, the nurse has conversations with many people: patients, family members, colleagues, and other health professionals. Some of these conversations are initiated by people who ask the nurse for information or advice. Sometimes the nurse initiates the interaction by offering information or opinions.

As nurses, we are taught to be conscientious and responsible about our communication with others, since often we are regarded as "experts" whose statements are especially meaningful. When a patient or family member asks us a question, we carefully respond with accurate information in a way that will be fully understood by the questioner. When we encounter someone who seems confused or upset, we try to help the person feel more comfortable by explaining to him or her what is happening. Although teaching may not be our primary goal in these kinds of unplanned conversations, we have the opportunity to affect the person's knowledge, attitudes, or skills.

As the nurse develops and practices her teaching skills, she will more easily recognize the learning needs presented in these ways. Her familiarity with planned teaching will make her more adept at purposely using her teaching skills in these situations.

> Good teaching goes beyond good communication. The communication process is the means the nurse deliberately uses to help a person learn, that is, help him to gain the knowledge, attitudes and skills that improve his ability to take action and solve problems.

In this book the emphasis is on learning teaching skills within the context of prepared teaching. As a more controlled situation, it provides the nurse with opportunities to carefully analyze her actions and the patient's responses. As she gains skill, she will begin to use the spontaneous opportunities to teach more frequently and more effectively. Chapter 7 focuses on spontaneous teaching, with special emphasis on identifying learning needs "on the spot."

Indirect Teaching

Sometimes a person learns from the nurse when she is not knowingly teaching, or even deliberately interacting with him. This usually happens when a person is anxious about the environment in which he finds himself or looks to the nurse as a role model. The "learner," in both cases, carefully observes the nurse's behavior and interprets it without further interaction.

> Whether or not the nurse chooses a teaching role, others often choose the nurse to help them learn.

It is important that nurses learn to identify those situations in which indirect teaching is occurring. Such awareness means that they can give conscious attention to their own behavior as it affects others or initiate direct interaction so that the situation becomes one of spontaneous teaching. The following cases are examples of indirect teaching.

Example 1.1   AN OVERHEARD CONVERSATION

It was a busy morning in the prenatal clinic. A nurse at the reception desk could be heard speaking on the telephone in an impatient and hurried tone of voice: "Look, the doctor is terribly busy. Can I answer your question?" A new patient in the waiting room might interpret this overheard exchange as follows: if you want a question answered, it's best not to call during morning clinic hours; nurses might be able to answer your questions.

Example 1.2   OBSERVATION OF A PROCEDURE

A nurse carrying a dressing pack walked into the room of a postsurgical patient. With a pleasant smile she said to the patient: "Mrs. Adams, I'm going to change your dressing now." After turning back the bedcovers and helping the patient adjust her position in bed, the nurse washed her hands thoroughly in the washbasin. The patient might interpret this event as follows: the nurse knows who I am; she doesn't mind changing my dressing; she is well organized; this is a clean procedure that necessitates hand washing first.

The interpretations made by the patients in these examples may or may not be correct, but their perception will be that they have "learned" these "facts." Such "learning" will probably result in an adjustment of their behavior, attitudes, or expectations.

It is a common human experience that when we are confronted by an unusual or anxiety-producing situation, we become extraordinarily alert to clues that will help us act appropriately and retain a measure of personal control. Although high levels of stress and fear inhibit learning and rational adaptation (see Section 2.5), the relatively mild anxiety produced by unfamiliarity stimulates increased awareness of the environment. Imagine yourself being interviewed for a job or visiting an attorney's office or going to a new dentist. Lack of familiarity and clear expectations makes one especially alert to the physical surroundings, the tone of voice and words of the receptionist, and the content of overheard conversations. One learns from these clues and adjusts accordingly.

Likewise, it is common experience that we are especially aware of the behavior of people we respect, admire, or like. If we observe them doing something that we will need or want to do in the future, they are likely to become role models for us. We learn from watching them and try to duplicate their behavior. Because of her knowledge, caring attitudes, and availability, the nurse is frequently a role model.

Recognizing that people are likely to look to her for clues· about their environment leads the nurse to more readily identify such situations as teaching opportunities and actively choose a teaching role. This understanding also encourages the nurse to periodically evaluate how her verbal and nonverbal behavior might be interpreted by others.

In summary, prepared, spontaneous, and indirect methods of teaching have been discussed in this section. The nurse's contribution to others' learning occurs not only in formally prepared lessons, but also as she converses spontaneously with them or is observed by them. *The nurse teaches constantly.*

The interpersonal communication that develops as part of giving and receiving nursing care is at the core of all three patient teaching methods. The challenge is to use the many opportunities that arise as a natural part of nurse-patient interaction to help people learn effectively.

1.2 NURSING PROCESS AND PATIENT TEACHING

Patient teaching is an important part of what a nurse does every day. The majority of the nurse's patient care activities can be organized using the steps of the Nursing Process. Within these pages, the point of view is taken that teaching is an activity that can benefit from the same kind of assessment and planning as coordination or physical care. Teaching is one of the nurse's options in choosing the interventions that will best meet patient needs.

Since first proposed in the early 1960s as part of the movement toward a scientific basis for nursing practice, the Nursing Process has offered a framework for the problem solving done by nurses. The division of the Nursing Process into a series of specific steps or phases has given nurses a way to make clear to others, and to themselves, just what they are contributing to patient care. Categorizing the specific actions of nurses has promoted the analysis and research of problems confronting nurses in everyday practice. By providing an organized approach to patient care, the Nursing Process has encouraged nurses to put relatively abstract concepts, such as "total patient care," into regular practice.

Some of the major reasons for using the Nursing Process are:

— it provides a method of organizing care so that the individuality of each patient and his full range of nursing care needs are recognized;
— it enhances the continuing interaction between nurse and patient and the coordination of care with other caregivers;
— it encourages active patient participation in care; and
— it promotes evaluation of the quality and effectiveness of care.

There is nothing mysterious about the form or intent of the Nursing Process. It is an adaptation of the "scientific method" of problem solving. A number of authors have written extensively on the parallels between scientific method, problem solving, and the Nursing Process (for example Yura and Walsh, 1983; Riehl and Roy, 1980). Because this comparative material is widely known and readily available in nursing theory and practice texts, it will not be reviewed here. In Figure 1–2 the four phases of the Nursing Process are reiterated and the terminology used throughout the book is specified.

Although the four phases are similar to those suggested by Yura and Walsh (1983), the details differ somewhat from other authors, and therefore bear explanation. Notice that I have used the word *phases* rather than *steps* in labeling the Process. This has been done to emphasize the fluid nature of problem solving where human problems are concerned.

The phases of the Nursing Process tend to blend and overlap as the dynamic relationship between nurse and patient unfolds.

For example, while determining approaches for meeting a particular goal, additional information about patient strengths may come to light. Or, the planned action may, for some unforeseen reason, be impossible to implement in the way intended, requiring a new plan. Evaluation of patient response in comparison with goals frequently results in the definition of new patient objectives or the choice of different methods of nursing intervention. The arrows in Figure 1–2 show the dynamic interaction between phases in the process, called "feedback" in systems terminology.

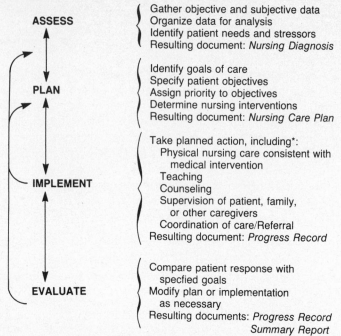

Figure 1–2. Phases of the Nursing Process. *See basic nursing texts such as Sorensen and Luckmann (1986) for a detailed description of nursing intervention methods and their place in the Nursing Process.

I have also used the words *goals* and *patient objectives* as the intended outcome of the Nursing Process, rather than *problem solution*. The emphasis on goals and objectives, rather than on problems, helps the nurse keep a broad perspective on patient care, taking into account both immediate treatment needs and longer-term health promotion needs. Although all of the agreed-on goals and objectives may not be met in the clinical setting, their identification will help both nurse and patient plan constructively for continued health as well as medical care.

Of the four phases of the Nursing Process, assessment is the most important. As Barbara Narrow (1979, p. 50) has phrased it, "the total process can only be as effective as its assessment phase." If the information gathered is incomplete, lopsided, or inaccurate, then the nursing care that derives from it will be of poor quality. In order to give nurses a way of approaching the sometimes formidable task of gathering relevant patient data, I have proposed a Health Balance model, which is presented in Chapter 4. This model involves the identification of the patient's unmet *needs* or deficits and the demands or *stressors* acting upon him as they are balanced by his internal *strengths* (physical, intellectual, motor, and affective) and external *resources*. Such a model helps the nurse identify a wide range of patient needs, not just those related to the person's present illness, and allows her to plan nursing interventions that will promote health as well as treat illness.

The assessment phase of the Nursing Process is the first step toward effective patient care. The Nursing Diagnosis, which summarizes the imbalances that have contributed to the patient's present distress, is followed by a plan whose goals and objectives are to restore and, if possible, improve the health balance. The nurse's intervention seeks to help the patient meet these goals and objectives and may include physical care, teaching, counseling, supervision, coordination of care, and referral. The effectiveness of these interventions is subsequently evaluated in terms of their success in meeting patient objectives.

Teaching and counseling have been described as processes with a number of phases similar to those of the Nursing Process but separate from it. However, for the nurse whose practice is already organized around problem solving and goal attainment, teaching and counseling are natural parts of the more comprehensive Nursing Process. The nurse does not stop doing "nursing" and begin doing "teaching." Rather, teaching is one of several interventions the nurse might choose to help her meet patient needs. It is as important to quality patient care as purely physical care interventions, such as giving a medication or turning a patient to prevent pressure sores.

> The nurse appropriately chooses a teaching intervention whenever the patient's health balance would be improved by gaining knowledge and understanding or developing new skills or attitudes. Teaching and learning are not separate from the Nursing Process; they are an integral and necessary part of it.

The following case example, although not described here in detail, demonstrates how the Nursing Process provides an important framework for care and how teaching forms an integral part of that process.

Example 1.3   AN EMERGENCY HOSPITAL ADMISSION

Jim Davis entered the emergency department at 3 p.m. accompanied by a co-worker. He had been experiencing severe, incapacitating right flank pain for the past hour. The doctor on duty tentatively diagnosed the problem as a kidney stone and arranged for Mr. Davis to be admitted. Susan Costa, R.N., received him on the surgical unit shortly thereafter. She reviewed his chart and completed a nursing assessment. The resulting nursing diagnosis included two items that required immediate attention. They were "acute pain probably due to kidney stone" and "acute anxiety associated with pain, uncertainty of diagnosis/treatment, and inexperience with hospital environment."

From these diagnostic statements, three objectives emerged that the nurse acted on immediately. One of these was for the patient to obtain relief from acute pain. Another was that Mr. Davis become acquainted with the hospital unit and be able to use its equipment, such as the signal light, appropriately. A third objective was that he receive confirmation of his diagnosis when his doctor visited that evening. This meant that several test procedures would need to be completed quickly. After defining these objectives as having priority, Ms. Costa proceeded to implement the following interventions:

Objective 1. Pain relief: Intramuscular analgesia was administered as per doctor's order.

Objective 2. Patient orientation: Once the patient was more comfortable, the nurse pointed out the various parts of the unit and demonstrated use of the signal light. She confirmed that she would be his nurse that evening and would be checking with him frequently.

Objective 3. Facilitate diagnosis: After telephoning the laboratory and X-ray departments to schedule the ordered diagnostic procedures as soon as possible, Ms. Costa explained to Mr. Davis the procedures for the tests and the nature of the information that would be gained from each of them.

In a short period of time the nurse had performed several nursing actions based on her Nursing Diagnosis and Care Plan: physical care (Objective 1), teaching (Objectives 2 and 3), and coordination (Objective 3). She recorded each action and, at the appropriate time, evaluated the patient's response.

Even though this nursing situation was uncomplicated, the nurse quickly identified her patient's need to learn and incorporated patient teaching into her overall care. As discussed in Section 1.1, teaching and learning occur in virtually all nursing care situations. By including prepared teaching as part of her planned nursing intervention, the nurse accepts the challenge and the opportunity to help patients effectively meet their learning needs.

In summary, the Nursing Process provides a framework for the nurse's organization and provision of patient care. Use of this framework encourages the nurse to identify a wide range of patient needs, including his need to learn. Having identified learning needs, the nurse can then plan, implement, and evaluate teaching as an integral part of nursing care.

1.3 ISSUES THAT INFLUENCE PATIENT TEACHING

A wide range of issues, concerns, and decisions by others influence patient teaching. Some of these seem to be far removed from patient-nurse interaction, yet they have an impact on how the nurse sees her role as teacher, what priority she gives teaching, how she justifies this use of her professional time and skill, and what methods and materials she uses in her effort to help others learn.

The issues discussed in this section are divided into legal, medical care, and administrative categories. Although it is beyond the scope of this book to explore these in detail, the purpose of the discussion is to alert the nurse to the kinds of influences that will shape her role as a nurse teacher. With increased awareness she will be able to identify important issues at an early stage and plan action appropriate to her own practice setting. The influence of these issues will vary according to the nurse's geographic location, her employer, the resources available to her, and the current status of legal and political decisions. The reader is encouraged to keep abreast of changes in these issues through regular reference to nursing journals and communication with professional nursing organizations.

Legal Issues That Influence the Nurse As Teacher

Two major sources of legal issues that influence the role nurses play in patient education are the Nurse Practice Acts in each state and the concept of informed consent.

Every state in the United States has adopted a nurse practice act. The major reason for these acts is to establish criteria for the licensing of nurses, thereby protecting the public from unqualified practitioners. Most of the documents approved by the states include a definition of nursing and a list of accepted nursing functions. Those that have closely followed the model Nurse Practice Act published in 1976 by the American Nurses Association (ANA) specify the nurse's functions as the "care, treatment, counsel and health teaching of persons." For nurses working in states whose practice acts are vaguely worded or contain no list of functions, the ANA's model serves as a reasonable guide, although not a legally binding one, for practice. It behooves every nurse to familiarize herself not only with the wording of the current practice act in her state, but also with any movements toward changing it.

The ANA has actively worked to support the role of nurses in patient education and encourage its legal recognition. The *Standards of Nursing Practice,* published by the ANA in 1973, outlines the responsibilities of nurses in planning care and "maximizing client/patient health capabilities." Two years later the ANA published a report entitled *The Professional Nurse and Health Education.* In it, the nurse's teaching role was described in detail.

> The 1975 ANA report states that the nurse's "responsibility [for the quality of nursing care] includes teaching the patient and family relevant facts about specific health care needs and supporting appropriate modification of behavior."

Some of the areas listed as being of special concern to the nurse teacher include preoperative and postoperative care, diagnostic preparation and treatment, and discharge planning and follow-up.

Although the nurse practice acts establish the major legal basis for the nurse's *general* involvement in patient education, the requirement of informed consent influences the *specific* content and timing of a large portion of patient teaching.

Informed consent is a legal term indicating that, on the basis of information provided to him, a person has given permission for certain other people to touch him. Without this permission, medical personnel could be charged with battery (Rothman and Lloyd, 1977, p. 159).

A person coming to a medical facility enters a contract with that facility to provide care for him. A provision of the contract is that the person's right to give informed consent will be protected. These rights are stated in the *Accreditation Manual for Hospitals* published by the Joint Commission on Accreditation of Hospitals in 1980. It states, in part:

> The patient has the right to reasonably informed participation in decisions involving his health care. . . . This should be based on clear, concise explanation of his condition and of all proposed technical procedures. . . . The patient should not be subjected to any procedure without his voluntary, competent, and understanding consent, or that of his legally authorized representative. Where medically significant alternatives for care or treatment exist, the patient shall be so informed. (pp. xiv-xv)

The same document goes on to say that the patient also has the right to expect that he will be given adequate instruction on how to care for himself between visits to caregivers.

As part of the contractual agreement between patient and medical care facility, patients or their family members are often given a copy of a Patient's Bill of Rights. This document is generally based on a version approved by the American Hospital Association. It summarizes the patient's legal right to information and confirms his role in making decisions about his care.

> Although the major legal obligation for seeing that the patient has adequate information and is able to make informed decisions about his care falls to the doctor, nurses are involved in the issue of informed consent in three ways: as a witness, as the doctor's agent, and as a teacher in her own right.

The nurse is often asked to witness the signature of the patient on consent forms. Her legal responsibility in such instances includes that she be able to certify that the patient is mentally competent, is able to read and understand the form, and is signing consent without coercion (see Rankin and Duffy, 1983, pp. 98-100). Although she has no legal role in determining the quality of the information given to the patient by the doctor before signing the consent, or evaluating the extent of the patient's understanding, these certainly are ethical issues for the nurse.

In many instances the doctor may delegate his informing or teaching role to the nurse. If the nurse is not very familiar with the doctor's attitudes and preferences, or if the order to instruct the patient is given verbally or written in vague terms, the nurse should take the time to clarify the doctor's expectations. Lack of complete communication between caregivers about information to be given to the patient can lead to increased legal liability, patient dissatisfaction, and strained working relationships (see Rosenthal, Marshall, Macpherson, and French, 1980).

To the extent that the nurse carries out treatment procedures, administers medications, and prepares the patient physically for a variety of medical interventions, she has an ethical, if not directly legal, responsibility to help the patient gain the information he needs to understand the process and consequences of treatment. This responsibility extends to helping the patient to understand the reasons for nursing procedures and learn how to deal with his immediate environment and prepare for predictable events. Teaching of this sort, initiated by the nurse, is one of the cornerstones of an effective nurse-patient relationship. The nurse has a legal responsibility to document patient teaching efforts and results in the medical record.

Although caregivers universally agree with the principle that patients have a right to information and a right to make decisions based on it, the problem of how best to impart adequate information continues to be a concern for all involved. As Davis and Aroskar (1978) point out, informed consent is not just available for the asking. Rather, a great many variables are involved in transmitting understandable information to another person. In addition, using that information as a basis for realistic decisions is a complex process.

The person who gives information to the patient may think that he or she has taught, but unless the patient has actually learned to the point of being able to take action or solve problems as a result of it, the criteria of informed consent have not been met.

One of the common ways in which information giving fails to result in learning is described by Davis: "To inundate patients with technical information that they are unlikely to understand is to essentially withhold information from them" (1985, p. 41).

Helping patients and their family members "translate" the information they have gathered about their condition, treatment, and prognosis into understandable form so that they can comprehend its meaning is an important aspect of the nurse's role in patient teaching. Performing this valuable function means that the nurse must confront a number of ethical as well as legal questions, such as those listed in Table 1–1.

TABLE 1–1. Ethical Questions Related to Informed Consent

How much information is enough? How much is too much?

To what degree should caregivers influence patients to make the "right" decisions, that is, those consistent with the values of the health professionals involved?

What is the nurse's responsibility when the doctor specifically does not want the nurse to teach?

What is the nurse's responsibility when the patient seems unable or unwilling to learn and actively make decisions about his care?

Should the nurse risk giving information that may lead to the patient's noncompliance with the wishes of his doctor?

These and the many other questions that arise as a result of patient teaching have no easy answers. In order to begin solving these kinds of dilemmas the nurse must first be aware of the questions and familiar with the factors that influence the specific situation. Nurses are encouraged to inform themselves about the expectations of their medical care team members and discuss legal and ethical issues with their nursing colleagues.

Medical Care Issues That Influence the Nurse as Teacher

The past 20 years have seen basic changes in the form and methods of medical care; the form has been influenced by increasing specialization and the methods, by developing technology. These changes have raised important issues for nurses who attempt to meet the age-old human needs of their patients while participating in the modern complexities of medical science.

The tendencies toward specialization and the use of technological methods in diagnosis and treatment are intertwined. On the one hand, vastly increased information makes it impossible for a single professional to have complete and current knowledge in more than a narrow field of practice. At the same time, specialization has added to the information explosion and technological development by encouraging the exploration of problems in great depth. Without the intense focus of specialists in cardiology, for example, it is unlikely that the knowledge and skills required for heart transplants would have developed to the extent they have in the past few years, or that cardiac monitors would now be so widely used for diagnosis.

Changes in medical practice have placed increasing demands on nurses in a number of areas. In order to participate knowledgeably in complex care, nurses must have a sound background in basics such as anatomy and physiology and up-to-date knowledge of technological advances. They must be able to use the equipment, information, and people resources available to them in the patient's behalf. They must balance complex procedures with human values such as comfort and safety. They must be able to communicate effectively with their medical colleagues. And they must be able to help patients and their family members understand what is being done to and for them and why, what they can realistically expect of the people and machines around them, and how they can participate in decisions about their care.

As the gap between specialized medical knowledge and the lay public's understanding has widened in many areas, the need for patient teaching has grown. The nurse, who is constantly communicating with both patients and medical professionals, is in an ideal position to coordinate care and teach. Making complex information and highly technical data understandable to those who do not have extensive scientific backgrounds is a daunting teaching challenge. Case example 1.4 illustrates some of the practical difficulties faced by nurse teachers.

Example 1.4   *GLAUCOMA TREATED WITH LASER SURGERY*

Mrs. Bensen, a 63-year-old native of Sweden, was hospitalized with a compound fracture of the femur. She progressed well physically after surgery, but she seemed tense and apprehensive. Her primary care nurse, Gayle Abbott, felt this was partly due to difficulty in communicating. Mrs. Bensen spoke heavily accented English in a soft voice. She seldom asked questions, and when she was offered an explanation of some aspect of her care, she just nodded. She had been hospitalized only once before when she was a child in Sweden.

On the morning of her third postoperative day, Mrs. Benson complained of extreme pain in the right side of her head and eye. Her vision was blurred, and the nurse interpreted the circles Mrs. Bensen repeatedly drew in the air to mean that she was seeing halos around objects. Ms. Abbott immediately notified the doctor of this turn of events and then summoned the ophthalmologist on call. He arrived within the hour and confirmed the nurse's suspicion that Mrs. Bensen was suffering from acute glaucoma. He scheduled her for emergency laser surgery.

Ms. Abbott remained in the room while the ophthalmologist described the procedure to the patient. She then went with him to the unit station, where she asked a few questions to clarify for herself what the patient might expect and why the use of laser was the treatment of choice. The doctor requested Ms. Abbott's assistance in helping the patient understand the reasons for the procedure and the need for urgency in making a decision to proceed. Given the communication difficulties involved, the nurse knew she would need to carefully repeat and clarify the information given by the doctor. The time available for this teaching effort was limited because any delay might result in damage to the optic nerve.

In this case example the nurse was presented with the need to quickly supplement her own knowledge of a complex and highly technical specialty in preparation for patient teaching. The teaching was complicated by the patient's language difficulty, her inexperience with hospital procedures, her present acute and frightening pain, and a severe time limit. Overcoming these difficulties in order to preserve the patient's rights and reduce needless anxiety was a considerable challenge to the nurse's commitment to teaching and to her teaching skills. Although the details of specific situations differ, the teaching challenges with which nurses are presented frequently include such complicating factors.

As in Mrs. Bensen's case, the specialization of health care providers has led to an increase in the number of people involved in the care of any one patient. Most have more than one doctor attending them, as well as an array of technicians and auxiliary personnel and several members of the nursing staff. The differing interests, backgrounds, and concerns of each of these people can lead to serious fragmentation of care and communication problems. Because of her interaction with the patient and his family members and her awareness of patient needs, the nurse is in an excellent position to take the lead in coordinating communication and reducing fragmentation of care. In many instances the coordination role involves helping caregivers understand the actions and priorities of their colleagues as well as the needs of the patient. Although directed toward other medical and health professionals rather than toward patients, this, too, is a teaching activity.

The nurse's use of teaching approaches and skills is an important contribution to her role as coordinator of patient care.

Once the patient leaves the clinical setting, he or his family members must be able to communicate his needs effectively to caregivers and solve problems of care fragmentation themselves. Helping the patient learn how to coordinate his own care is an area of patient education that has not yet received a great deal of attention. Although doing this effectively may mean teaching complex knowledge and skills, the alternative is that patients return home without the ability to manage their health problems or make realistic decisions about asking for professional help. With fewer community health personnel available to help with coordination of care on an outpatient basis, it is even more important to use the opportunities for teaching which exist in clinical settings (see Waring and McLennan, 1979, Ch. 2).

Administrative Issues That Influence the Nurse as Teacher

Rapidly rising costs have brought permanent changes to health and medical care organizations. Administrators within such organizations are increasingly pressured to keep costs to consumers down while maintaining the same quality of service and the financial health of the facility. In order to do this, they must look carefully at the cost-effectiveness of activities carried out by personnel in all classifications.

In past years nurses have sometimes tried to pretend that economic concerns did not exist or were openly hostile to administrators who wanted them to justify their services in financial terms. Recently, however, the advent of diagnosis-related groups (DRGs) in the payment that hospitals receive for Medicare patients and the trend toward itemizing charges for nursing care on patient bills have clearly focused attention on what nurses do and how they spend their time. Nurses are now faced with showing their contribution to the profitability of the organizations who employ them or risking restrictive nursing budgets. As a result, nurses at all levels are looking closely at the components of quality nursing care (see McKibbin, 1985).

Nurses who attempt to protect their role as teacher from financial cutbacks or extend it to help patients learn in new areas are caught in a dilemma. The beneficial effects of patient teaching are often regarded as impossible to measure with validity. In addition, nurses themselves sometimes assign teaching a low priority, seeing it as something extra they will do "if they have time." On the other hand, there are good legal and public relations reasons for encouraging nurses to teach. Sometimes negative attitudes are the result of seeing patient teaching only in terms of formal, time-consuming educational programs with long-range goals. Both nurses and administrators may fail to identify and acknowledge the multitude of incidents of teaching that occur in the normal course of patient care. These everyday instances of teaching are much less time-consuming, usually have much more specific and time-limited goals, and are more validly evaluated within the clinical setting than are extended, formal programs.

While administrators and nurses may wonder whether a teaching role is valid use of nursing time, patients and their families want and need information, understanding, and skills that are available only if the nurse does take time to teach (see Mumford and Skipper, 1967; Rosenthal et al., 1980).

> Patients are being discharged from acute care sooner and sicker than in years past. Their learning needs are more pressing because they are faced with assuming responsibility for their care earlier in the course of their illnesses.

Because hospital stays are shorter, nurses working in acute care settings have less time to help patients learn. If they are to help the patient understand his illness, learn how to manage its residual effects, and prepare for discharge, nurses must begin patient teaching very early in acute care. This requires careful planning and skillful teaching. In order to be successful, nurses need administrative support and a commitment to teaching that includes a willingness to improve teaching skills and practice them diligently.

Increased patient needs for help with learning are evident in nonacute settings as well. Nurses working in skilled nursing facilities and home care agencies are increasingly called to fill in the learning gaps left by confusion about instructions, concerns about prognosis, and continuing questions about patients' acute care experience. Harron and Schaeffer (1986), for example, report a fivefold increase in the need for support and twice as much need for teaching among patients admitted to a skilled nursing facility after, as compared with before, the advent of DRGs.

Patients clearly do have learning needs and, as discussed previously, a right to information. As medical and health care organizations face the realities of

TABLE 1-2. Preparing for Discussion of Patient Teaching Role

Examine your own definition of patient teaching. Does it include informally giving information to patients and their family members? Does it include activities such as helping patients make decisions and solve problems? Together with nursing colleagues, write a comprehensive description of the teaching role of nurses in your unit.

Estimate how much time you actually spend helping others learn. Do not forget to include the time taken to teach family members and other caregivers as well as patients. How much of this time is planned and how much teaching is spontaneous and informal? To what degree are teaching activities encouraged by your immediate supervisor and nursing colleagues? What do you think are the patient care benefits of teaching?

Examine the record-keeping procedures in your facility. Are nurses encouraged to chart their specific activities, including patient teaching? Together with nursing colleagues, make a list of ways in which the recording system could be improved to better reflect nursing roles generally and patient teaching specifically.

Look up the policies and procedures of your facility and identify objectives, definitions, or descriptions of quality care and statements about priorities. What kinds of information must the facility legally provide patients?

Discuss what you find out about facility policies with administrators or supervisors on a one-to-one, informal basis in order to more fully understand the views, attitudes, and priorities of the leaders in your facility. How do they see various nursing roles contributing to the overall objectives of service? What kinds of economic issues do they see affecting administrative decision making?

Investigate the kinds and content of your facility's public relations efforts. What does the organization tell the community about its benefits and services? How important is public good will to the facility's functioning? Discuss your findings with the person in charge of public relations in order to more fully understand facility plans in this area and the priority given public relations activities. Have studies of patient satisfaction with services been conducted? What implications do results have for nursing care?

---

economic issues, nurses must be prepared to justify, without defensiveness, their roles in communication, coordination, and teaching. This means that nurses themselves must be convinced of the value of these activities and be willing to document them. At the same time, administrators must try to see quality care in terms of human responses as well as technology and appreciate the economic advantages of patient satisfaction and good public relations.

The resolution of these kinds of issues and the clarification of priorities are essential to positive relationships between administrators and nurses and, consequently, between nurses and patients. Nurses may need to take the lead in opening up discussion of the issues. To be successful, such discussions should represent a mutual attempt to understand the concerns of all parties and a willingness to talk about them openly. In preparation for such discussions, nurses must first clarify their own attitudes about nursing roles and then try to understand some of the administrative problems and concerns facing the organization. The activities listed in Table 1-2 are suggested as ways of helping nurses prepare for effective dialogue with administrators about the role of teaching in patient care.

These kinds of activities will provide the nurse with basic understanding of the structure and priorities of the facility and background information about how administrators see nursing roles.

Helping an organization clarify policies or bring about changes begins with finding out how that organization currently functions, appreciating the pressures that are

operating on it and making an honest attempt to understand the points of view of the leaders within the organization.

Although the scale of activities is different, helping with an organization's change process is similar to helping an individual learn, grow, and change. In both cases basic information that allows the helper to assess needs and plan objectives is crucial to success. An attitude that is positive and optimistic toward the organization's willingness to change, rather than aggressive and confrontational, is also important. The nurse involved in organizational change may want to consult management texts (e.g., Rakich, Longest, and O'Donovan, 1977), texts on the change process (e.g., Bennis, Benne, Chin, and Corey, 1976), and texts on nursing leadership.

Regardless of long-term organizational objectives, it is important that nurses themselves recognize the extent of their teaching activities. Part of this awareness comes from diligently recording all teaching activities, including informal information giving to patients and their family members. By doing a better job of charting such activities, nurses can clarify for themselves the contribution they are making to patients. Seeing teaching activities noted can also be a revelation to medical colleagues. In addition, teaching that is carefully documented is powerful evidence when helping administrators better understand why this is such an important nursing role.

In summary, a number of legal, medical care, and administrative issues that influence the nurse's role as teacher have been discussed in this section. The goal has not been to give nurses answers about resolving these issues, but to increase awareness of the questions that continue to be raised. These issues, for the most part, are controversial; attitudes will continue to change. It is important that nurses keep themselves informed of developments and decisions that will influence their roles and the quality of patient care they are able to give. It is also important that nurses be willing to be involved in the decision-making and change processes.

1.4   A HISTORICAL PERSPECTIVE ON PATIENT TEACHING

The present-day teaching role of nurses is supported by a long and distinguished history of helping others learn. In this section some of that history is reviewed in order to give the reader a historical perspective on patient teaching.

Organized attempts to provide humane care for the sick and injured long predate the work of Florence Nightingale in the mid-1800s. For example, European monasteries are usually credited with establishing the first hospitals by offering care to pilgrims during the Crusades. In 1610, St. Francis de Sales and Madame de Chantal organized home nursing care in a town in eastern France. Care was provided by a special order of nuns. These and other early nurses saw it as their duty to teach as well as to comfort and care for their patients (Leahy, Cobb, and Jones, 1977, Ch. 11). Although the wisdom contained in this early teaching was not "scientific" by modern standards, the instruction often included valuable information about cleanliness, disease prevention, and early remedies.

In the mid-1700s a major shift occurred in what had been the largely rural populations of Europe and Britain (Hobson, 1975, Ch. 1). During what came to be known as the Industrial Revolution, thousands of people poured into urban areas seeking jobs. The cities were ill-equipped to handle their housing and sanitation needs. Wave after wave of disease epidemics ravaged the densely clustered populations. For nearly a hundred years attempts were made periodically to teach people the relationship between filth and disease, but it was not until word of the discoveries of Pasteur and Koch spread that this relationship became clear and health teaching became more focused and successful (Gordon, 1976, Ch. 10). During this period, nursing care was still provided by the religious orders, but because of the overwhelming need, large numbers of other women were recruited to do nursing tasks. Many of these women were poorly educated and untrained for their patient care duties.

In 1853 the outbreak of the Crimean War gave impetus and public attention to Florence Nightingale's crusade for respectability and discipline in the practice of nursing. As well as giving what physical care they could, Nightingale's nurses tried to help their patients understand that poor hygiene and the lack of sanitation lead to infection and illness. Even in those desperate circumstances they demonstrated the use of primitive sanitation techniques. The idea of disease prevention through teaching was an important part of Nightingale's philosophy (Nightingale, 1859). After the war her nurses shifted their teaching focus to maternal and child health in the belief that improved hygiene in caring for infants would reduce the high infant mortality rate (Cohen, 1984).

In the United States the early 1900s saw an increasing awareness of nurses' needs for educational preparation in addition to apprenticeship training for their roles in patient care and teaching. This led to the inclusion of academic subjects in nurse training programs. Following Nightingale's lead, American nurses learned to teach hygiene and disease prevention as well as give patient care in these early programs. In the years before World War I, leaders such as Lillian Wald, a pioneer in community health nursing, and Edith Abbott of the Children's Bureau, helped to establish and confirm the nurse's role in health teaching. The newly formed American Red Cross introduced rural community health nursing and health teaching. Nurses conducted courses in maternal and child health as part of their services (Leahy et al., 1977).

After World War I, professional nursing associations provided a forum for a growing group of nurse authors and theorists and took public stands on nursing issues. In 1918 the National League for Nursing Education went on record as supporting the role of nurses as health teachers and warned nurse educators that they must not focus their programs exclusively on disease (p. 6).

At the same time there was increasing concern about the quality of nursing education and the preparation nurses were receiving for their expanding roles. The establishment of the Yale School of Nursing as a collegiate school by Annie W. Goodrich in 1923 was an important step in confirming that nurses should and could have a broad scientific basis for their nursing practice.

By the time World War II broke out, nurses had become an organized and professionally prepared group of caregivers who were ready to make their contribution to the war effort. The war experience gave nurses a sense of kinship with nurses from many parts of the world and a self-esteem born of public recognition of their service to their countries.

After the war there was a surge of interest in a wide range of medical and health services and, consequently, a rising demand for nurses. Progress on such issues as the quality of nursing education, appropriate nursing roles and functions, and professionalism became urgent. The 1948 report by Ester Lucille Brown, *Nursing For the Future*, was one of a number of studies that raised pertinent questions about the preparation of nurses and the distribution of nursing services. The team concept of health care delivery and the more widespread inclusion of natural and social sciences in nursing curricula were two outcomes of this postwar period.

The dramatic changes in nursing patterns and roles that have been initiated since the end of World War II reflect equally dramatic changes in medical science and technology. Nursing theory has changed as well, paralleling trends in philosophy and the behavioral sciences. One way to make sense of the complex and increasingly rapid changes that have taken place in nursing practice is to view them within the context of a few basic principles or ideas that have influenced nursing throughout its history.

Three principles that emerge from a study of nursing history as having consistently affected nursing practice are:

— that nursing care is appropriately based on the needs of the patient,

— that each person is a unique individual, and

— that the caring, helping, teaching relationship that the nurse has with the patient makes a unique contribution to health and medical care.

Keeping these ideas in mind, we will look briefly at some of the changes in nursing theory and roles that have come about since the end of World War II.

During the 1940s and 1950s the idea of the patient's *needs* as the basis for nursing care was emphasized. This idea had been introduced by Nightingale many years before, but now it gained credibility from the newly developing field of psychology. Abraham Maslow (1943) and Erik Erikson (1950) were early leaders in developmental psychology, stressing changes in a person's needs as he or she matured and pointing out how needs could be altered by emotional or physical trauma. Nursing care was described as therapeutic in a broad sense and as a "maturing force" (Peplau, 1952). The concept of total patient care was developed which was to continue as a focal goal of nursing practice until quite recently, although with some differences in definition. When first introduced, total patient care referred to the activities of the nurse in meeting a wide range of patient needs (Yura and Walsh, 1983, p. 4).

Within the context of helping the patient meet his needs, teaching was clearly identified as a valuable, even indispensable, role for the nurse. The nurse was recognized as instrumental in helping the patient develop the knowledge and skills needed to reach his full potential for health.

The late 1950s were also years of exciting changes in public health. The availability and widespread use of antibiotics dramatically reduced deaths from such killers as tuberculosis, while new attenuated vaccines proved effective in preventing a number of other communicable diseases. The virtual eradication of infantile paralysis within a few years through massive immunization programs is one of the dramatic successes of medical advance. Nurses took a lead in helping to educate the public about the effectiveness of the new vaccine and assisting with its distribution. The number of polio cases in the United States declined from more than 18,000 in 1954 to 19 in 1971 (Smolensky, 1977, p. 257).

By the 1960s psychologists and social scientists had turned their interest toward the dynamic, communicative, interactional aspects of human functioning. Influenced by them and the existential philosophers, nursing theory of this period emphasized the interpersonal aspects of nursing care. Orlando (1961), Wieden- bach (1964), and Travelbee (1966) wrote from this point of view and had great impact on the profession. A major concept presented was that the nurse combines scientific knowledge with a "therapeutic use of self." The *relationship between nurse and patient* was seen as distinguishing nursing as a profession and as a unique contribution to patient care. There was decreased emphasis on the nurse as a generalist and an increased awareness that the nurse should take into account each patient's unique combination of attitudes, values, knowledge, and skills. The phrase "total patient care" was still used but was now interpreted to mean that the nurse should relate to the patient as a total, multidimensional, *unique person.*

Theories of human motivation recognized that most people will not change their behavior unless they learn how and why the change is important to them. Because medical and health care so often require changes in patient behavior, the teaching role for health professionals was emphasized. Teaching was a natural extension of the "therapeutic relationship" between nurse and patient.

Starting in the late 1960s and extending throughout the 1970s, changes in medical care delivery begun as a result of World War II and the Korean conflict, such as coronary and intensive care units, were joined with such technological advances as positive-pressure respirators and cardiac monitors. As care became more complex, doctors and nurses became more specialized. It was no longer possible for health professionals to know even a little about "everything" as the generalists of the past had done. Nurses were directly involved with the use of technology in the continuing care of patients. At the same time, nurses were gradually recognized as valuable partners in medical decision making with unique knowledge of their patients. Their expanding role as teachers now included crisis intervention and helping people cope with acute care as well as helping them prepare for self-care.

By the mid-1970s more and more patients who just a few years earlier would have died were now being saved by new surgical techniques, new approaches to cardiac treatment, and new drugs. This ability to treat the seriously ill raised unprecedented ethical issues for the whole medical community. Nurses wondered whether the very young deformed infant and the very old should be resuscitated. They wondered how a nurse could help the family of a patient who was being kept alive by life-support systems. They examined nursing theory and found that patient needs were still a good guide to nursing care but questioned whether the uniqueness of the individual was being lost among the machines.

Nurses also found that with increasing technical demands and earlier patient discharges, they often no longer had time to establish the "therapeutic relationship" in the same way that they had in the past. During this period there were major transitions in the nature of nursing care and in the nature of the satisfactions and rewards derived from nursing practice.

By the late 1970s and into the 1980s certain social changes began to have an increasing impact on the nursing profession. Because nursing was largely a female occupation, the women's movement contributed to some basic changes in the way nurses thought about themselves, both as individuals and as professional women. There was a general social revaluing of the role of working women; two-income families and single-parent families became common. The staff in many medical facilities included more part-time and "per diem" nurses. Nurses again raised the issue of adequate pay for their highly developed professional skills, this time with more enthusiasm and aggressiveness, and perhaps less defensiveness, than in years past.

Meanwhile, the burgeoning computer industry was beginning to influence medical care in diverse ways. What had been an accounting and, in some institutions, a research tool was introduced to the nursing station for record keeping and information processing. Computers also increasingly became part of complex imaging procedures for diagnosis and treatment. The role of electronic equipment will undoubtedly continue to expand into all areas of patient care for years to come. The potential of computer technology in the area of patient education has yet to be fully realized but should, in future years, become a powerful resource for nurse teachers.

As discussed earlier in this chapter, perhaps the social change that has had the most impact on nursing practice is the rising cost of health and medical care. The introduction of DRGs by Medicare in 1983 and the movement toward "pre-authorization" of hospitalization by insurance companies in an effort to contain costs have inspired a variety of changes in patient care. Reductions in nursing staff, the increased acuity of patients, and shorter hospital stays have perhaps had the most impact on day-to-day nursing practice. At the same time hospitals are now more likely to overtly compete for patients in the community. In addition to advertising, they are increasingly offering educational programs and auxiliary services, such as home care, to attract patients. New patterns of nursing management that give nurses greater financial responsibility have emerged and are being tested in many centers (see, for example, *American Journal of Nursing*, vol. 86, no. 4). These kinds of developments provide new opportunities and challenges for nurses.

In summary, teaching has long been an accepted and expected role for the nurse. Although the terminology has changed, certain principles have appeared consistently throughout our professional history. The concepts of patient need as the basis for nursing intervention, the importance of the nurse-patient relationship, and the recognition of patients as unique individuals continue to be central to nursing theory. Social changes, advances in the control of communicable disease, economic concerns, and technological developments have changed the shape of nursing practice, but the principles on which quality nursing care is built continue to function as its heart. Nurses now have new opportunities for helping people learn how to maintain their health and prevent illness. They are challenged to help an increasingly large elderly population learn how to manage chronic diseases and disabilities. They have the chance to use new technology to help people understand developments in patient care. Patient teaching has even more to contribute to quality patient care today than it ever had in the history of nursing.

SUMMARY

In this chapter we have explored four factors that have a major impact on patient teaching. Nurse-patient interaction is described as being at the core of effective teaching. Because communication skills are so important to patient teaching, Chapter 3 is devoted to a discussion of these skills. Patient teaching has been emphasized as an integral part of the Nursing Process, one of several interventions the nurse might select in meeting patient needs.

The teaching role of nurses is also influenced by factors outside the immediate nurse-patient relationship. Current issues within the areas of legal obligation, changing forms and methods of medical care, and administrative concern for delivering cost-effective care to the community all act to shape nursing roles and teaching priorities. At the same time the long history of nurses as teachers supports the nurse in her effort to help patients learn.

These four influential factors provide a way in which to present the general context of the nurse's role in patient teaching. With these ideas as an introduction, we will go on to look at the patient as a "learner" in Chapter 2. In doing so, we will return to the three philosophical principles summarized in the Introduction and show how these influence the learning process.

Study Questions and Exercises

To derive maximum learning benefit from the study questions and exercises included at the end of each chapter, discuss your answers and experiences with your classmates or nursing colleagues. This kind of sharing helps all participants to clarify their thinking on the issue, consider alternative ideas, and see the issue with a broader perspective.

1. Spend at least 10 minutes talking with a soon-to-be-discharged patient or a member of his family. Ask what he thinks he has learned about his illness, treatment, and so on during his hospital stay. Discuss with him what he thinks he may still need to learn before going home. Write a summary of this conversation and share it with classmates or other nurses. Referring to Figure 1-1, identify examples of the four factors shown that influenced this patient's teaching.

2. List the instances of patient teaching you have observed within the past few days. Note whether the teaching was planned, spontaneous, or indirect. Did you notice opportunities for teaching that were bypassed? What might have been done to take advantage of these to help people learn?

3. Sit in the reception area of a clinic or medical unit for 15 to 20 minutes. Pretend that you are a new patient and unfamiliar with the surroundings and procedures. Make

notes about what you hear and observe. What conclusions might you come to on the basis of these observations? Do you think what you "learn" this way is accurate? Share your experience with colleagues or classmates.

4. How does the patient record system in your facility make use of Nursing Process? In what ways does the system used differ from that presented in this book? (See Figure 1–2.) How is it similar, although perhaps with different labels (as in the Problem-Oriented Medical Record system)? What are the major advantages and disadvantages in using such a system on a regular basis?

5. Review the nursing or "progress" notes on several patient records. Is there evidence that patient teaching has been done? Do you have a clear idea, from the recording, of the goals involved in the teaching, the methods used, and patient responses?

6. Obtain a copy of the Patient's Bill of Rights used in your facility. Discuss with your classmates or a colleague your responsibilities for teaching that are implied by the Bill.

7. Discuss with classmates or colleagues some of the ethical questions raised in Table 1–1. What has been the experience of other nurses with regard to ethical or legal issues raised by the principle of informed consent?

8. Choose and carry out several of the activities shown in Table 1–2 in order to familiarize yourself with the concerns and priorities of your facility. If you are a student, small groups might be formed to investigate various aspects of your organization and report back to the class. How do the attitudes and priorities of administrators differ from your own and those of other staff nurses? What implications do these differences have for patient care?

9. Note briefly some of the changes in status and functions that have occurred in nursing within your knowledge and experience. Ask two nursing colleagues to identify some changes of which they have been aware. Discuss and compare these viewpoints with classmates or other nurses. What impact do you think computers will have on patient teaching in the next 10 years?

10. Watch the local newpapers for articles about developments in medical care and the cost of medical and health care. Discuss these articles with classmates or colleagues. How are patient needs or expectations likely to be affected by such articles? How might nursing care be affected?

2

THE PATIENT AND THE LEARNING PROCESS

This chapter focuses on the learner and some of the factors which influence him as he participates in the teaching-learning process. To this end, a few relevant ideas from the fields of educational theory, educational psychology, motivational psychology, and stress theory have been chosen for exploration. The selected topics give only a brief introduction to the wealth of material of practical use that is available to the nurse teacher. The reader is encouraged to pursue these in greater depth to enrich her personal resources as a teacher. The major points contained in this chapter are as follows:

- Learning takes place within three major categories or domains: knowledge, attitudes, and skills. (Introduction)
- Learning is preceded by a preparation or readiness phase and results in the ability to change behavior. (Section 2.1)
- Factors that influence learning include previous experiences, perception of need, nurse-patient interaction, the sociocultural context within which it occurs, and the stress response level of the learner. (Section 2.1)
- The nurse's role in helping the patient get ready to learn is an important first step toward effective teaching. (Section 2.1)
- A person's experiences with modeling, trial and error, and problem solving help prepare him for new learning. (Section 2.2)
- Previous experience provides the foundation on which more complex learning can be built. (Section 2.2)
- A person's perceived problems, goals, concerns, and interests reflect unmet needs. (Section 2.3)
- Subjective perceptions about one's ability to control situations and about health risks play an important part in one's motivation to learn and change. (Section 2.3)

- A person's primary social relationships, secondary social influences, and ethnic patterns strongly influence his self-concept and his perception of needs. (Section 2.4)
- The support and encouragement of those in the learner's primary social group are important for successful behavior change. (Section 2.4)
- Stress is a normal physiologic response to change in the internal or external environment, the effects of which may accumulate over a period of time. (Section 2.5)
- In order for learning to be effective, the nurse teacher must recognize the effect that stress levels have on the patient and plan her intervention accordingly. (Section 2.5)

Learning takes place within several broad categories. The ancient Greeks recognized that there were different kinds of learning, each requiring the learner to use different mental processes. This notion was refined and expanded by Benjamin Bloom, an early learning theorist. His *Taxonomy of Educational Objectives* (1956) continues to strongly influence educational practice. He outlined three "domains" of learning: the cognitive domain, or knowledge; the affective domain, or attitudes; and the psychomotor domain, or skills. Within each domain Bloom identified a number of learning levels arranged in hierarchy of complexity. This hierarchy, as it applies to planning teaching, is discussed in Section 2.2 and again in Chapter 4.

> Throughout this book, learning is referred to as belonging to three domains: knowledge, which is informational and concerned with facts; attitudes, which involve feelings, beliefs, and values; and skills, which involve mental and motor abilities.

Besides providing a convenient way of labeling different kinds of learning, these categories remind the teacher that her approach, choice of teaching methods, and manner of evaluation of learning will differ according to the category of learning involved.

As an illustration of how these labels might be used to differentiate kinds of learning, let us take the example of a nurse who wants to learn how to teach patients more effectively. The nurse will need to gain *knowledge* of how to identify learning needs and what to teach. She will need to develop a positive *attitude* toward teaching, which will include a willingness to take the time to plan and carry out a teaching function. And finally, the nurse will need to learn teaching *skills*, such as how to make a lesson plan, how to conduct a discussion, and perhaps how to operate audiovisual equipment. Categorizing learning in this way helps us see clearly what needs to be learned so that we can plan our teaching accordingly.

Section 2.1 contains an overview of the learning process, together with a conceptual model of the factors that influence it. In Sections 2.2 through 2.5 some basic learning principles are explored as they relate specifically to patient teaching.

2.1 AN OVERVIEW OF THE LEARNING PROCESS

It has been said that a human being's ability to think about thinking is what distinguishes him or her from the animals. Learning is an aspect of thinking that has intrigued philosophers, as well as teachers, throughout the ages. The ability to repeat or modify their behavior based on their experiences allows humans to exercise control over their world, for good or ill. In this historical sense, learning theory is as old as humankind itself. It is indeed presumptuous for us to imagine that ages of wisdom can be condensed into a single chapter. At the same time it is essential that the student of learning have a place to begin. With the intent of providing such starting points, we begin with a conceptual overview of the learning process.

> Learning is a dynamic process consisting of three basic phases: readiness to learn; acquisition of new knowledge, attitudes, or skills; and a resulting ability to change behavior.

These three phases occur in sequence but may overlap to a greater or lesser degree. They may occur quickly or take place over an extended period.

Lewin's Model of the Learning Process

In the mid-1940s Kurt Lewin, psychologist and educator, proposed a simple model for understanding learning and change (1947a). His terminology for the three phases of the learning process were "unfreezing," "moving," and "refreezing." If one imagines an ice cube, the meaning of these stages becomes clear. Faced with a need to learn, the person affected must first "unfreeze," that is, become aware of the need and be willing to think through the consequences of the resulting change. This is followed by the "moving" phase, in which one learns how to change and tries out new behaviors. Finally, if the change is to be adopted, new habits and patterns including the changed behavior "refreeze" in the new mold.

It is not by chance that the model implies that a greater expenditure of energy is required for thawing and reforming than for moving. Lewin was especially aware that teachers often are so focused on the "moving" aspect of learning that they fail to give appropriate attention to the other two phases. Nurses, too, are at risk of failure to take the whole learning process into consideration and instead become absorbed in the technical aspects of teaching.

Because the duration of a nurse's interaction with a patient is often short, the nurse may feel a sense of urgency in getting important information to the patient. She seldom sees the behavior that is the target of her teaching effort, much less the completion of the "refreezing" phase. For this reason it is difficult for the nurse to maintain a broad perspective on the whole learning process (see Mc-Govern and Rodgers, 1986). Such a perspective is necessary, however, if teaching is to result in learning. Awareness of the patient's readiness to learn allows the nurse to time her teaching well and carefully match it with his concerns and needs. Awareness of the "refreezing" phase allows the nurse to prepare the patient, his family, and his environment to support the whole process.

> The goal of teaching is learning. A broad understanding of the learning process helps the nurse teach efficiently as well as effectively.

Factors That Influence the Learning Process

Theorists from many disciplines have contributed to the investigation, analysis, and description of learning as a process. As a framework for this discussion, a number of factors that influence learning have been identified. Exploration of these factors cuts across several disciplinary boundaries to include ideas from motivational and educational psychology, sociology, and stress theory.

> Learning is a multidimensional process influenced by a person's previous experiences, his perception of his present needs, the social and cultural context within which learning takes place, and his present level of stress. Through her interaction with the patient, the nurse has the opportunity to influence these factors so that effective learning is encouraged.

In Chapter 1 a number of factors that influence the nurse as a teacher were explored. A diagram of these factors was presented initially as a way of illustrating their interaction (see Fig. 1–1). In this chapter some of the factors that influence the patient as a learner are also described initially in terms of a diagram, in Figure 2–1, to help the reader conceptualize their interaction. Two-dimensional paper is, of course, limited in its ability to convey dynamic relationships. For this reason we begin with an illustration of an ideal situation, one in which all factors are in place to promote the learning process.

The person who is ready to begin the process has had *experiences* that prepare him for new learning. He is aware of a *need* that can be fulfilled by learning. The *social and cultural context* within which he finds himself supports, rather than obstructs, learning. And his *stress* response levels are neither so high that learning is inhibited nor so low that he lacks motivation. Finally, a *resource* exists to help him learn—in this case, the nurse.

The diagram shows that learning takes place at the intersection of experiential

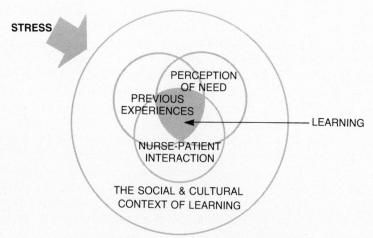

Figure 2–1. Factors influencing the learning process.

preparation and perception of a need to learn. These two factors are essential to a person's readiness or preparation for learning. The interpersonal relationship that the nurse develops with the patient and with family members involved in his care gives her the opportunity to assess learning readiness, influence the interaction of learning factors, and plan and carry out teaching interventions that will lead to effective learning.

In the two case examples that follow, the nurse is in the second, or influencing, stage of the process; she has determined that a learning factor is not yet playing a significant part in the patient's readiness to learn. In interaction with the patient she promotes awareness of the missing factor so that its influence can help prepare the patient to learn. In the first example the nurse is concerned with the "previous experience" factor; in the second, she helps the patient with the "perception of need" factor.

Example 2.1   AN APPARENT LACK OF RELEVANT EXPERIENCE

Mrs. Andrews was admitted for a series of diagnostic procedures. In talking with her the nurse discovered that she had never been hospitalized before, and, although she was aware of her need to understand what was to be done to and for her and was eager to learn, she could not see where to begin or what questions to ask. The nurse spent some time with Mrs. Andrews exploring her previous outpatient experiences and identifying some similarities in procedures. The patient recalled that she had visited a friend who had been a patient on another unit several years ago. In interaction with the nurse the patient began to appreciate how she could use these previous experiences as resources on which to build present learning.

On a conceptual level, the nurse had helped the patient bring her perception of need and her previous experiences together so that she was ready to learn. The learning factor model shown in Figure 2–2 has been modified to reflect this particular situation. The arrow indicates the major focus of the nurse's interaction with the patient.

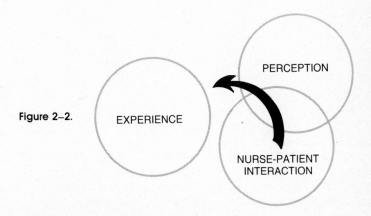

Figure 2–2.

EXPERIENCE

PERCEPTION

NURSE-PATIENT INTERACTION

Example 2.2   HELP WITH RECOGNIZING A NEED TO LEARN

Mr. Baxter, age 56, came to the clinic for an annual physical examination. He complained of frequent episodes of indigestion. He also stated that he had not had as much energy in the past year or so as he had previously. He had given up playing tennis regularly. Examination showed that Mr. Baxter was 25 pounds overweight but otherwise, he was a healthy man with normal electrocardiogram and blood pressure. In consultation, doctor and nurse concluded that patient teaching in the area of diet and nutrition was appropriate.

The nurse initially encouraged the patient to tell her what he normally ate and what foods he especially liked. He reported that he was fond of the spicy Italian dishes his wife prepared so well. Through careful use of questions that encouraged him to explore the subject, Mr. Baxter began to see a relationship between his increased weight, decreased energy and exercise, and indigestion and his eating patterns. Within a short time he was asking the nurse questions and seemed interested in learning how he might modify his behavior toward healthier patterns.

In this situation the health professionals uncovered what they assessed to be a learning need. Teaching was not attempted, however, until the patient shared this perception. By exploring some apparently unrelated experiences, the nurse helped the patient become aware of a problem area that was affecting his health. Problem identification was the first step in helping Mr. Baxter perceive a need to learn. The factors affecting the learning process in this case are diagramed in Figure 2–3.

In these two situations the nurse took an active part in helping the patient get ready to learn. In other situations high stress levels or unsupportive sociocul-

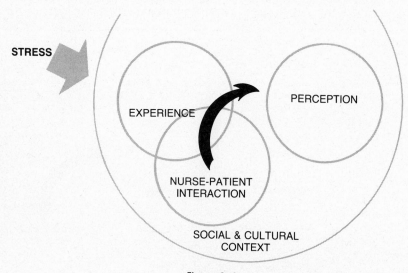

Figure 2–3.

tural factors may present as much of a barrier to learning as lack of relevant experience and need perception did in these cases. Within the context of nurse-patient interaction, the nurse's objective is to reduce the effect of barriers to learning while promoting supportive and helpful factors.

An important aspect of the model presented in Figure 2–1 is the interdependence of the five factors; each has an impact, positive or negative, on the others. For example, as in the case of Mr. Baxter, sociocultural considerations may play a part in how a person perceives a need or whether he follows through on a learned behavior. Similarly, high stress response levels may change a person's interpretation of an experience or block his ability to acquire new knowledge or skills. Nurse-patient interaction can also have either a positive or a negative effect; it can either stimulate learning or, through a negative attitude or impatient behavior on the part of the nurse, present a barrier to learning. Exploration of some of the principles of learning will help us to better understand these dynamic relationships.

Principles of Learning

Many rules, or principles, govern how the factors identified in the model influence learning. Ten are especially relevant to patient teaching. Each factor, along with its related principles, is discussed in the next four sections of this chapter and in Chapter 3. Learning principles and factors that influence the process are summarized in Table 2–1.

TABLE 2–1. Learning Principles and Factors That Influence Learning

Learning Principle	Related Factor
1. A wide range of experiences contributes to one's resources for further learning. 2. Learning progresses from simple to complex.	Previous experience
3. Learning is motivated by perceived problems or goals arising out of unmet needs. 4. A person's beliefs and values affect how he perceives problems and what priority he places on learning.	Perceived need
5. Verbalization assists the progress of learning. 6. The trust relationship provides an environment in which change can take place.	Nurse-Patient interaction
7. The network of sociocultural relationships that surrounds a person determines his perception of learning needs and his willingness to begin the learning process. 8. The behavioral changes that result from learning are most likely to occur when they are supported by those with a primary social relationship to the learner.	Social and Cultural context
9. Stress may promote learning or act as a barrier to it. 10. Learning and change are themselves stressful.	Stress

2.2 EXPERIENCE AS A FACTOR IN LEARNING

Life is a continuous series of experiences. We refer to these experiences in a variety of ways, indicating our pleasure or displeasure with them, our sense of control over them or our sense of frustration. Consider the following statements:

"I've just discovered the most wonderful thing..."

"What a frustrating experience that was!"

"I learned a lot from that experience."

"I hope I'm never subjected to that kind of experience again!"

"I really enjoyed doing that. Maybe we can do it again."

"That was an unexpected pleasure."

Each statement suggests an attitude toward an experience and implies that future behavior will be guided by it. The speaker in each instance has "learned" something that will be applied to future experiences he identifies as being similar.

In this section we will explore two basic principles that relate to learning through experience.

LEARNING PRINCIPLE 1: A wide range of experiences contributes to one's resources for further learning.

LEARNING PRINCIPLE 2: Learning progresses from simple to complex.

How Experience Teaches

By the time the nurse becomes involved in helping an adult patient learn, the patient already has a wealth of life experiences, as well as formal educational experiences, that have led him to develop ideas, beliefs, values, and approaches to problems that work for him. He calls on these experiences whenever he encounters a new situation or a problem to solve. As Malcolm Knowles, an authority on adult education, shows so conclusively, the accumulated experiences of adults provide an invaluable resource on which further learning is based (1984, Ch. 4).

Experiences from which one learns are acquired in a number of ways or as a result of different strategies.

Three strategies by which both children and adults learn through experience are modeling or example, trial and error, and problem solving.

A person's background of experiences plays a large part in his readiness to learn and is important in determining what and how the nurse should teach.

Learning Through Modeling or Example

In Section 1.1 I noted that some of the teaching done by nurses is indirect; people observe their behavior and learn by their example. In these instances the nurse is used as a "model" by the learner. Although we often think of learning through modeling or example as being confined to childhood, it is actually an important strategy for learning throughout life. It is particularly useful when skills are being learned; we watch the behavior of someone else and then attempt to duplicate it. The child learns to tie her shoes, button her buttons, and brush her teeth by watching and being helped by a parent. The teenager learns to perform the latest dance movements by watching others. The nursing student imitates the instructor in giving an injection; the employee may use his boss as a model of success; the hostess attempts to duplicate the valued graciousness of a good friend.

If someone is regarded by others as having special expertise, that person's behavior is a powerful example from which others may learn. The neat, clean uniforms of nurses provide a concrete example of basic principles of personal hygiene for all who regard nurses as having special knowledge about health.

As teachers we can consciously use modeling or example as a strategy for helping others learn. In a planned teaching session one might demonstrate the preparation of an insulin syringe or the technique of walking with crutches as an introductory lesson, with the aim of helping the patient do these things himself. Likewise, a counselor may model good listening behavior for a client before helping the client learn these skills and their application in other relationships.

While modeling or example is most useful when applied to specific behaviors or skills, such as nursing procedures or physical movements, attitudes are also imitated when the person demonstrating them is held in high regard or when the attitude is expressed by a valued group. If both caregivers and family members, for example, believe that a patient can get well and take care of himself again, the power of this modeled attitude is bound to have a positive influence on the patient.

Learning Through Trial and Error

A second strategy we use as adults to learn by experience is trial and error. Whenever we attempt to solve a problem with which we have had no previous experience and no helpful model is present, we have no choice but to try something and see whether it works. As adults, this kind of learning, especially when there are time limits or excellence of performance is demanded, is usually frustrating.

A family recently acquired a home computer. They rapidly discovered that the manuals accompanying the machine were woefully inadequate, leaving them no choice but to "play with it" and learn about the capabilities of the computer by trial and error. Some people have justified this approach to learning by saying that we learn best from our mistakes. This view seems not to be borne out by research. (See, for example, discussion of stimulus-response learning in Lefrancois, 1975, Ch. 2.) We do remember our mistakes more vividly, but there is little evidence that the frustration and feelings of helplessness generated by failure are beneficial to the learning process.

In our complex modern lives few decisions are clearly good or bad, black or white. To this extent we continue to discover, by trial and error, a "good," or at least "satisfactory," way to solve a particular problem. We learn only later, with the clear vision of hindsight, whether our choice was the best one possible. Two examples of this continual search by trial and error for the "best" solutions are job decisions and relationship decisions. In neither case can we possibly know all of the consequences of a particular decision. So we are compelled to accept the new job or allow a close relationship to develop based on currently available, but incomplete, information even while accepting the risk of later regretting the decision.

In a clinical setting people are also learning by trial and error. When patients are hospitalized for the first time, they may have little or no knowledge about how they are expected to behave. Some patients try out behaviors, such as compliance or demandingness, until they can find out whether it works for them. Other kinds of trial-and-error learning range from selecting a doctor to discovering what kinds of insurance documents should have been brought along to the hospital.

> Under normal teaching circumstances, one would like to minimize instances of trial-and-error learning, since it is time consuming and frustrating for the learner.

Purposely setting up this kind of learning situation for someone may seem highly manipulative and may generate a great deal of anger.

Learning Through Problem Solving

All kinds of experiences may contribute to learning, but the best opportunity occurs when a person can effectively solve a problem of concern to him. Helping a patient, a family member, or a colleague identify a specific problem and work through the steps of investigating alternatives and taking planned action is a useful approach to learning by experience. The participation of the learner makes the learning truly "his," not something imposed upon him by the teacher or by unforeseen circumstances, as in trial-and-error learning. The benefits of helping people learn through the experience of problem solving are emphasized in a discussion of teaching methods in Chapter 5.

One of the reasons problem solving is so effective in producing learning out of experience is that by the time a plan is made and action is taken, a person has progressed from a simple formulation of the problem to a complex understanding of it.

How Learning Progresses from Simple to Complex

There are two visual images that have been used to describe the principle that learning progresses from simple to complex. One is to imagine learning to be like a tower of blocks, each layer built on the preceding layer, and the other, to visualize learning as an ever-rising spiral, each rotation connected to earlier turns. Although the principle of learning progression seems self-evident from everyday experience, it has implications for the conduct of teaching far beyond common sense. It applies both to the learning ability of the individual as he develops from infancy to intellectual maturity and to learning developed within a particular subject area (Darkenwald and Merriam, 1982).

The progression from simple to complex is most easily seen in the development of learning ability in children. The first learning done by infants is simple, even primitive. They respond to sounds and events in their environment, soon learning to organize their responses to meet their needs for food, comfort, and attention. Then, as the child becomes able to use language, learning takes on new dimensions of complexity. Learning ability progresses from the use of simple sentences to express needs and interests to the use of complex language constructions to express principles, concepts, and abstract ideas.

Many developmental psychologists have studied the intellectual development of children, but no one has surpassed the impact that Jean Piaget has had on school programs in the United States and elsewhere. He proposed that learning be classified into four basic stages, beginning with the simple sensorimotor period of infancy and progressing to the period of formal operations in the early teen years when the child is able to manipulate abstract concepts (Furth, 1970; Inhelder and Piaget, 1958).

The nurse who frequently works with children or the intellectually handicapped will find it helpful to familiarize herself with these ideas, since recognizing a child's capabilities for thinking at certain stages will help her communicate more effectively. For example, a 5-year-old child, representing Piaget's stage of intuitive thought, described her experience of anesthesia as "I disappeared." An 8- or 9-year-old who is within the stage of concrete operations, would be able to understand an explanation of a recovery room as "a big room with lots of beds and bright lights," since this is an extension of his own concrete experience with beds and lights. He would not, however, be able to relate to being told that after surgery, he would wake up in a "special place where people will take good care of you," since this more abstract explanation would be beyond his ability to understand.

A summary of the developmental stages described by Piaget is shown in Table 2–2.

The principle that learning progresses from simple to complex also applies to a person's learning about particular subjects. One needs some background of information before one can reach a decision or discuss a subject in detail. For example, a nurse needs to know about aseptic technique and be able to handle a syringe without contaminating it before she can correctly administer a parenteral medication. Another way of stating this principle is to say that all learning depends on some previous learning.

> A challenge for the nurse teacher is to identify what progression of learning will be needed to reach a particular goal and what experiences the learner already has available to build on.

The following case example demonstrates this point.

Example 2.3 TWO PATIENTS WITH HYPERTENSION

Jennifer Dole was caring for two patients, both of whom, on entry to the hospital for other medical problems, had been diagnosed as having hypertension. Part of her Nursing Care Plan for each of them was to help the patient learn what risk factors were associated with hypertension and how diet and stress management could augment medication in lowering blood

TABLE 2-2. Piaget's Stages of Cognitive Development

Stage	Age	Characteristics
1. Sensorimotor	0–2 years	Develops concept that objects have permanence and an identity of their own. Begins to use symbols to represent activities.
2. Preoperational A. Preconceptual	2–7 years 2–4 years	Use of concepts is incomplete and illogical. Reasoning is "transductive," going from one particular instance to another particular instance without linking them logically.
B. Intuitive	4–7 years	Thinking is dominated by perception rather than reason. Events are interpreted only from the child's point of view (egocentrism).
3. Concrete Operations	7–11 years	Can apply rules of logic to classes of objects and their spacial relationships and to numbers, but not to objects or events that are not "concrete," i.e., those within his own experience or ability to imagine.
4. Formal Operations	11–15 years	Able to reason from the hypothetical to the real or from the actual to the hypothetical. Imagination and idealism are characteristic of stage.

Source: Lefrancois, G. Psychology for Teaching, 2nd ed., Palo Alto, Calif.: Wadsworth, 1975, pp. 206–228.

pressure. One of her patients, Mr. Egan, was a computer technician; the other, Ms. Franklin, was a dietitian. In initiating teaching on this subject, the nurse's first action was to assess what each patient already knew that might apply to the learning objective. By talking with them she found out that Mr. Egan had had a basic biology course in college and had recently seen a television program on the link between stress and high blood pressure. He had little knowledge of diet. Ms. Franklin, on the other hand, had a secure understanding of a low-sodium diet and the potential physiologic benefits of following such a diet. This knowledge was expected by the nurse but not assumed. Having made this assessment, Ms. Dole's teaching was planned to take each patient's previous learning into account and build on it to meet the present learning objectives.

In this case example the nurse took the time and care to fully assess each patient's background of learning. Our everyday experiences make it clear that we progress in learning from simple to complex; and it is almost automatic to check with children to find out what they already know. It is surprisingly easy, however, to become contaminated by our own understandings and forget that other intelligent adults might have background knowledge and attitudes that are quite different from our own. In order to be effective teachers, we must teach ourselves to be alert to this problem.

In his exhaustive work on identifying levels of learning, Bloom (1956) made the principle of building on previous learning abundantly clear. He also gave us a way to express exactly what we mean when we assess a person's current level of learning and identify learning objectives. In Table 2–3 a simplified form of a learning hierarchy is shown. Within each domain or category of learning, five levels of complexity are named and described. Number 1 is the simplest and number 5, the most complex.

TABLE 2–3. Levels of Learning

Knowledge

1. Remember	To recall information
2. Understand	To grasp the meaning
3. Apply	To use the information
4. Analyze	To understand the underlying principle
5. Evaluate	To judge value and compare with other known information

Attitudes

1. Recognize	To be aware and give attention
2. Respond	To react and give feedback
3. Verbalize	To be able to explain attitude
4. Utilize	To take action demonstrating attitude
5. Conceptualize	To make attitude part of one's larger value system

Skills

1. Perceive	To be aware of component parts and their relationship to one another
2. Manipulate	To be able to handle parts appropriately but separately
3. Combine	To put parts together for coordinated action
4. Perform	To carry out sequenced actions and complete total task procedure
5. Adapt	To modify procedures to fit circumstances

Taking the example of Mr. Egan, he may be able to "remember" some facts about the physiology of the cardiovascular system from his biology class. This is certainly a starting point, but his nurse would like him to "apply" this knowledge to his own situation. From watching the television program, the patient may "recognize" that stress affects blood pressure, but the learning objectives in this case might well be for him to develop more complex abilities, such as being able to "utilize" these attitudes in his life and "perform" relaxation techniques. If Mr. Egan is to modify his future behavior for the benefit of his health, he must be helped to progress from his current simple levels of prior learning to more complex ones.

The concept of levels of complexity in learning is also explored in Chapter 4, with a discussion of how to write learning objectives.

In summary, in this section we have discussed previous experience as it influences the learning process. Some ways in which a person learns through experience have been described in terms of modeling or example, trial and error, and problem solving. The principle that learning progresses from simple to complex has been explored using Piaget's stages of learning development and Bloom's taxonomy of learning complexity.

The previous experiences of patients are of major importance to the nurse in planning teaching intervention.

> By organizing her teaching so that it builds on the patient's previous experience, the nurse increases learning effectiveness and efficiency.

For the nurse teacher, utilizing previous learning as a resource on which to build means taking the time to explore these with the patient, being alert to the several ways in which people learn. It means not making any assumptions about the patient's background knowledge, attitudes, or skills. It means being willing to adjust the content of her teaching so that it has relevance to the patient and his world of experience. And it means discovering that people learn more quickly and effectively when the nurse is able to prepare teaching in this way.

2.3 PERCEPTION OF NEED AS A FACTOR IN LEARNING

Just as one must identify a problem before being able to solve it effectively, so one must perceive that a need exists before one can be motivated to learn. The connections between perception or a mental awareness of a need, the intention to fulfill it, and the willingness to change behavior as a result of learning have concerned educators and social scientists for many years. This interest has led to a wealth of scientific study as well as creative speculation.

Although the mental process involved in perception, motivation, and changed behavior is complex, its importance to learning is clear. In this section we will explore some ideas about needs, beliefs, and values as they affect a person's perceptions and, consequently, his motivation to learn. The following two learning principles are the basis for our discussions.

> **LEARNING PRINCIPLE 3:** Learning is motivated by perceived problems or goals arising out of unmet needs.
>
> **LEARNING PRINCIPLE 4:** A person's beliefs and values affect how he perceives problems and what priority he places on learning.

Two general concepts are implied by these principles. One is that perception of a need, goal, or problem precedes learning. A second is that the perception must be the learner's own, not someone else's. In helping a patient become ready to learn, or "unfreeze," the nurse must first assist him to arrive at his own perception of the need or reason to learn. Only then, like Mr. Baxter (Example 2.2), will he be motivated to acquire needed knowledge, attitudes, or skills.

We will first look at the relationship between unmet needs and motivation by exploring the work of Abraham Maslow and then proceed to some ideas about personal beliefs and values as they affect readiness to learn.

How Needs Affect Motivation

Abraham Maslow pioneered in the identification of needs and their relationship to motivation. His work, which spanned three decades, made an outstanding contribution to the understanding of human behavior (1943, 1962, 1970). The ideas he presented are easily understood and readily applied to patient teaching situations.

Maslow suggested that everyone has some general needs that they seek to fulfill. These *unmet needs* motivate behavior. Maslow saw these general human needs as arranged in a hierarchy of complexity with the simpler, more elementary needs at the base, progressing through a number of successive steps to the higher, more complex needs, as shown in Figure 2–4. Once a particular need is fulfilled, another, higher need takes its place as a motivator. The ways in which this theory supports the principle that learning progresses from simple to complex are clear.

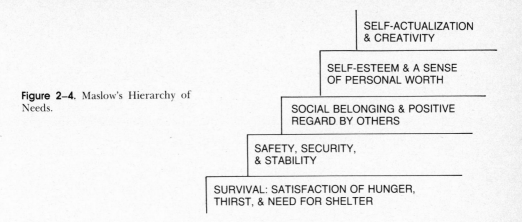

Figure 2–4. Maslow's Hierarchy of Needs.

Maslow would add to it by suggesting that each level of fulfilled need provides the vantage point from which one can perceive that more is available and within reach.

The behavioral stages of human development provide an example of this model, just as Piaget's stages (Table 2–2) are an example of progressive cognitive capability. During infancy the child is totally dependent on others for *survival*. His behavior reflects his needs for food, water, warmth, and physical protection. As the child's awareness increases, the need for a stable, close, nurturing relationship becomes paramount. He needs to feel *safe and secure* in his environment. Then, during the school years, his personal world expands; he needs *social belonging* and acceptance by others. Although he does not stop needing food and safety, his behavior reflects more concern for this emerging and as yet unfulfilled need. The school-aged child, for example, is particularly interested in learning something new if his friends are also involved.

The person moving into the adolescent years needs to develop feelings of *self-worth* if he is to have the confidence to take on adult responsibilities. Finally, the mature person needs to feel that his contribution to life is *unique and creative;* he strives toward fulfilling the level of his greatest potential.

In addition to describing the maturational sequence of behavior changes, Maslow's theory of a needs hierarchy contains some important concepts affecting the motivation of adults. These are summarized as follows:

- Unmet needs are reflected in a person's interests and concerns, his perceived problems and goals.
- A person is motivated to fulfill the highest unmet needs within his perception as long as more basic needs are met at a satisfactory level.
- The person whose dominant needs are self-esteem and self-actualization continues to be motivated by these throughout life; they are never completely fulfilled.
- At a time of high stress or personal reverses, such as during ill health, a person experiences needs in more basic areas, such as survival or safety.

The higher needs that motivated him before his illness continue to concern him, but the majority of his energy will be used to meet the more urgent, elementary needs.

Job satisfaction is an example of Maslow's hierarchy of needs model applied to the everyday experience of adults. A manager who analyzes the needs of a job applicant as reflected in his interests and goals would be in a good position to decide how a particular job would fit the applicant's needs and motivate him. In general, one feels satisfied with one's job if (a) it provides enough money to ensure survival, (b) there is job security, and (c) one feels a part of a supportive work group. These aspects of a job would meet the first three basic needs described by Maslow. If, in addition, one's accomplishments on the job were noticed and publicly acknowledged by the supervisor, this would fulfill a need for self-esteem and self-confidence.

In a study of registered nurses Longest (1974) found that self-actualizing factors (the worth of the work itself and a sense of achievement) were major motivators. Also important to nurses was good interpersonal relationships. Longest suggests that this concern, reflecting the less complex need for social belonging, might motivate nurses because satisfaction in this area has often been lacking, making them more aware of it as a need. In such a situation, a lower level need that is temporarily not being met is a powerful motivator until it is again fulfilled.

Patients demonstrate this principle every day. When physical survival and psychological safety are jeopardized by injury or illness, meeting these most basic needs overwhelms all other motivational factors. The following case example shows how a nurse was able to interpret a mother's concerns and apparent perception of problems as a reflection of needs and plan care accordingly.

Example 2.4   A MOTHER'S MOTIVATION TO LEARN

The Jackson family's ordeal had started on a chilly Saturday evening. Four-year-old Angela was standing close to a gas heater when her nightgown caught fire. Her sudden scream brought her mother running from another part of the house. She wrapped Angela in a blanket to smother the flames and then tried to put out a fire that had spread to some papers. The fire department and an ambulance arrived within minutes, but to Mrs. Jackson, it seemed like they had waited for an eternity. The Emergency Department staff immediately began treating Angela's legs and back which had suffered second- and third-degree burns. She was admitted to the burn unit and placed in isolation. Mrs. Jackson was treated for first-degree burns on her hands and arms.

For Mrs. Jackson, the next few days passed in a blur of telephone calls, considerable pain, and near panic over Angela's condition. She spent long hours at her daughter's bedside trying to comfort her. Angela had regressed to wetting the bed and using baby talk. She screamed when her mother left, even for a few minutes.

Mrs. Jackson religiously followed the isolation procedure each time she entered or left Angela's room. She hadn't had the energy to understand the reasons behind the procedures; she just followed them by rote. Julie Evans, R.N., had been there when Angela was admitted and continued to care for her almost every day. She had explained the isolation procedures to Mrs.

Jackson, emphasizing that by putting a germ barrier between Angela and the outside world, Angela would be protected from infection and have the best chance of full recovery. Mrs. Jackson was thankful for the large sign posted by the door outlining the procedure for gowning that she could follow step by step. She worried that she would accidentally forget something and jeopardize her daughter's recovery.

As Mrs. Jackson became better acquainted with Ms. Evans and the other staff, she began asking questions and they took the time to explain Angela's treatment and progress. She noticed that Angela had gradually become less demanding of her time and attention and that she greeted Ms. Evans literally with open arms. It seemed like a great weight had been lifted from her shoulders to know that Angela was getting good care from warm, competent people.

Several days after Angela's admission Ms. Evans told Mrs. Jackson about a group meeting for patients' relatives and other concerned visitors that was held on the unit twice a week. During the informal meeting people could ask questions of the doctor or nurse who was present. Mrs. Jackson attended regularly. Not only did she learn about physiotherapy and some of the care Angela would need at home, but she also had the chance to talk with other people who shared her feelings of guilt and confusion and worry.

In reviewing Angela's case with her supervisor, Julie Evans identified three "needs" that she felt had been met in addition to quality nursing care for the patient. At the time of crisis, when Mrs. Jackson was too overwhelmed by events to be able to think clearly, she was offered simple explanations of Angela's care and condition and step-by-step instructions. Because she was able to stay with her daughter during the crisis, she helped to calm the child and felt *reassured that she would survive* and receive the best possible care. Consistent staff assignments allowed both mother and child to develop trusting relationships with a small number of people which contributed to their sense of *safety and security.* Finally, the group meetings gave Mrs. Jackson a chance to learn many things she needed to know about Angela's care and to become *part of a group* that shared her feelings and valued her as a participant. She found that she was not alone.

In this case example Julie Evans and her colleagues recognized the importance of identifying the needs of both mother and child. They then tailored their interaction with them to help meet these needs. An involved explanation of asepsis as Angela was being admitted would have been inappropriate and time-consuming. Instead, a simple explanation focused on Angela's future well-being was understood and heard as reassuring. By later helping Mrs. Jackson meet her need for safety and security, Ms. Evans set the stage for being able to help her learn about Angela's treatment and, eventually, how to give care at home. Although Mrs. Jackson may not have been able to say, "I need safety" or "I need a sense of social belonging," her interests, concerns, and questions were interpreted by the nurse as perceptions that reflected her needs.

The perceptions that people have of problems confronting them reflect their most urgent needs. Actively helping people meet basic needs allows them to learn and participate in care more quickly.

Table 2–4 lists some actions that might be taken by the nurse teacher in an effort to help the patient meet basic needs and encourage learning.

TABLE 2–4. Helping to Meet Patients' Basic Needs

Need	Suggested Action
Survival	Keep instructions and explanations simple. Provide structured environment. Reduce environmental stress. Make goals clear and short-term. Encourage trust and reassure appropriately.
Safety and Security	Respond to questions quickly and matter-of-factly. Help patient take actions to help himself and become less dependent. Keep lessons practical and goals clear.
Social Belonging	Include family members in teaching. Encourage open discussion of feelings as well as facts. Include information with implications for future care/health in learning goals.

The nurse's awareness that, in the face of a medical crisis, elementary human needs are not being met in a usual way also helps her understand and have patience with seemingly demanding or attention-getting behaviors. Assisting the patient to feel secure and participate in decisions about his care is often a successful way of handling what may seem to be childish behavior.

How Beliefs and Personal Values Affect Motivation

Values and beliefs are convictions that a person carries with him throughout everyday life. They give emotional color to events and provide some shortcuts for making sense of them. They are a kind of mental catalog that allows us to decide quickly how we should react to a given circumstance. Values and beliefs are products of our past experiences influencing our present perceptions. When supported and encouraged by others who are important to us in our immediate social world, they become part of a value "system," or set of internal rules, by which we conduct our lives. The following examples illustrate how beliefs and values may affect the interpretation of current events and, consequently, behavior.

- A person passing by a war memorial in a park where the American flag is displayed pauses, standing at attention with his right hand over his heart. A short conversation with him reveals that he served his country during World War II. He values democracy and believes that it is every citizen's duty to be patriotic.
- A person at the checkout of a grocery store becomes loudly angry when he perceives that the clerk has overcharged him on an item. He states: "You people try to cheat me every time I come in here!"

The people in these examples were acting on beliefs that reflect deeply held values concerning democracy and fairness. Their immediate perceptions were colored by these beliefs and expressed emotionally as attitudes. Previous experiences helped to shape them.

An interesting aspect of beliefs is that the person holding them generally regards his own set as true and absolutely valid. As Muldary (1983) has phrased this observation: "We believe that what we believe is true. We take it for granted that our beliefs are correct, because we have an ultimate belief in the reliability of our own senses" (p. 208). In terms of emotional response to situations, what we perceive, is. A problem arises when perceptions and beliefs about an event are not shared between people who are attempting to communicate with one another. We return to this point in Chapter 3, in a discussion of how the nurse's values and beliefs may affect the quality of nurse-patient communication. For now, the focus is on patients' beliefs about health and how these affect both their attitudes toward illness prevention and medical care and their motivation to learn.

One large group of beliefs that have major implications for medical and health care delivery focuses on how an individual sees his ability to control events and environments. A great deal of research has been conducted on people's *locus of control* (e.g., Phares, 1976; Lau, 1982). Beliefs about control are best represented by a continuum. At one end are those peoples who perceive that their behavior influences events in their lives; they believe that one "makes one's own luck." They are said to have an "internal" locus, or center, of control. At the other end of the continuum are those who think that their lives are controlled by outside forces: God, luck, or fate, for example. They believe that their behavior has little impact on events in their lives. They are said to have an "external" locus of control (Rotter, 1966).

Most people's personal beliefs fall somewhere between these two extremes and may vary according to the circumstances in which they find themselves. Although the sources of one's perceived locus of control are not clear, the experience of poverty, repeated discrimination, or long-term disability seems to correlate with an "external" orientation (Lefcourt, 1982). In addition, events in which a person feels out of control for an extended period, such as serious illness, can result in a general shift in beliefs toward the external end of the scale. This finding is consistent with Seligman's work (1975) on learned helplessness.

A person's beliefs about his degree of personal control over his life's events determine, to a large degree, his willingness to participate in care and his motivation to learn. The more internally focused the person is, the more interested he is likely to be in making behavioral changes that will benefit his health. Alternatively, the strongly externally focused person may well feel that the effort to learn and change is pointless. A series of statements is shown in Table 2–5 which reflect either a strongly internal or strongly external point of view about health matters.

Those who have chosen careers in the health field typically have an "internal" orientation toward health beliefs. As a result, they find themselves in conflict with patients who tend toward the opposite end of the belief continuum.

> When the nurse does not share the patient's beliefs concerning control over health matters, ignoring the conflict or attempting to argue the person out of them will not be effective.

A more effective approach includes the following steps:

- Assess the patient's *beliefs* about locus of control through open-ended discussion of issues such as those suggested in Table 2–5. The nurse will

TABLE 2–5. Beliefs About Control Over Health

Persons with these kinds of beliefs have a strongly *internal* locus of control:
1. I am basically responsible for my own health.
2. Proper nutrition, exercise, and sleep keep me healthy.
3. When I become ill, I know it is because I haven't taken proper care of myself.
4. The more I learn about my body, the better prepared I am to get well and stay healthy.
5. It's important that I work hard at getting well and staying well.

Persons with these kinds of beliefs have a strongly *external* locus of control:
1. Whether or not I become ill is a matter of luck.
2. The doctor knows best how I should take care of myself; I must do exactly what he tells me to do, even though I don't understand why.
3. Some people just catch everything that comes along no matter what they do.
4. If you're meant to stay healthy, you will.
5. If I become ill, all I can do is hope I get well soon.

Based on Wallston, B. S., K. A. Wallston, G. D. Kaplan, and S. A. Maides: Development and validation of the health locus of control (HLC) scale. *Journal of Consulting and Clinical Psychology*, Vol. 44, No. 4 (1976), p. 581.

need to estimate not only the internal-external dimension of beliefs, but also whether they are the result of current circumstances or part of a long-term, pervasive belief system.

- Determine what health problems or *concerns* are most important to the patient. Although the nurse may not share the patient's sense of urgency about them, the key to helping the patient learn and change is to start with *his* perception of the most troubling problem.
- Work with the patient to determine a realistic approach to minimizing or solving the problem. Clearly identify *short-term objectives* and the steps necessary to achieve them. Joint objective setting allows the patient to participate actively in planning the change process.
- Recognize that your goal is to help the patient experience *personal control* over an aspect of his health behavior, no matter how minor. It is important that he achieve success within a supportive environment. (See discussion in Section 9.1 on use of feedback.) Involve others of significance to the patient in planning, encouraging, and supporting changes.
- Be aware that helping a person change a belief system is a long-term project. Usually all that can be done in the clinical setting is to help him open the previously closed door a mere crack. Become familiar with helping/support resources in the community because the strongly "external" person will need *continued encouragement* to change health behaviors.

In addition to general systems of beliefs about the controllability of life events, a person develops a range of beliefs that have an impact on his health related behavior. One area of great interest for health professionals is what influences people to seek help with a health problem or engage in preventative action. Out of investigation of this area the Health Belief Model was developed by Rosenstock in the 1950s. He identified a number of perceptions or beliefs, all of which must be present before a person is motivated to take action (Rosenstock, 1966, 1974, 1980). Becker and Maiman (1975, 1980) did additional work with the model, showing how it applies to sick role behavior as well as to preventive behavior. The elements of the Health Belief Model are listed and described in Table 2–6.

TABLE 2–6. Elements of the Health Belief Model

Element	Description
Perceived susceptibility	Belief that one is in danger of contracting a given disease. When illness is present, belief in accuracy of diagnosis.
Perceived severity	Belief that the disease would/will have serious consequences for one's health, well-being, and/or daily life.
Perceived effectiveness of proposed action	Belief that a given action will be beneficial in preventing the disease or controlling its negative impact.
Perceived ability to overcome barriers to action	Belief that barriers such as cost, inconvenience, and effort are realistically surmountable.
Existence of a cue	An event, interest, or active concern that helps motivate action.

In addition to the elements in Table 2–6, factors that seem to influence motivation for an action include a person's perceived relationship with the health care provider, previous experience with the illness or the proposed action, and the presence of social or cultural supports for the action (Becker, 1974). The following example shows how perceptions work together to influence action.

Example 2.5   BELIEFS ABOUT AIDS

In early 1982 the first newspaper reports began to appear about a "new" disease, Acquired Immune Deficiency Syndrome or AIDS. The cause of the disease was unknown, and it seemed to block the body's natural defenses to infection, making it vulnerable to certain rare forms of skin cancer and pneumonia. There was no known treatment. Mortality rates were extremely high. At first, AIDS was largely a disease of male homosexuals, apparently transmitted sexually. Then it was discovered that AIDS could be transferred through blood from affected donors.

Surveys of male homosexuals in the San Francisco area indicated that many believed that:

— their sexual preferences and activities made them *susceptible* to AIDS,

— the disease was *serious* and likely to be fatal within a short time of diagnosis, and

— the most *effective preventive action* available was to reduce exposure by limiting sexual partners.

Many believed that the *barriers* to action, such as change of life-style, could be satisfactorily overcome, since increasing numbers of homosexuals reported taking action to reduce exposure (*Time* magazine, 12 Aug. 1985).

Cues that may have increased motivation to take action include the death of a friend or associate who had AIDS and the death of movie star Rock Hudson.

In this example the subjective perceptions that make up health beliefs about AIDS influenced the behavior of members of a high-risk group in reducing exposure to the disease. Other factors that may have played a part in decisions about this health-related behavior include the social supports for change within the homosexual community, the strength of cultural discrimination against homosexuals, and the degree to which the person has an "internal," versus "external," locus of control.

Although the Health Belief Model has not been reliably predictive of particular health actions, it clearly shows the significance of perceptions and beliefs in motivating behavior.

The Health Belief Model suggests that the nurse teacher include a careful assessment of the patient's subjective beliefs and perceptions, as well as more objective data, in her determination of the patient's readiness to learn and change.

The model also indicates that the nature of the relationship between patient and health professional is important in the formation of beliefs and subsequent decisions about action. This point is taken up again in Chapter 3. Some interesting parallels between health beliefs and stress as a motivating factor are discussed in Section 2.5.

In summary, this section has focused on some of the internal and subjective perceptions that influence a person's motivation to learn and change. Maslow's hierarchy of needs has been discussed as a way of better understanding the priorities that people place on their interests, concerns, and activities. Some general beliefs about a person's ability to control events and his environment were explored in terms of their impact on a person's willingness to take beneficial health actions. These ideas were then developed further through presentation of the Health Belief Model. If teaching is to result in effective learning, the nurse must take all of these factors into consideration as she assesses the patient's readiness to learn. She also must appreciate the potential impact her interaction with him can have in improving his motivation to learn. Most important, the nurse must approach the teaching-learning process with a willingness to find out what factors are currently influencing the patient's motivation to learn and then begin her teaching with these.

Because the quality and nature of nurse-patient interaction are so important to the teaching-learning process, a separate chapter has been devoted to the subject. Chapter 3 explores ways in which the nurse can effectively establish a basis of communication with the patient and his family members. Contained therein is a discussion of Learning Principles 5 and 6.

2.4 THE SOCIAL AND CULTURAL CONTEXT OF LEARNING

In this section we proceed to the next factor shown in the model of factors that influence the learning process (Fig. 2–1).

Every person, even those who live "alone," is immersed in a network of relationships with other people. This network provides each individual with continuing feedback about reality and how one fits into the group, the society, the culture. A person's self-concept is shaped by the sociocultural group to which he belongs, and its values continue to influence him throughout his life. At the same time any distinct change in the individual's behavior affects those around him, just as a pebble thrown into a pool of water creates ripples far and wide (see Rogers, 1970).

Let us look briefly at the reciprocal relationship that exists between an individual and the social and cultural groups to which he belongs. The give-and-take nature of this relationship is reflected in the two learning principles that provide the framework for our discussion.

LEARNING PRINCIPLE 7: The network of sociocultural relationships that surrounds a person determines his perception of learning needs and his willingness to begin the learning process.

LEARNING PRINCIPLE 8: The behavioral changes that result from learning are most likely to occur when they are supported by those who have a primary social relationship with the learner.

How Sociocultural Values Influence Perception

The individual who comes to a clinical setting for help with a health problem brings his whole network of social and cultural relationships with him. For

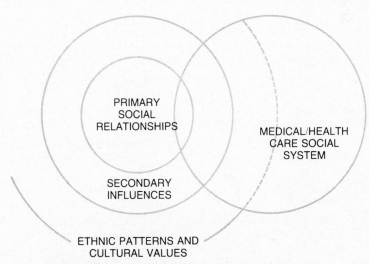

PRIMARY
SOCIAL
RELATIONSHIPS

MEDICAL/HEALTH
CARE SOCIAL
SYSTEM

SECONDARY
INFLUENCES

ETHNIC PATTERNS AND
CULTURAL VALUES

Figure 2–5. Components of a patient's social world.

discussion purposes, I have divided this network into three general components: primary social relationships, secondary social influences, and ethnic patterns. These components are represented conceptually in Figure 2–5.

The diagram suggests that a person is surrounded by his "world" of relationships with other people and cultural values. He conducts his life largely within this system. Because familiar, comfortable relationships are usually given preference, a person's social system insulates him, to some extent, from contact with other, dissimilar, or "foreign" systems.

Social System Components

Primary Social Relationships. These relationships are closest to us. The people who populate this component of our social system characteristically know many aspects of our personality and are familiar with the way in which we play many of our life's roles. Because of this familiarity, these people are influential in how we perceive ourselves and interpret life events (Goffman, 1971). Although we usually think of a person's primary relationships as being largely composed of his family, this cannot be assumed. A family member may not be close enough to an individual to have much influence, whereas a good friend may be extremely important.

A key factor in the assessment of a patient's learning needs and his motivation to meet them is knowledge of the people who are part of his primary social relationships, his "micro-social world."

> Knowing the people and some of the attitudes that most directly influence the patient in his everyday life helps the nurse determine the extent of the patient's personal resources and strength of support for change.

Secondary Influences. These relationships are with those people who typically know only one or two dimensions of our personality. We may have frequent interaction with them but within only a limited number of roles. For example, co-workers know us professionally and may have knowledge of some aspects of our personal lives, but unless they become good friends, they have a secondary social relationship with us. They may influence our professional behavior but have limited impact on our lives generally. Nurses usually have a secondary relationship with patients; they know them within the "sick" role and, consequently, may influence their behavior within the clinical environment. If behaviors that result from learning are to have a more general impact on a patient's life, the nurse will need the help and support of the patient's primary social group in sustaining changes.

Ethnic Patterns and Cultural Values. These provide the underlying structure to life. They provide us with general rules about our behavior toward other people, giving us a sense of what is "right," "proper," and socially acceptable to others of our group. Patterns and values include such things as language, religion, dress, and food and drink. They determine our roles according to status, age, and gender; rules for displaying emotion, sexual rituals, and perceptions of attractiveness; codes for nonverbal behaviors and their interpretation; and many other aspects of social conduct. An ethnic or cultural group may be nationally or racially oriented, or it may occupy a minority position within a dominant culture. For example, teenagers tend to belong to a special subgroup that has its own rules of social and sexual conduct, language, music, and food patterns.

> Because ethnic patterns and cultural values are so deeply entrenched and so pervasive in a person's life, it is important that they be identified, acknowledged, and accepted by the nurse before she begins teaching.

The nurse who does not do this will have little credibility as a teacher. At the same time an attempt to bring about changes in behavior that are counter to ethnic patterns is seldom successful.

Medical and health care are also conducted within a social system. The system's relationship components are based on a hierarchical "class" system, as well as on friendship, respect, and frequency of communication. Because of its special language, rituals, values and priorities, it is experienced by many patients as being "foreign," and therefore anxiety-producing. In Section 1.1 the extent to which nurses teach "indirectly" was discussed. A major reason for this kind of teaching is that nurses provide role models to patients and their family members of acceptable behavior within the medical subculture.

The potential for conflict between the patient's social system and that of the medical subculture is great. The following are just a few examples.

- A Vietnamese patient's family brings him special foods with "healing" properties without regard for his strict hospital diet.
- A German woman insists that the door of her room be kept closed.
- A doctor doubts that a patient's wife understood the directions he gave her about her husband's care at home because she did not look at him during the entire conference. She is Japanese.
- A low-income family repeatedly comes to the busy Emergency Department of a large hospital for care for minor medical problems even though the family members have been told that this is inappropriate.
- An Iranian woman begins to wail in a high pitched cry when told that a relative has died.

These kinds of situations reflect culturally determined perceptions of need and appropriate behaviors. Patients and families generally try to fit in with the sociocultural demands of the medical community but are disadvantaged in this effort by the lack of specific information and their state of physical and mental distress. They do, however, acutely feel the rejection of caregivers when their behavior is deemed unacceptable.

Caregivers are usually alert to religious differences but may not consider how social relationships and ethnic patterns affect:

— need for privacy,
— acceptability of physical contact with another person,

— experience of and outward response to pain,
— expression of anxiety and mental distress,
— reactions to diagnosis and adaptation to disability,
— patterns of growth and development, and
— attitudes toward death and dying.

Social relationships and ethnic patterns give a person a background of experiences that shape his perceptions. Medical care may interrupt some of these patterns but will seldom change them dramatically.

> Giving attention to the patient's sociocultural system helps the nurse to understand the context within which the patient identifies his needs and plan teaching so that it builds on the patient's previous experiences in a positive way.

Recognizing the sociocultural system of patients is examined further in Chapter 3, in the discussion on how the nurse can encourage a relationship of trust.

How the Sociocultural Context of Learning Affects Behavior Changes

If social relationships and ethnic patterns are a major influence in determining a person's readiness to learn, they are equally important in determining the extent to which he will alter his future behavior as a result of learning. It is in evaluating behavior changes and the "refreezing" process that the reciprocity of social relationships is especially evident.

> A person is willing to change elements of his behavior if he anticipates support and acceptance from those in his primary social world.

At the same time family members sometimes fail to fully realize the extent to which a patient's changed behavior will have an impact on their lives as well. The following case demonstrates such a situation.

Example 2.6   FAMILY ACCEPTANCE OF NEW BEHAVIOR

Mr. Innes was a hardworking, successful executive. During an annual physical examination, his doctor recommended that he pursue some form of regular physical exercise. After giving the idea some thought over several weeks and telling his family of his plan, Mr. Innes decided to start jogging after work each day. He purchased some good shoes and began his new ritual. Much to his surprise, he quickly became the target of teasing comments about his physique made by his children and a few work colleagues and complaints from his wife about having to delay dinner for the whole family. His family had always thought of him as basically sedentary and found this new image difficult to accept, even though they knew it was good for his health. Mr. Innes, however, was thoroughly committed to the change and persevered until his new behavior finally became established as "normal."

If Mr. Innes had had a less secure self-perception or a dimmer view of the risk to his health by not exercising, the lack of support from those close to him would have undermined his attempt to change.

Benne (1976) has pointed out that therapists, counselors, and teachers often forget about the importance of a person's primary social world to the refreezing process. They leave the burden of adjustment and adaptation to life outside the clinical situation entirely to the patient, sometimes returning him to the same environment that caused his difficulty in the first place. Most caregivers can think of many examples of this oversight involving people with drug or alcohol dependencies, mental illnesses, or physical handicaps. Such people may be labeled noncompliant without an appreciation of the social complications that result from a major behavior change.

> Compliance with medical advice is not a one-time decision, but a continuing decision process that is influenced by, and in turn influences, those in one's primary social world.

Recognizing the importance of the patient's primary social world to any behavior change will lead the nurse to consider one of the following options for her teaching.

- She can include the people closest to the patient in the teaching, helping them as well as the patient to learn.
- She can help the patient form new strong relationships with people who will be able to support a change in behavior, such as a self-help group or a counselor.
- She can help the patient prepare to "teach" those who are close to him about the change and why it is so important to him.

Or she may choose a combination of these methods to ensure adequate refreezing. Mr. Innes' change in behavior would have gone more smoothly had he been able to help his family learn some new attitudes before he took up jogging. Telling them his plan was clearly not sufficient. In addition, had he been able to discuss with another jogger the difficulties he encountered, he would have felt more supported during the transition period of his new behavior.

Even though the nurse is often not in a position to directly help with changes in behavior that result from her teaching, she has a crucial role to play in helping the patient organize his defenses against negative influences. She can do this most directly by assisting the family to give active support to change and by identifying sources of help and support outside the clinical setting. After all, if the patient is unwilling or unable to change his behavior as a result of teaching, the time and effort involved have been wasted.

In summary, a number of ideas about the social and cultural context of learning have been explored in this section. The sociocultural "world" in which a person lives has been described as being composed of primary social relationships, secondary social influences, and ethnic patterns. The influence of this "world" is especially marked in the unfreezing and refreezing portions of the learning process. It is essential that the nurse carefully consider the social and cultural world of the patient and recognize areas of conflict with her own values and beliefs and with those of the medical/health care social system.

Effective teaching includes an assessment of how the patient's sociocultural system will influence learning and a plan for maximizing support for behavioral changes.

2.5 STRESS AND ITS EFFECT ON LEARNING

In the past decade stress has become a popular and somewhat overused term. It has been named as the cause of behaviors ranging from hysterical joy to homicide and as an explanation for athletic achievement, artistic creativity, divorce, sexual deviance, and mental illness. Stress is, indeed, common to all of us. It is a natural response to the changes that surround us. Its effects may be positive or negative, motivating or disabling, stimulating or overwhelming.

Patients are especially vulnerable to the negative consequences of stress as they experience unusual environments and expectations, unfamiliar procedures, and the physiologic changes that accompany their illness. In this section we will look at how a patient's response to stress influences his motivation and ability to learn as well as his success in incorporating positive behavioral changes into his life. The following principles will provide a framework for our discussion.

LEARNING PRINCIPLE 9: Stress may either promote learning or act as a barrier to it.

LEARNING PRINCIPLE 10: Learning and change are themselves stressful.

How Stress Affects the Individual

A first step in understanding stress as an important influence on learning is to define the term. As Sorensen and Luckmann (1986) point out, usage of the word *stress* has changed over the years and still tends to have quite different definitions, depending on the author's orientation.

Hans Selye (1974), a physician and pioneer in stress research, defined stress as the "non-specific response of the body to any demand made upon it." This response involves stimulation of the hypothalamus, resulting in release of adrenocorticotropic hormone by the pituitary. By "non-specific" Selye meant that any demand, or "stressor," results in hormone-induced changes to the cardiovascular, respiratory, and gastrointestinal systems, thereby affecting the entire body. This response represents the body's normal attempt to adjust to the demand and preserve its balance, or homeostasis. Selye particularly emphasized that both pleasant and unpleasant events cause a stress response and that the body's physiologic reaction is the same. Tears of joy and of sorrow are, physically, very much alike.

A principally physiologic definition of stress is useful because it focuses on the individual experience of stress rather than on the many variables that might contribute to it. For our purposes here, then, we shall differentiate between a stress response and a stressor, using the following definitions:

Stress is the physiologic response that an individual has to a change in his internal or external environment. Any change that requires energy for adaptation or readjustment is a *stressor.*

By itself, stress is neither good nor bad; it is simply a mechanism used by the body to cope with its environment. As such, it is a normal and universally experienced response. Without some stress reflecting changes in our lives, we would be bored, static, and unmotivated to achieve or create. On the other hand, too much stress that overwhelms a person's ability to adapt is incapacitating. Selye calls this latter experience "distress." At any given time each individual seems to have an optimum range of stress tolerance that stimulates and motivates without upsetting the health balance.

People are often unaware of the physical effect that environmental stressors are having on them. The stress response may intensify so gradually that it is not until the person feels tired or irritable at the end of a day that his now high stress level becomes apparent.

> Stress can accumulate over a period of time with both major and minor stressors, good and bad events contributing to one's current stress response level.

Holmes and Rahe (1967) showed that a major stressor may adversely affect an individual for two or more years, long after the actual stress event occurred. Chronically high levels have been implicated in cardiovascular disease, vulnerability to infection, and psychological disturbances.

A further factor in understanding the effect of stress is that a single stressor might cause responses of different intensity in different people, or even in the same person at different times. For example, a heavy rainstorm might cause annoyance in one person and near panic in someone else. The variation in response depends on previous experience with similar events, the importance and meaning of the stressor to the person, and his already-present stress level. This makes it difficult for a nurse to assess a patient's stress response level accurately without more information than just identification of current stressors.

> Knowledge of a stressor does not allow one to predict the intensity of an individual's stress response level.

Sections 4.1 and 4.2 contain discussions of how the nurse can gather relevant information about a person's stress response level and how this knowledge can help her in planning patient teaching. In the following case example the patient's behavior suggested to the nurse that stress response levels needed to be investigated further. The situation involves Ms. Franklin, the dietitian described in Example 2.3 as one of two patients with hypertension.

Example 2.7   STRESS INFLUENCES ATTITUDES TOWARD LEARNING

Jennifer Dole, R.N., had had a chance to assess Ms. Franklin's background knowledge and experiences about hypertension earlier. She had learned, for example, that Ms. Franklin knew that diuretics and a low-sodium diet were often prescribed for patients with hypertension. The patient said that she had been on a self-imposed low-sodium diet for years because there was a history of heart problems in her family. In response to other questions asked by the nurse, Ms. Franklin said that she knew "all about" the risks of high blood pressure and that, although she was aware of various stress management techniques, she figured they were just a way of "entertaining psychiatrists and hippies." She went on to say that the only thing she was interested in was getting out of the hospital as quickly as possible. (She had had elective orthopedic surgery.)

As the nurse talked with Ms. Franklin, she had become increasingly aware of the patient's clipped, hurried manner of speaking and frequent use of nervous gestures. Despite the negative attitude expressed, the nurse felt that stress management was an area of great importance to this patient's control of her hypertension. Before she could do any teaching on the subject, however, she would have to help Ms. Franklin identify high stress levels as a problem for her. She decided to give the patient more opportunity to talk about herself and her goals. This would give the nurse more information and encourage a more trusting relationship.

During the next two days, as Ms. Franklin learned to walk with crutches, she told the nurse that she was anxious to get back to work because she had recently taken unexpected time off to attend the funeral of her mother, who had died of a stroke. She confided that her diagnosis of hypertension frightened her. She described herself as a disciplined and organized person who didn't like to "waste time." This was all important information to the nurse as she planned how to help the patient learn to better deal with the stress in her life. Although Ms. Dole was tempted to teach her relaxation techniques, she also realized that this would be ineffective unless and until Ms. Franklin saw this as a need for herself. The nurse decided that the best way to proceed was to encourage discussion of the patient's desire to be disciplined and organized and help her think through how these demands on herself, in combination with the other stresses in her life, could be affecting her blood pressure.

In this case example the nurse gave her attention to both the physical evidence of high stress levels (e.g., the patient's manner of speaking) and the diagnosis of hypertension. She took the time to discover how Ms. Franklin perceived the events in her life as contributing to her total stress response. The nurse's approach to teaching began with helping the patient develop awareness of a problem and perception of a learning need.

How Stress Response Varies

In helping nurses and other caregivers understand some of the major principles of stress theory and its implications for patient care, I have found a continuum model useful (Waring and McLennan, 1979). The continuous scale of the Stress Gauge, shown in Figure 2–6, suggests that the buildup of stress can be gradual and that there are no clear divisions between levels.

Although a person's stress response level cannot be quantified like his blood pressure, the symptoms of stress that the person exhibits and the knowledge of stressors that may be affecting him provide clues for the nurse. Each of the four levels of stress shown on the Stress Gauge represents a grouping of commonly experienced responses to stressors of increasing intensity.

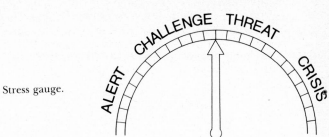

Figure 2–6. Stress gauge.

The stressors that produce an *alert* response are relatively minor, commonly occurring events. Their presence has enough impact to stimulate a person's awareness and make him feel temporarily anxious, unsettled, or pressured, but accommodation to such events requires only a straightforward problem-solving effort. Stressors that might produce an alert response include changes in the weather requiring an alteration in clothing, inability to meet a previously planned time schedule, a temporary change in eating or sleeping pattern, or a minor physical complaint, such as a headache or mild dysmenorrhea. Each of these events would cause a normal physiologic stress response, alerting the person to a higher-than-normal state of tension. As a result, the person would be stimulated to take action to minimize the disruption caused by the stressor; he would put on a sweater, make a telephone call, take a nap, or take an aspirin. If all of these stressors occurred in a single day, however, the person's accumulated stress response level would be high enough to make him much more aware of his stress and somewhat uncomfortable. Consequently, the actions taken might be less effective and the person might begin to show his stress by nervous gestures or inability to concentrate.

Advertisers are aware of the usefulness of everyday, minor problems in focusing attention and stimulating interest in a better solution. Many commercial dramatizations portray just such a stressor being dealt with effectively by use of a certain product. Likewise, teachers can often make effective use of the minor concerns experienced by their students as a starting point for a lesson. Sometimes changes in usual procedures are introduced by a teacher in order to stimulate students' alertness and interest. Films, learning games, and discussion groups, as alternatives to explanation or lecture, are useful for this purpose.

The next level on the continuum model is *challenge*. A stress response at this level may include excitement, apprehension, and some temporary doubts about one's capabilities. Stressors that are likely to produce a challenge response are marriage, the birth of a child, a new job, or a move to a new community. Typically, these stressors challenge one's former roles in relation to other people or some aspects of life-style. They may present an opportunity for new accomplishments or creativity and, in so doing, help a person meet the higher-level needs outlined by Maslow. Because a great deal of energy is required to meet the demands of these stressors, the problem presented takes a central place in the person's life. People often actively seek information or skills to improve their adaptation.

The challenge of solving a significant problem presents an ideal opportunity for effective learning.

Alert and challenge stress response levels are confronted optimistically. There is no serious fear that one will be unable to meet the demands involved, although one may need to work unusually hard to accomplish the task of adjustment. This is what Selye calls good stress, or "eustress."

At a point approximately midway on the Stress Gauge, the optimistic viewpoint gives way to a very real fear that one may not be able to maintain control over one's life and circumstances. The upper end of the continuum is divided into two areas: threat and crisis. Others, such as Gerald Caplan (1964), use the term crisis to include a number of different stress levels and some popular writers refer to stress only as a negative and destructive entity.

A *threat* response occurs when the demands placed on the individual by events or stressors are so great that they upset normal functioning. Stressors that may, by themselves, stimulate such a response are a serious illness, surgery, loss of a job, or family discord. Unlike the stressors that cause challenge, those that are threatening come on one uninvited, and often unexpectedly. They threaten some of the more basic human needs, such as safety and social belonging. The responses they evoke may lead to loss of appetite, depression, inability to concentrate, anger, guilt, or general anxiety. The person experiencing threat feels like he is under attack. When a medical problem is involved, he may seek help and willingly comply with treatment or, in an effort to flee from the problem, he may inappropriately avoid care.

People entering a hospital for care are certainly experiencing threat if not crisis. Their personal resources are mobilized to fight off the "attack" of the stressor. Whatever caregivers can do to relieve the impact of additional psychological or sociocultural stressors will free the person to use more of his energy to deal with the physical problem. Information about what is happening and what to expect, recognition of individual needs, reassurance about the quality of care, and allowing family members to show their concern and support all help the patient focus his energy on the medical problem at hand. (See discussion of basic needs in Section 2.3.) Patient teaching that helps the patient understand his diagnosis and treatment makes it possible for him to participate in care earlier and avoid being overwhelmed by a sense of powerlessness. For some people even a short period of lack of control is extremely upsetting and raises stress response to high levels (Houston, 1972; Janis and Rodin, 1979).

Many studies have shown that efforts to reduce patient stress to or below the threat level are important to the patient's acceptance of treatment, confidence in his caregivers, and compliance with medical advice (Elms and Leonard, 1966; Johnson and Leventhal, 1974; Ridgeway and Mathews, 1982). Sime (1976) and others have identified some of the benefits of stress reduction as decreased need for anesthetic and pain medication and apparently improved healing.

Finally, *crisis* is a response to distress that overwhelms a person's present capacity to adapt and adjust. Stressors that cause a crisis response usually represent a sudden, traumatic loss, such as loss of personal possessions through fire or flood, loss of self-esteem through failure, loss of the relationship with a beloved person through death or separation, or loss of bodily functioning through mutilating surgery or stroke. The feelings engendered by such losses are helplessness, disbelief, shock and panic, or intense anger and guilt.

Any situation involving loss may mark the onset of a crisis response.

A great deal has been written about crisis responses, especially those prompted by death and dying. Consequently, we understand a good deal about the response mechanisms and stages of coping with this stress level. Elisabeth Kübler-Ross (1970, 1975) has been a major contributor to this understanding through her work with dying patients. A number of general principles that have evolved from this work are summarized below:

- Early identification, or anticipation, of a crisis allows help to be *immediate*. Once a person develops a maladaptive way of coping with a crisis, his healthier responses are undermined. Such a coping method is difficult to change and can lead to permanent emotional dysfunction.
- A person in crisis needs support *through* the situation rather than assistance in avoiding it. Renewed strength and growth can occur only if a person confronts and fully experiences the reality of the crisis situation.
- A person in crisis should be encouraged to *express* the very strong emotions he is probably experiencing. Such expressions, which might include heart-rending grief, explosive anger, or wild fantasies, help the person begin to come to terms with painful reality rather than deny it.
- A person in crisis is especially *susceptible* to influence by others. Although caregivers should avoid giving offhand advice or offering personal opinions in place of information, they do have an opportunity to help the person accept additional help or otherwise get started on a healthy resolution of the crisis.

The early identification of a crisis response and actions based on these principles will give the patient the best chance of emerging from the crisis with his coping mechanisms intact, or even strengthened. In the following case example the nurse acted on her suspicions and was able to give the patient the support and help she needed at a time of crisis.

Example 2.8   A CRISIS OF ACCUMULATED STRESS

Mrs. Klein, aged 58, had been recuperating well from gallbladder surgery 5 days ago—so well in fact that she was hoping to be discharged this afternoon. Nancy Fowler, her nurse, had noticed, however, that Mrs. Klein had a slightly elevated temperature at 7 a.m. She went back into the room to check the patient's temperature before the doctor was scheduled to make rounds. It was 101.4°F and Ms. Fowler warned Mrs. Klein that the doctor would probably not discharge her as long as she had a fever. Although she said that she was disappointed, the patient did not seem to be upset by the news.

About 45 minutes later Mrs. Klein put her call light on and requested pain medication. The following conversation ensued:

NURSE: You had a pain pill only about an hour ago, Mrs. Klein. Is something wrong?

PATIENT: Oh I don't know.... (In a louder, angry voice, tears welling up in her eyes) Yes, everything's wrong.

NURSE: (Pulling up a chair by the bedside) Can you tell me about it?

PATIENT: (Crying now) So much is going on, so many changes in my life. I just don't know what to do.

NURSE: I'd like to hear about what's happening to you, Mrs. Klein. There are a couple of things I must do first, but suppose I come back in, say, ten minutes. We can go down to the conference room where we can talk privately. Okay?

A little later, as planned, Ms. Fowler escorted the patient to the conference room. Mrs. Klein talked willingly about the recent events in her life, saying that "everything has been bottled up inside of me until I felt like I was going to explode." She explained that, in addition to not feeling well for several months before her surgery, a good friend had died of cancer. Mrs. Klein said that she had almost been in a state of panic for several weeks, sure she also had cancer. Then her youngest son had announced his plans to marry in a few weeks and move to a city several hundred miles away. She was glad for him, but this meant that her three children would be widely scattered. On top of finding out that she wouldn't be going home today, her husband had telephoned to say that he had finally decided to accept his company's early retirement plan and would be retiring the first of the year. He had expected her to be happy about this, but all she could do was cry.

Although Mrs. Klein wept steadily throughout the conference, she ended by saying, "Thank you for listening. I really feel better now." Nurse and patient agreed to talk again the next morning about who Mrs. Klein might be able to share her feelings with once she went home.

In this case example the patient had experienced a series of what might otherwise have been "good" stressors: she did not have cancer, there was to be a wedding in the family, and she could look forward to her husband's retirement. Taken one at a time, each of these might have been met with a challenge response, but now they came on the heels of the much more stressful event of her friend's death and her own feelings of severe threat about cancer. The accumulated effect for this patient was a crisis. The nurse recognized intuitively that physical pain was not the reason for the patient's request for pain medication. She invited Mrs. Klein to talk about what was troubling her in a private environment, even though she had to delay the conference briefly. In this unhurried setting the patient was able to express her feelings and at the same time begin to sort out the reality of her situation by hearing herself explain it to a concerned listener. The nurse effectively helped the patient cope with the immediate stress situation and furthered the patient's trust relationship with her. The nurse also successfully "taught" the patient that it was all right to express her strong feelings, that having such feelings in the circumstances was normal, that talking about her state of crisis was helpful, and that caregivers are concerned about more than just physical care.

How Stress Affects Learning Readiness and Resistance

Behavioral scientists who have studied the nature of learning and change agree that people both seek and resist change; they welcome change when it provides a solution to a problem or promotes growth but resist it when it threatens their system of beliefs, values, and interaction with others. Because learning results in changes to one's attitudes, knowledge, skills, and, ultimately, behavior, it places a demand on the individual to give up practiced, predictable ways and devote energy to the new and unfamiliar.

Learning can be both a remedy for a stressful situation and a source of stress itself.

As discussed in Section 2.3, before learning can occur, a person must perceive a need or identify a problem. This perception is itself a source of stress. Without it, one has no motivation to move or change. As we saw with the Health Belief Model, certain kinds of perceptions are especially helpful for the unfreezing process that leads to learning, change, and action. The nurse often finds herself in the paradoxical situation that in order to help a person successfully deal with a problem and avoid future threats or crises, she must sometimes raise his stress level by helping him identify a problem outside his present awareness.

When the learning required to solve a problem is simple, the resources are readily available, and the change involved is relatively minor, new knowledge, attitudes, and skills are welcomed. For example, a person wanting to buy a particular kind of shoes is ready and willing to learn which store carries the brand he is looking for. He is motivated to acquire this new knowledge because of his perception that a problem exists. The stress caused by learning that he must go to an unfamiliar store for the shoes represents a simple state of alert on the Stress Gauge and is met with simple problem-solving behavior.

When events present a person with a challenge, a common response is to consciously make learning part of one's attempt to solve the problem. Although such learning tasks may require concentrated effort and may themselves be stressful, the person is usually aware that accomplishing them will lead to increased self-esteem, a sense of satisfaction, or an improved life-style. Learning how to use a computer to record patient data or learning how to drive a car involves a complex mix of knowledge, attitudes, and skills and is therefore stressful, but unless the process becomes mired in frustration, it is approached positively.

Going beyond the positive, future-oriented end of the Stress Gauge, the person who feels threatened by stressors in his life is likely to seek out learning only when he perceives that it will *reduce* his stress level. Presented with learning that is itself stressful, the person may resist participation. The resistance most commonly takes the form of not hearing, not paying attention, or not remembering information offered. A person who is already in a state of threat is unlikely to add to his stress by attempting to change his present beliefs, values, or social system. For example, many patients resist learning self-administration of medications, since it threatens their self-image as "well" people, not dependent on drugs. As Knowles (1984) points out, once an adult has formed a self-concept as an independent, self-directed individual, learning that is contrary to this concept will be met with resistance.

Certainly many, or even most, of the patients the nurse attempts to help with learning are already in a state of threat because of their ill health. Teaching that calls a person's self-esteem, social adaptation, or sense of security into question will be experienced as unduly stressful.

> A patient with an already high stress level will find it difficult to learn effectively unless the nurse teacher reduces his overall stress level and approaches teaching in such a way that his self-esteem is not threatened.

Helping to reduce a person's overall stress level gives him more flexibility in meeting new, potentially stressful situations. At the same time teaching that recognizes the patient's individuality, invites his participation, and builds on his previous experiences reinforces self-esteem. Some of the specific steps the nurse might take to encourage learning are to:

— reduce the impact of other stressors in the environment that are adding to the patient's stress level, such as noise, confusion, or lack of privacy;

— focus teaching content on the immediate concerns of the patient and the practical application of new knowledge or skills; and

— help the patient understand how learning can reduce his urrent stress level through participation in decision making and resumption of control over aspects of his life.

Faced with the realities of shorter hospital stays and the discharge of sicker patients, the nurse finds that she must teach more quickly and more extensively than ever before. Unfortunately, the conditions that create stressful time limits for the nurse also create resistance to learning for the patient. A condescending or overtly aggressive approach to patient teaching or lack of consideration for patient needs and concerns can push a "threatened" patient to the brink of crisis.

For the person experiencing a crisis response because of traumatic life events, any learning that does take place will be distorted by the crisis. For example, it is common for explanations and information about potentially life-threatening diagnoses to be misunderstood by the affected patient and his family members. This is not surprising, given that such a person may already have a distorted perception of reality and an inability to think logically because of the severe stress response of a crisis. Although an extensive teaching program is inappropriate at this time, the nurse does have the opportunity to reduce current stress levels and help the person begin to prepare for effective learning later. This can be done by giving emotional support, encouraging the expression of feelings, and assisting the person in taking active control in some area of his life.

The intense crisis response is resolved slowly with gradually diminishing stress levels. In effect, the person goes through each of the stages on the Stress Gauge until the former crisis becomes a series of challenges that are amenable to problem solving. This "healing" process takes one to two years, depending on the significance of the loss to the person.

Although the ability to learn is severely limited by the immediate presence of extreme stress, the person who has faced and is beginning to overcome a crisis may be unusually open to learning and change. Having already confronted a dramatically changed situation and recognized that his life will not be quite the same because of the crisis experience, he is likely to try out new patterns of behavior. This gives the nurse teacher an unparalleled opportunity to offer help with the knowledge and understanding the patient will need in order to choose and plan these new directions and behaviors. If the nurse has been able to offer the kind of support and caring that Nancy Fowler gave Mrs. Klein during her crisis experience (Example 2–8), she will be able to anticipate the patient's learning needs and prepare for her teaching intervention.

There are, basically, only two possible outcomes to the experience of a crisis response: either the person learns and grows through the crisis, acquiring a higher level of personal strength and flexibility, or he fails to grow and learn and instead becomes emotionally impaired (Caplan, 1964). The importance of the nurse's support and guidance early in the crisis experience is that it helps to make the positive outcome much more likely.

In summary, we have discussed the fact that stress is a normal response to changes in one's environment and that people experience stressors with a high degree of individuality. A Stress Gauge model was used as a guide to the four major levels of stress response. Each of the levels was discussed in terms of its characteristics and its role in promoting learning readiness or resistance. The identification of a patient's stress response level helps the nurse plan teaching intervention and meet the challenge of helping people learn effectively in spite of potential barriers to that process.

SUMMARY

In this chapter five major factors that influence the learning process have been identified. Previous experience, perception of need, the sociocultural context of learning, and the role of stress have been explored in detail. The fifth factor, the nurse-patient relationship, is the focus of Chapter 3.

The intent in exploring this theoretical material has been to show that patient teaching occurs within a much broader context than the immediate clinical environment. An understanding of the many factors acting on the learner allows the nurse to more fully assess the learner's needs and motivation and plan her own teaching intervention. The challenge and the opportunity for the nurse teacher are to appreciate the complexities of the learning process and the individuality of the learner while helping him adopt behaviors that will benefit his health.

Study Questions and Exercises

Maximum learning benefit is derived from these questions and exercises when your answers and experiences are shared with classmates or colleagues.

1. In order to learn how to quickly identify the category of learning applicable to particular situations, listen to five television or radio commercials. List the advertiser and then note whether the commercial has given you facts or *knowledge* about the product, influenced your *attitude* by prompting an emotional response, or demonstrated a *skill* or how to do something.

2. List two things that you do now that you did not do a year ago. Identify the factors that contributed to your change in behavior. What, in particular, led to your "unfreezing," or readiness to change? What resources did you use during the "moving" phase? What conditions assisted you to "refreeze"?

3. Identify some instances of learning by example or modeling, by trial and error, and by solving a problem that you have experienced in the recent past. How is your behavior likely to be affected in the future? Are there any differences in your feelings about these learning experiences?

4. Observe a child at play. Using Piaget's stages of development (Table 2–2), identify his characteristics. What practical evidence do you have of his stage? What previous learning is the child using in his play activities?

5. Choose two patients with whom you have had recent contact and identify what you think their needs are right now (refer to Section 2.3). What evidence do you have for this judgement?

6. Ask two friends to identify something that they know they should do for their health or well-being (such as have a medical checkup, go on a diet, exercise) but have not yet been motivated to do. Try to discover why they are unmotivated in terms of health beliefs, previous experience, or interference from other people.

7. List the people who have a primary social relationship with you. Note your reasons for including them. List the people or groups that you consider to be within your secondary influential group. Why have you included them in this category? Now list some of the values and traditions of your ethnic background that continue to influence you. In what ways are these similar to or different from those of the "majority" culture? Have you experienced conflicts when differences were not recognized?

8. Imagine that the medical/health facility in which you work is a small country. List the rules, values, beliefs, and relationships that set it apart from the larger society and culture. How do people (patients, family members, and new staff) learn the rules of conduct in this "country"? What happens when there are conflicts?

9. Keep a log of stressors in your life for 2 days. Start by listing all of those things that are "chronic" stressors, that cause stress repeatedly over a period of time (such as "getting child to school on time" or "conflict with a colleague"). As events occur during the day (such as "late and hurried lunch" or "three admissions arrived at the same time"), jot them down on your list. Review the list and reflect on your physical response to each event and on what you feel is your overall, accumulative stress level. How do you generally handle high stress levels? How can you tell when you begin to exceed a positive level? What do you do to reduce stress in your life?

10. Think of two or three situations you have observed in which someone has faced a crisis. Analyze how the situation was handled by other people. What did they do that was helpful? Unhelpful?

11. Think of two formal learning situations in which you have been a participant. Was there any evidence of resistance to learning in yourself or others? Was this recognized by the teacher? Was it overcome? How?

3

THE NURSE-PATIENT RELATIONSHIP AND TEACHING

Patient teaching is distinctively a communicative process with nurse-patient interaction at its core. In Chapter 2 this interaction was identified as one of the major factors that influence learning. Through interacting with and relating to the patient and his family members, the nurse has the opportunity to assess learning needs, influence readiness to learn, act as a resource for learning, and guide the learning process toward effective behavior changes. The skills involved in constructive relationship development and interpersonal communication are so important to the nurse teacher that this chapter is devoted solely to this learning factor.

The chapter begins with an overview of two basic roles of the nurse and proceeds to a discussion of the personal characteristics that encourage the development of patient trust. This is followed by two sections that deal with the application of relationship skills and, finally, some ideas about how personalities can interact to influence the nature and quality of the teaching-learning process.

James P. McLennan, a counseling psychologist and longtime teacher of relationship skills for nurses, has made a major contribution to Sections 3.1 through 3.3.

The main points contained in this chapter are as follows:

- The nurse carries out both an "instrumental," or physical care and technically oriented, role and an "expressive," or communicative, role within the context of nursing care. (Introduction)
- Although the "expressive" role is part of all nursing functions, the quality of counseling and teaching interventions are most dependent on it. (Section 3.0)
- Effective teaching shares with counseling interventions the prerequisite of

a trust relationship in which feelings as well as facts can be communicated. (Section 3.1)

- The effective use of the nonverbal communication skills of "attending" is as important to the nurse-patient relationship as the effective use of verbal skills. (Section 3.2)
- "Open" responses invite the learner to focus on his experience and freely express his feelings and priorities. (Section 3.3)
- Before effective teaching can begin, the nurse must learn about the patient. Active listening and open responses assist her in doing this. (Section 3.3)
- Understanding how personality characteristics might influence a person's learning priorities can add to the nurse's teaching effectiveness. (Section 3.4)

Communication and relationship skills have always occupied a central place in nursing practice. Of all the people on the health care team, the nurse spends the most time with the patient, talks more with him and his family, and is in the best position to coordinate information between the medical care delivery system and the patient. The performance of nursing care also requires that the nurse have a high level of scientific knowledge and technological skill. These two general nursing roles have been described by Sorensen and Luckmann (1986) as the "expressive" and "instrumental" roles, respectively, of the nurse. The first involves motivation, understanding, and goal-oriented communication; the second involves scientifically based technical skills. These authors emphasize that "instrumental and expressive functions complement each other. No matter how efficiently a nurse performs instrumental tasks, their effectiveness will be reduced if she does not practice expressive roles in a sensitive and caring way" (1986, p. 24).

Over the whole range of nursing activities, it is evident that these two general roles combine in different ways. For example, the assessment phase of the Nursing Process (see Figure 1–2) depends on the quality of information obtained directly from the patient and indirectly from his family and his medical records; this is clearly a communicative process. Judgments about nursing needs, however, are based on clinical knowledge and expertise: an "instrumental" role.

Similarly, in the planning phase, there is interaction between these two basic nursing roles. The nurse calls on her "instrumental" knowledge of the medical care delivery system, specific disease entities, and treatment methods in order to plan nursing intervention even while communicating information to the patient and his family. The nurse's ability to quickly establish a relationship of trust with the patient allows the patient to participate in planning and setting goals at an early stage of his treatment.

The diagram in Figure 3–1 represents the involvement of these two nursing roles for each phase of the Nursing Process, beginning with first contact between nurse and patient and proceeding through a variety of intervention activities. The expressive role forms the foundation for the more technical, or instrumental, role throughout the Nursing Process. Counseling and teaching share an especially high component of the expressive role.

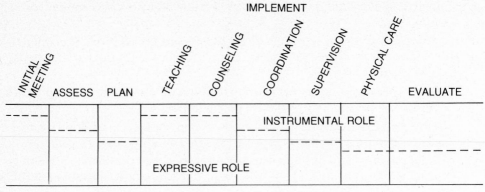

Figure 3–1. The expressive and instrumental roles of the nurse.

> The quality of counseling and teaching interventions depends directly on the quality of the nurse-patient relationship.

These two kinds of nursing intervention share a group of interactive skills that will be explored in more detail in the next three sections of this chapter. Providing the framework for this discussion are two basic principles of learning. (See Table 2–1 for a list of other relevant principles.)

LEARNING PRINCIPLE 5: The trust relationship provides an environment in which change can take place.

LEARNING PRINCIPLE 6: Verbalization assists the process of learning.

This material is presented to show how the nurse teacher can use nurse-patient interaction most effectively to stimulate and encourage the learning process. More comprehensive material on relationship development can be found in most basic nursing texts or in special texts such as those of A. J. Davis (1984) or Robinson (1984). The remainder of this chapter contains practical suggestions for the nurse teacher as a supplement to other learning resources. In doing this I have drawn especially from the fields of counseling and educational psychology.

3.1 HOW TO ENCOURAGE TRUST

Any student of human nature knows that few people have simple, straight-forward life situations. When problems arise, the concerns they have and the conditions they experience are, as Gerard Egan (1975) expressed it, "messy." They are messy partly because feelings are such an important part of a person's functioning. Emotions such as anxiety, sadness, anger, guilt, and resentment interfere with rational thinking and problem solving as well as with physical functioning. As discussed in Section 2.4, other people contribute complexity to a person's problem situations. Few experiences of acute or chronic medical difficulties are not "messy."

A major impetus to the nurse's use of the expressive role is her awareness that patients, if they are to cope with their present circumstances and prepare for responsible self-care, must begin to sort through the complexities and identify realistic goals early in their care. Two interventions frequently selected by the nurse to help further this process are teaching and counseling.

> Effective teaching and counseling occur within a climate of trust in which the patient is able to share his feelings as well as the facts of his situation with the nurse.

From the patient's point of view, this level of trust does not occur automatically. He probably assumes that the health professionals involved in his care are "trustworthy," in the sense that they will not do anything injurious to his well-being and will respect the confidentiality of information related to his case. He may expect to be asked probing questions that will reveal some personal facts and experience some invasion of his physical privacy. He may not, however, expect that he will be invited to share the complexities of his problem situation with his nurse; nor should the nurse expect that such sharing will come easily to the patient.

> It is difficult for many people to accept help with any problem, even a purely physical one. For them, admitting that a problem is beyond their control or arouses strong feelings signifies a kind of personal failure or shortcoming.

Help involving the realm of feelings is always approached with some misgivings, as Brammer notes:

1. It is not easy to receive [this kind of] help.

2. It is difficult to commit one's self to change.

3. It is difficult to submit to the influence of a helper: help is a threat to esteem, integrity and independence.

4. It is not easy to trust a stranger and be open with him.

5. It is not easy to see one's problems clearly at first.

6. Sometimes problems seem too large, too overwhelming, or too unique to share easily (1973, p. 49).

7. Some cultural traditions deprecate giving and receiving help outside the family (1973, p. 49).

To make things even more difficult, medical care usually takes place in an environment that is distracting and "foreign" to most patients and their families. This combination of environmental, social, and psychological factors may, understandably, make the patient reluctant to share all the facts of his situation with the nurse, much less the feelings engendered by it. To not share completely, however, prevents him from receiving the kind of help that would make him a real participant in his care.

> It is the nurse's responsibility to initiate a relationship in which trust can be developed.

She must not only listen effectively, but also actively encourage the kind of sharing that makes effective counseling and teaching intervention possible.

In initating a relationship of sharing and trust, the nurse uses specific nonverbal and verbal skills to communicate that she cares about the person and is trying to really hear him and his concerns. These skills are discussed in Sections

3.2 and 3.3. The nurse also presents herself to the patient as a multidimensional person with subjective attitudes and values as well as professional knowledge and expertise. She risks the exposure of her attitudes and beliefs so that the patient can also interact as a whole and multidimensional person. The nurse's attitudes are communicated to and experienced by the patient as her personal characteristics. They help him decide to what extent he is willing to begin a working relationship with her and allow her to become temporarily part of his "primary social world" (see Section 2.4).

Clinical and counseling psychologists have identified a number of characteristics that, when communicated by a helper, promote the development of trust (see, for example, Rogers, 1961; Egan, 1975; Muldary, 1983). Here I use the terms *warmth, respect, empathy* and *genuineness* for the characteristics that are especially important for establishing the kind of relationship in which learning and change can take place.

The Quality of Warmth

Warmth is a quality that helps others feel accepted.

The nurse who communicates warmth is willing to extend herself to other people with openness, expressing her own feelings appropriately. Rather than being cold, expert, or disapproving, she acknowledges her own and other people's humanness. This behavior reflects an attitude of self-respect, self-acceptance, and genuine concern for the welfare of those in her care. Others respond by feeling that they can safely be themselves in her presence.

The Quality of Respect

Respect means treating another person as a worthwhile and unique individual, giving consideration to his personal attributes, such as his personality, preferences, culture, and opinions.

Respect shares with warmth the valuing of other people as equals. This means that a person is accepted as a unique individual even though his characteristics, opinions, and background are quite different from one's own. To respect does not necessarily mean to like, but to accept and value. Carl Rogers (1961) captured the essence of this quality by calling the effective helper's attitude toward others "unconditional positive regard." By this he meant that the helper should value others without any "strings attached," viewing their capabilities optimistically. For the nurse teacher, respect involves believing in the patient's self-responsibility for his own problem solving, even though his decisions or actions might not be what she herself might do.

An attitude of respect is reflected in a variety of ways, some of which are simply politeness. Addressing people who are older than oneself as Mr., Mrs., or Ms. until invited to use their first names denotes respect, as does ensuring physical privacy when possible and avoiding the use of jargon or abbreviations that are possibly not known to the person.

Within a clinical setting, nurses and other health care personnel do have the power to insist that things be done their way, on their time schedule, and with

their priorities, regardless
avoiding "overpowering" t
only when an adequate exp
events in his care, or even ju
being respected and treated
entity.

The Quality of Empathy

Empathy means helping a pe

The empathic nurse susper
and instead tries to think and f
word *empathy* derives from the G
This means actively tuning in to th
gestures so that the whole picture
It also means letting go of stereoty
view of the person. Some of the ex
section at the end of the chapter will   that could
be interpreted by a patient as lack of

Empathy is an essential ingredient   relationship. If the patient feels
that he is understood, he is much more likely to hear information presented to
him. Real awareness of what the person is experiencing allows the nurse teacher
to present information in a way that will make sense in his frame of reference.

There are two ways in which busy nurses can be entrapped by a patient's
expression of feelings and fail to show empathy. One occurs when the patient's
feelings about the situation seem irrational to her. It is tempting, but not helpful,
to tell him what he should be feeling or what other people have felt in similar
situations.

Another trap occurs when the nurse identifies closely with the feelings
expressed by the patient. In this instance it is tempting to say, "I know how you
feel!" when she actually does not. Rather than feeling understood, most people
who are told this by a well-intentioned helper mentally respond: "No, you don't!"
Demonstrating empathy means being willing to be involved with people and
willing to exert the effort of concentration to really hear them without demanding
that they feel as you imagine you would in the situation.

The Quality of Genuineness

Genuineness or congruence is a quality that helps a person feel that he is interacting
with a "real" person whose interest and care he can trust.

Two aspects of the elusive quality of genuineness are especially important to
the nurse-patient trust relationship. One is that the nurse avoid "playing games"
with people by attempting to manipulate the situation and their responses.
Inappropriate joking, making light of a serious situation, and coldly professional
and efficient busy-ness are examples of ways in which nurses and others sometimes
avoid real, caring contact with people. Although she cannot always be intense and
serious and sometimes must, in fact, put procedures before people, the self-aware

...re or, in general, why people behave as they do?
...ple have?
...people have problems and need help?
...goal of the nurse teacher?
...st suited to be an effective teacher?

...these behaviors are appropriate and when they signify avoid-

...er aspect of genuineness has to do with being consistent. Parents know
...ildren are good at picking up discrepancies between the verbal and
...verbal messages of adults. For example, the parent who says no in a pleading
...one of voice or with a smile is seldom obeyed. Likewise, when concern is voiced
by the nurse but she fails to make eye contact with the other person, the verbal
message may be disregarded or judged "put on," whereas the nonverbal message
of emotional distance is considered "real."

People in stressful and threatening situations are more alert than usual to
any lack of congruence in communication. Developing trust means that the patient
can rely on the nurse to mean what she says and say what she means. The nurse-
patient relationship depends on tactful honesty and a willingness to share oneself
with others.

The questionnaire in Table 3–1 is useful for helping nurses clarify the values
and beliefs that are reflected in their communication with patients. There are no
right or wrong answers.

In summary, the characteristics of warmth or openness, respect, empathy, and
genuineness or congruence reflect some basically positive attitudes and values
about people. Communicating them to others demands that the nurse be self-
aware and self-confident in her interaction. The nurse's willingness to extend
herself, her time, and her interest to another person and actively help him share
both the facts and the feelings of his situation is the basis for building trust. Out
of this beginning an effective working relationship can develop within which
learning and change can occur.

3.2 HOW TO USE NONVERBAL COMMUNICATION SKILLS

Nonverbal behavior often communicates more "loudly" than the words that
accompany it. As discussed in the preceding section, it is important for the
development of a trust relationship that the nurse's nonverbal communication be
congruent with her verbal messages. It is also important that the nurse use
nonverbal communication skills as a deliberate adjunct to verbal exchanges in her
effort to establish clear and effective communication.

When people are troubled, anxious, or uncertain they depend much more
than usual on feedback from others. They need to be reassured that they are
worthwhile, important, and accepted by the nurse before they risk verbalizing
their real concerns. A natural response by a caring person to the needs of others
is to give them his or her full attention. A combination of nonverbal actions and

words convey the message that the caregiver is interested in them and regards what they have to say as important. Sending this kind of message to a patient early in nurse-patient interaction provides the feedback necessary to begin building trust and gives the nurse the opportunity to begin learning about the patient. Counselors use the term *attending* to refer to the nonverbal component of this message. In this section we will review four aspects of attending: centered attention, appropriate responses, relaxed posture, and eye contact.

> The most important ingredients of attending to a person and their concerns are summarized by the mnemonic C-A-R-E:
>
> C–ENTERED ATTENTION
>
> A–PPROPRIATE RESPONSES
>
> R–ELAXED POSTURE
>
> E–YE CONTACT

This mnemonic provides a kind of checklist for the nurse who is purposefully communicating attention and concern to another person.

Centered Attention. When a nurse wants to let a person know that she is attending to them, she stops doing other tasks and makes them the center of her attention. She also mentally focuses on what the person is saying *here and now*; she does not try to anticipate what they might say or follow her own train of thought. This kind of concentrated listening is difficult for nurses to do for a number of reasons—many of them environmental. Distractions to the listener include a high noise level, movement of other people in the immediate vicinity, lack of privacy for confidential conversation, and a variety of interruptions.

Sometimes nurses feel defensive about "only" talking with a patient. Given other pressures on her for her skill and attention, it is easy for the nurse to avoid spending time on attentive communication. Sometimes nurses are tempted to pretend that they are listening carefully, hoping that the person will not continue for too long or say anything of importance. Such a pretense is seldom convincing. It is more open and honest to say something like: "I can see that this is important to you and that you would like to talk about it. Right at the moment I cannot stop and really pay attention. I'll finish what I'm doing and come back at 10 o'clock so we can talk then." Just as in the case of Mrs. Klein (Example 2.8), this kind of statement is generally well accepted. The nurse indicated that the patient's concern was valid and that she was worth paying attention to. The delay seldom interferes with the helping relationship unless, of course, the nurse does not return as promised!

Appropriate Responses. Full attention is usually accompanied by some sounds, even if not complete sentences, by facial expressions and gestures. These responses are not intended to interrupt the flow of the speaker's words or thoughts, but merely to let him know that you are hearing what he says. This kind of feedback is powerful encouragement for him to continue. Counselors have come to call these responses "minimal encourages to talk" (Ivey, 1971). They include such paralingual responses as "um-hmmm," repetition of a significant word, and one-word questions, as well as nonverbal actions such as nods of the head, reflection of the general feeling tone in the listener's facial expression, and various gestures. These, in combination, give the message "I'm hearing you; it's all right to continue."

Relaxed Posture. Stiff, tense, or rigid postures, collapsed or withdrawn postures, turning away from the other person, nervous squirmings, and agitated movements all communicate that the would-be listener is uncomfortable, would rather not be there, and may disappear from the scene at any moment. Good attending behavior requires a relaxed, balanced, open posture. Most people feel at least a little anxious or tense when discussing their feelings or emotional events with someone. The listener must not contribute to this tension by also showing discomfort and anxiety. Some nurses are in the habit of placing their hands on their hips when standing still; this posture can be construed as disapproving and impatient.

The best listening position is one in which patient and nurse are physically at the same level. For the nurse working in clinical settings, this usually means sitting down so that she does not tower over the person lying in bed. In most Western countries the appropriate distance between people who are communicating is approximately arm's length. At this distance the listener can lean forward a little without invading the other person's "personal space." Comfortable distances do, however, vary with culture. Southern Europeans position themselves more closely for talking than do Americans, for example. The nurse needs to familiarize herself with these kinds of cultural expectations for the groups with which she regularly works. (See Davis, 1984, Ch. 3, for a discussion of "Space and Communication.")

Associated with the concept of social distance is the relative comfort with which a person accepts the touch of another. In clinical situations nurses and patients generally disregard conventions about touch in order to give and receive physical care. When discussing an emotional topic, however, touch takes on a different meaning. The nurse may pat a shoulder, stroke an arm, or hold a hand, intending to comfort the person; however, there is at least a possibility that these gestures may be considered intrusive or condescending. The nurse must use her own sensitivity and what "feels right" at the moment as a general guide to her behavior, while making no assumptions about the other person's comfort with touching.

Eye Contact. When you attend to someone that person occupies the middle of your field of vision and you establish eye contact with him. Some people feel less comfortable than others about being looked at. As with social distance, eye contact is subject to cultural variation; if a woman meets the eyes of an Oriental man, this can be interpreted as lack of respect. The appropriate amount of eye contact is enough for the nurse to communicate her sincere effort to understand the person and hear his concerns, but not so much as to seem intrusive. Looking at the floor or gazing past a person's shoulder indicates lack of involvement. For the patient not to meet the nurse's eyes may indicate that he is uncomfortable or embarrassed about the topic of conversation and needs extra assurance of the nurse's acceptance.

Nurses are educated observers of people and their surroundings. It is tempting, when talking with someone, to visually survey the room, mentally noting the availability and status of any equipment present. During verbal communication this behavior is the equivalent of glancing frequently at one's watch or at the door and indicates a definite lack of attention.

Although it is desirable for caregivers to fully attend to all communication, this is simply not possible. There are certain times, however, when the messages given by attending are especially important. Two of these are illustrated by the following case examples.

Example 3.1   ADMISSION FOR EXPLORATORY SURGERY

Mrs. Carla Mason, aged 48, had just been admitted for an exploratory laparotomy after discovery of a large abdominal mass. Nurse Deborah Graham, her primary care nurse, greeted Mrs. Mason briefly and told her that she would return in 20 minutes to do a full admission assessment. Mrs. Mason's nonverbal behavior suggested that she was tense and anxious. She apparently had come to the hospital unaccompanied. The nurse made mental note of these observations and decided to give herself plenty of time to do the assessment. She would give special attention to Mrs. Mason's awareness of a possible malignancy and any communication about her family or supportive friends. The nurse knew that by using good attending behavior, especially related to these subjects, she would be able to give her patient the messages that she was concerned about feelings as well as facts and that her interest in Mrs. Mason extended beyond her physical ailment. By attending to this patient, Ms. Graham wanted to begin a nurse-patient trust relationship that would provide the basis for patient teaching and postoperative emotional support as well as clinical treatment.

Example 3.2   A DISTRESSING DIAGNOSIS

Barry Nelson, aged 30, had been a patient on Deborah Graham's unit for several days while undergoing various neurologic test procedures. As Nurse Graham passed by his room she noticed that he was sitting on the edge of the bed in a slumped posture, apparently deep in thought. This was quite a departure from his usual display of nervous energy. As soon as she had a few minutes that were unlikely to be interrupted, Ms. Graham went to his room, closing the door behind her, and sat down next to the bed. It was a minute or so before Barry even seemed to notice that she was there. When he looked up she could see that his eyes were red. She waited another moment and then asked gently, "Tell me about it?" The patient responded, "Yeh," and then told her that the doctor had just confirmed a diagnosis of multiple sclerosis. Barry continued to talk for some time without intervention by Nurse Graham except attentive listening. Her impression was that he felt comforted by being able to say out loud the many things that were going through his mind about the likely effects of the disease on his life and his concern about his wife and young children. The nurse knew that this was not the time to teach; that would come later. Right now her patient was in a state of crisis and needed good support and listening while he talked through his concerns.

In these two cases the nurse consciously used good attending behavior in order to convey particular messages to her patients and meet their emotional needs. She also paid special attention to the messages given by the patient's nonverbal behavior. On the basis of these clues, for example, she planned to give

Mrs. Mason the opportunity during the assessment procedure to talk about her feelings and social supports as well as her symptoms. This was intended to lay the groundwork for a good working relationship by, in effect, saying to the patient, "I am interested in and concerned about you as a person, not just as a patient." In the second example Ms. Graham responded to the patient's crisis by encouraging him to talk through some of the feelings surrounding his situation, knowing that the clinical aspects could be dealt with later. In both cases the nurse recognized the principle that being able to verbalize the feelings as well as the facts of their situations would prepare these patients to learn the new knowledge, attitudes, and skills that would allow them to grow beyond this experience.

In the following paragraphs we will explore some of the specific behaviors that promote this kind of verbalization.

When to Attend to a Patient

There are a number of times when it is especially important that caregivers give full attention to a person's concerns. These include:

— the *beginning* of a nurse-patient relationship. This helps to establish the trust that will later be important to teaching and other kinds of nursing care.

— when the person is experiencing a *crisis*. A person in crisis especially needs the support of good listening in order to get started on resolving the crisis (see Section 2.5).

— when *reinforcement* is needed. By being given "permission" to talk about a topic of concern by the nurse's willingness to listen carefully, the person is encouraged to focus his own attention on it and think more deeply about it.

— when a person is relating something that is of *special significance* to him. The nurse's warm acceptance by listening attentively confirms the strength of the nurse-patient relationship.

Gerard Egan has summarized the reason for using good listening skills this way:

> Effective attending makes the counselor [or nurse] an *active* listener. . . . What is the helper listening for? Feelings and content. He wants to know about the experience and behavior of the client and the feelings that suffuse them. His ability to listen underlies his ability to understand the client from the client's frame of reference (1975, pp. 69–70).

The attending behaviors of C-A-R-E help the nurse establish and maintain a good working relationship of trust with patients, family members, and others. They contribute to the kind of understanding that forms the basis for effective teaching.

3.3 HOW TO USE QUESTIONS EFFECTIVELY

Questions and answers are a major part of all communication with others. Some questions are part of social ritual, such as "How are you?" Some questions inquire, probe, challenge, quiz, interrogate, and suggest advice (You are going to . . . aren't you?) Some questions confirm the authority and knowledge of the questioner and others establish mutuality in seeking an answer. Some questions demand one-word answers and others invite open-ended exploration of a problem or concern.

Types of Questions

Counselors speak of two basic kinds of questions: *closed* questions, which seek specific information, and *open* questions, which promote self-exploration by the person answering. Some parallels exist between the instrumental and expressive roles of the nurse and these two kinds of questions.

Closed Questions. Within the context of the instrumental role, the nurse seeks to discover information applicable to clinical treatment for a medical problem. She gathers data for both medical and nursing diagnoses. When specific information is required, closed questions are often appropriate: What medications are you taking? When did the pain begin? Have you been in the hospital before? When did you last have anything to eat? These questions can be answered in a few words and are efficient for obtaining critical information. Asking closed questions establishes the questioner as the one in control of the situation.

Open Questions. Within the context of the expressive role, the nurse is more interested in gaining understanding than in collecting specific information. Her goal is forming a working relationship with the patient and significant others. She may still use questions to focus attention on a concern, to give a person "permission" to talk about his thoughts and feelings, and to encourage him to think through the situation for himself. Open questions are appropriate in accomplishing these goals: How did this all start? Could you tell me a bit more about ——? What are you most concerned about right now? How do you think this is going to affect you? Such questions are less time efficient than closed questions but the answers are much more revealing about the person as well as his medical condition. Open questions are followed by active listening and C-A-R-E-ing. They establish a partnership in dealing with problems and concerns. Because effective learning requires a partnership between teacher and learner, the skills of asking open questions and good listening are basic to effective teaching. In the following case example the nurse teacher uses open questions to get to know the patient and his wife, to ascertain what needs to be learned, and where teaching might begin.

Example 3.3 COMMUNITY CARE FOR A PATIENT WITH ALZHEIMER'S DISEASE

Julia Hernandez, P.H.N., had been referred to the Owens family by George Owens' doctor, who had recently diagnosed the patient as having early

Alzheimer's disease. The doctor believed that Mrs. Owens would need guidance in caring for her husband at home.

On her first home visit, Ms. Hernandez introduced herself to the Owenses. Mr. Owens, aged 55, is well groomed and distinguished looking. Shortly after she arrived Mr. Owens excused himself, saying that he was going to take a nap. Part of the subsequent interaction between Mrs. Owens and the nurse is recorded here. An analysis of the nurse's responses is shown at the right.

NURSE: Can you tell me a bit about how you discovered your husband has Alzheimer's disease?

WIFE: Well, about six months ago George began being so forgetful. He says now that it probably started before that but that's when we first noticed. And he got more and more irritable. He didn't want to be around people anymore, not even the children.

The nurse asked an open question so that the subject of Mr. Owens' illness might be explored. People often find it less threatening to start with historical or other factual information than with subjects of highly emotional content.

NURSE: That must have been very difficult for you.

WIFE: Yes it was ... because what can you say. He hadn't had a physical exam for a long time and I finally convinced him he ought to go have one. We've known the doctor for a long time, so I called him before George's appointment and told him I was worried. I think George was worried by then too.

Here the nurse uses a short sentence to reflect the feeling tone conveyed by Mrs. Owens. Like a "minimal encourage" response, it did not interrupt the flow of Mrs. Owens' thoughts, but it did effectively give the message that it was all right to talk about feelings.

NURSE: What happened then?

WIFE: He saw George and then asked us both to come in to talk with him. That's when he told us about this disease that George has. At the time it was almost a relief to know there really was something wrong and wasn't just our imaginations. (Said with sadness and a sense of irony.)

Combined with carefully attentive listening, this open question helps Mrs. Owens move forward in her story.

NURSE: (Reflecting nonverbal behavior) But it doesn't feel good anymore.

WIFE: No, it sure doesn't.... It seems pretty hopeless.... (Long pause while she seemed to be sorting through her feelings.) I want him to stay at home for as long as possible.

The nurse uses an open response, although not a question, to reflect the feeling implied by Mrs. Owens. By doing so she accepts the complex emotions of the situation and invites further exploration. Mrs. Owens names her feeling of hopelessness but seems unready to explore it now.

NURSE: You said the doctor had talked to both of you. Can you tell me what he discussed with you?

WIFE: He told us that the disease was progressive and there was no cure. He said it was like being very old much too early. That's about all, really, He said you would be visiting and could answer our questions and help me figure out how best to care for George.

The nurse does not push Mrs. Owens to further discuss her feelings right now. In this response the nurse returns to a comment she noted earlier as having possible significance. This is called "following." She asks an open question to redirect Mrs. Owens' attention.

There followed a discussion of the kinds of things Mrs. Owens felt she needed to know and questions that had occurred to her. During this visit the nurse did not try to do any extensive teaching except for answering some specific questions. Instead, she focused on Mrs. Owens, encouraging her to express some of her concerns about the situation. In so doing, the nurse established a supportive relationship with Mrs. Owens, letting her know that she was interested in the welfare of both husband and wife. She also learned something about family relationships and the background of information that the Owenses already had.

This nurse-client interaction demonstrates the principle that open responses, either questions or reflective statements, give a clear message that the nurse cares about feelings as well as facts, and that she is willing to join with the patient in exploring them. An example has also been given of "following." This technique is useful for bridging the natural gaps that occur in any conversation and keeping attention focused on the person and his or her concerns. In order to follow well, the nurse must be paying close attention to both the content and the feelings being expressed.

In summary, we have explored two basic aspects of nurse-patient interaction in the two preceding sections: attending and use of open responses. The skills described here are at the core of patient teaching. They help the nurse establish a bond of communication with the patient while allowing her to assess the patient's perceptions and explore his previous experiences—critical factors in determining his readiness to learn. They are the basis of "discussion" methods of teaching (Chapter 5) and are essential to effective "spontaneous" teaching (Chapter 7). The use of these skills encourage the patient to participate actively in his care and communicate freely, thereby increasing his ability to anticipate the consequences of behavior changes.

Skillful communication is at the heart of the nurse's ability to teach effectively.

The kinds of skills required go beyond conversational abilities; it cannot be assumed that concerned caregivers automatically have them. Like any skill, they require conscious attention, practice, and regular self-evaluation.

3.4 HOW PERSONALITIES INTERACT

One aspect of interpersonal communication that has intrigued theorists for many years is the distinctive mix of personal characteristics and preferences called "personality." This factor is not commonly mentioned within the context of the teaching-learning process, and yet one's personality does influence the way in which one solves problems, including how and what one learns. Although it is not possible to completely survey the field of personality theory, an introduction to one particular theory is offered here—that of Carl Jung—since it seems to have special relevance to nurse-patient relationships and is easily put to practical use.

There is no such thing as a theory of human behavior that explains all events or leads to a comprehensive understanding of all people. Rather, each theory, at best, makes some aspects of life a bit more understandable by presenting a generalization.

Carl Jung, famous psychologist and philosopher, became interested in the relative similarities and diversities in people quite early in his career. In 1923 he proposed a theory of four personality types, or dimensions, that attempts to explain how people can have so much in common and yet function so differently. Jung's ideas were later elaborated on by other authors (Myers, 1962; Keirsey and Bates, 1978).

> Each of the four dimensions described by Jung is a pair of opposite characteristics, representing a continuum. A person shares the four basic dimensions with all other people but has a unique blend of relative strengths for each characteristic.

Jung strongly believed that one's inclination toward one or the other end of each continuum is determined at birth but that personality continues to develop and change throughout life (Schultz, 1977).

The four basic personality dimensions proposed by Jung, with some modification of terminology,* are:

EXTROVERT———INTROVERT

CLOSURE———NONCLOSURE

SENSATE———INTUITIVE

ANALYZER———PERSONALIZER

In the following paragraphs each of the dimensions is described briefly along with some of its implications for teaching and learning.

Extrovert———Introvert

The common use of extrovert and introvert to mean liking or disliking people does little justice to what Jung had in mind. He saw these characteristics as determining how the individual defines reality as well as how he relates to his social world (Schultz, 1977).

For the *extrovert*, the reality of daily life is basically external to himself. Its

---

*I am indebted to Dr. William Yabroff, Professor of Counseling at the University of Santa Clara, for suggested changes in the terminology for the second and fourth dimensions. In the former case, Jung used the words *judgmental* and *perceptive*, which have since acquired distinctly "bad" and "good" implications. Likewise, Jung called the fourth pair *thinking* and *feeling*, words that are limited in their descriptive value for the characteristics involved.

major influences are the desires and expectations of other people. For this reason, the strong extrovert may be at risk of making decisions based on what is expected and acceptable to other people and only belatedly consider his own preferences and needs.

For the extrovert, energy is gathered from contact with other people, who give meaning and inspiration to his life. Rapport is readily established with caregivers, since extroverts are both verbally and emotionally responsive. This responsiveness in the strong extrovert can be misleading. He may appear to understand information and instruction more completely than he actually does so as not to seem socially inept or the cause of extra work for the nurse teacher.

For the *introvert*, reality is rather like a little house inside himself. If the house is tidy and the introvert really trusts someone, that person will be invited to "visit," sharing the ideas and feelings that furnish the internal reality. The introvert is sometimes seen by others as being uninvolved in a situation, since he seldom publically displays emotion. He may take much longer than the extrovert to make a decision, since each major decision must be tried out in his "house" of reality, much like a new piece of furniture. A decision for change will be made on the basis of whether it seems right for the person rather than whether others think it is a good idea.

Most people are combinations of these two characteristics, with few occupying the extreme ends of the continuum. Unfamiliar situations in which there is considerable stress, such as becoming a hospital patient, can act to polarize personality dimensions, however. That is, the person who is normally somewhat extroverted may act much more so because of his alertness to the apparent demands of others. He may appear inappropriately cheerful and superficial in his responses. The person tending toward introversion, faced with the same stress, may appear withdrawn and emotionally distanced from his circumstances. In both extremes the reluctance to share deeply felt emotions, such as grief, fear, and anger, is a psychological defense mechanism that helps protect the self-concept of the person under stress.

Whereas the extrovert is relatively easy to involve in a conversation and is likely to respond to open questions, the introvert may give the nurse little verbal feedback about his needs and concerns. Faced with a patient who appears unwilling to interact, the nurse may become anxious and impatient and repeat information over and over or ask a long series of closed questions in an attempt to elicit some response. She may also feel anger or disappointment at the end of such an encounter.

> Apparently superficial verbal behavior or withdrawn lack of verbal response may signal a person's high level of stress.

The nurse may be able to reduce the impact of some environmental stressors that are contributing to the patient's discomfort. She can also alleviate some stress by helping the patient understand what is being done to or for him and what he can expect to happen in the immediate future. She will want to use simple, unrushed explanations and give him ample opportunity to ask questions.

When planning teaching for the extrovert, the nurse might consider using a group setting, since this learner will be influenced by the attitudes of others and will generally be active in the learning process. The introvert will be more comfortable with an individual learning situation; however, a group is often beneficial to this person as well, since it allows him to hear the concerns and approaches of others even though he may be unable to share his own. Finding out that one is not alone with a problem is reassuring, whatever one's personality structure.

Generally, the strong extrovert will relate well to auditory and kinetic teaching methods because of a higher level of interactive skills, whereas the introvert may prefer visual methods. (See deTornyay and Thompson, 1982, pp. 126–127, for an annotated list of tools for determining learning style.)

Closure————Nonclosure

The closure-nonclosure dimension of personality has to do with how people deal with the tasks and decisions of their lives. Although few occupy the extreme ends of this continuum, the tendency toward one or the other of these character-istics is usually clear to the sensitive observer.

Some people feel better if tasks are completed as they arise, decisions are made promptly, and their world of many roles is kept tidy. These people have a personality characteristic called *closure*. At the extreme the closure person can be fairly compulsive. It greatly annoys this person to have a decision unmade or a project uncompleted. The strongly closure person can feel so driven to complete tasks efficiently that sometimes he takes over control of a problem from others who are less anxious and organized. Viewed negatively, the closure person can be seen by others as being inflexible, unwilling to change, insensitive, and unneces-sarily aggressive.

By contrast, the *nonclosure* person prefers to carefully gather all relevant information before making a decision, even if it means a delay in completing a task; for the nonclosure person, a decision made is a door closed. He is not made uncomfortable by several things going on simultaneously, none of which may be finished within a predictable time span. This person may be viewed as being lazy or unmotivated by the strongly closure people in his life but may be appreciated for his ability to be spontaneous and flexible by those with a more positive view of him.

The results of surveys of more than 300 nurses show that the great majority (85%) regard themselves as having strongly closure characteristics. It is not surprising that nurses at least behave as though they were closures because of the diverse roles and tasks of nursing and the approval given to those who are well organized and accomplish a great deal. This characteristic that helps nurses cope well with the diversity of their jobs may make it more difficult for them to teach well. Strongly closure nurses may feel so pressured by the instrumental role and all its tasks that they fail to take the time necessary for the expressive role. They may find it difficult to sit by a bedside listening attentively to a patient's response to an open question. Likewise, they sometimes become impatient with the process of finding out what the patient feels he needs to learn and allowing that to direct the teaching effort. Instead, they may decide in advance what will be taught and then rush the learner through the prescribed material.

Determining whether a person leans toward the closure or the nonclosure characteristic is often possible just from informal conversation about life-style and preferences. The closure person is more likely to tell stories about organizing, cleaning, and deciding, while the latter will tell of spontaneous leisure activities.

> Closure people often suffer even more than nonclosure people under the indignities of reduced privacy, feelings of helplessness, and loss of control that may accompany a medical crisis.

Their relationship with the nurse will be improved if care is taken to supply current information and include the patient in decision making as much as possible. If the nurse tells a closure patient that an event is to occur at a specific time, he is likely to be upset over an unexplained delay.

Nonclosure people are easier to get along with in a time sense, except when it comes to decision making. The highly stressed nonclosure patient will probably find it hard to make decisions. He may be especially vulnerable to feelings of helplessness and of adopting an external locus of control if unduly pressured or controlled by impatient caregivers (see Section 2.3).

Both closure and nonclosure learners benefit from having the learning task broken down into relatively short-term and easily accomplished steps. The feedback that the teacher can give the learner for completing each step assists both patient and nurse to feel rewarded. The closure person will especially relate to the organization of such a scheme and the sense of completion that accompanies each step. By contrast, if learning tasks are presented to the nonclosure learner as a lengthy outline of steps to be taken, he may regard this as a control attempt and resist involvement. Instead, the nurse will first want to discuss with him possible approaches to the learning task so that he maintains a sense of participation in the plan.

When teaching involves the patient's spouse or a close friend, the nurse may well find that this other person tends toward the characteristic opposite to that of the patient. Research has shown that, with this dimension in particular, the old adage that opposites attract does apply (see Keirsey and Bates, 1978, Ch. 3).

Sensate————Intuitive

The sensate-intuitive personality dimension relates to a person's priorities and mental functions. As such it has strong implications for the teaching-learning process. Research indicates that far more people are strongly sensate than are strongly intuitive (Bradway, 1964).

The term *sensate* derives from the same root word as *sensible*. The *sensate* person is focused on the here and now of reality. He knows that life is lived one small step at a time and is content with this. Sensates are practical, often efficient people who pride themselves on solving the problems of today without worrying especially about the distant future.

The word *intuitive* is somewhat misleading because people with a strong intuitive characteristic are not necessarily more sensitive to other people, the common usage of the word today. They are, however, capable of intuition, meaning that they can easily grasp the overall picture, even in a complex situation. Strongly *intuitive* people are basically future oriented; they are interested in what can become and what is possible in a situation. Their lives are often cluttered with unfinished projects (unless they are also strongly closure) because it is the vision of what can become that is more important than actually finishing the product. Intuitives are idealists, philosophers, business leaders, and, often, teachers.

From a practical standpoint, the nurse teacher can assume that the majority of people she encounters will be sensate. Because they assimilate knowledge *starting with the specific and working toward the general*, they need to be given information about what will be done to and for them in the next short period of time. They relate well to examples, cases, and demonstrations. By contrast, intuitive people assimilate knowledge *from the general to the specific*. They want to know the principle or process involved before they deal with the details. They would relate well to a nurse teacher who begins with an overview of what diabetes is and the general goals of insulin control before teaching them how to give their own injections.

Intuitive people seem especially subject to depression and demoralization when faced with helplessness and a negative view of their personal futures. They are likely to be encouraged by a conversation with someone who has overcome their particular malady, since this gives them a positive vision to grasp. Although the sensate may be overwhelmed by a similar encounter, he will probably be willing to "plug along," taking one day at a time, if he is given encouragement and continuing emotional support.

Analyzer———Personalizer

The final dimension of personality—analyzer-personalizer—has to do with how one uses new information and the relative importance accorded facts and feelings. *Analyzers* think of information within discrete categories. They are the list-makers of the world. When confronted with an unfamiliar or ambiguous situation, the analyzer depends on factual information, initially in a rather unemotional way, attempting to categorize it on the basis of what is already known. He prides himself on logic and organizational ability. An analyzer suffering a heart attack will want to know the facts of his situation before he will be able to talk about his feelings.

By contrast, the *personalizer* is likely to apply any information or experience to himself first in a fairly emotional way before coming to terms with the "cold" facts. Given an unfamiliar or ambiguous situation, the personalizer will trust his gut reaction and respond with awareness of feeling.

In sociological terms, it is interesting that the characteristics of the analyzer are identified as valued male traits, while women are often chastised for having more emotional or personalizing traits. A note of caution, however: not all women are personalizers in Jungian terms, or all men analyzers. Beware also of judging an extrovert to be a personalizer or an introvert an analyzer without additional information.

Careful listening on the part of the nurse during introductory conversations will provide clues about whether the person leans toward analyzer or personalizer characteristics. If he asks or talks about facts, he is probably the former; if he talks about how the present situation makes him feel, he is probably the latter. In terms of planning teaching, an analyzer is more likely to trust and relate easily to a nurse who is able to start by giving him verifiable data about his condition. He may be more comfortable with an initial discussion of the relevant anatomy and physiology or with information about medications, rather than having to focus immediately on feelings. For the strong analyzer, the expression of feelings denotes a personal weakness that will be revealed only within a secure, trusting relationship. The personalizer will be relatively more aware of his state of confusion and uncertainty and will respond well to the nurse's use of open responses. The nurse's acceptance of both positive and negative feelings is especially important to this person.

In summary, Jung's theory of personality dimensions has been presented here to help the nurse identify some common themes in human personality and give her a way to communicate about some otherwise elusive information and observations. There is an obvious danger, however, in overgeneralizing or applying

TABLE 3–2. Summary of Jung's Personality Dimensions

Dimension	Some Major Characteristics	Useful Teaching Approaches
Extrovert*	Sociable; easy to engage in conversation; has many visitors	Include significant others in teaching sessions; use group approaches and refer to support groups.
Introvert	Seems quiet and introspective; may especially seek privacy; has few visitors but they come frequently	Start with individual approach, encourage trust by stable staff, and show personal interest; use reading materials as basis of discussion in early teaching.
Closure	Values organization, decisiveness, punctuality; anxious to get back to work/routine	Use structured, task-oriented approach; divide learning into smaller steps.
Nonclosure	Values spontaneity, adaptation to circumstances; willing to take some time off to recuperate	Use open, discussion approach; connect teaching with present concerns and goals.
Sensate*	Values experience and practical problem solving; concerned with present reality	Start with specific and practical; use examples and concrete illustrations.
Intuitive	Values imagination, insight, and speculation; lives in anticipation of the future	Start with principles and long-term goals; use behavior rehearsal and discuss consequences of action.
Analyzer	Interested in facts, standards, rules; uses few "feeling" words	Start with facts; build credibility and trust before approaching emotionally charged issues.
Personalizer	Interested in people, social values; uses "feeling" words easily	Build trust by good listening and reflection of feeling; allow application of learning to own situation.

*According to Keirsey and Bates (1978), there are many more people with this characteristic (3:1) than with the companion characteristic.

stereotypes to unique individuals. Perhaps the most useful aspect of this theoretical material will be to help the nurse identify, at least in retrospect, why certain interpersonal approaches sometimes are successful and sometimes not; why she sometimes relates immediately to a patient or instinctively feels that there is a barrier to trusting communication with him.

In Table 3–2 the four dimensions discussed in this section and their major characteristics are summarized, along with some suggested teaching approaches. It is important to remember that an individual's personality is a combination of characteristics of varying strengths. Distinct traits may not be identifiable. Like a jar containing different colors of paint, one color may be visible from one angle, yet another from a different angle; some may blend together and defy description.

SUMMARY

In this chapter we have focused on the nurse-patient relationship and its place at the center of the teaching-learning process. After a description of the qualities that promote trust, the skills of attending and use of open responses have been reviewed. The effective use of these skills and behaviors requires practice. Likewise, considerable introspection is required in order to come to terms with one's own attitudes and value system. Some ways in which the reader might develop these skills are suggested in the Study Questions and Exercises portion of this chapter. The best learning of this type occurs in a group of four to eight persons who develop a trusting relationship with one another so that they can "risk" trying out behaviors and receive nonthreatening feedback. The reader is encouraged to participate in such small-group learning experiences.

In the final section of the chapter, material was introduced on Jung's theory of personality dimensions and its application to teaching and learning. The usefulness of such theoretical constructs in promoting understanding was pointed out, while warning the reader of the dangers of overgeneralization.

This chapter concludes the discussion of learning principles and the factors that influence the teaching-learning process. We will now proceed to an examination of how the nurse can apply these principles to effective teaching. The following chapters are arranged in approximately the order in which the nurse makes decisions about patient teaching paralleling the steps of the Nursing Process.

Study Questions and Exercises

Feedback from others is an important part of the learning process, especially when learning communication skills. If a formal learning group is unavailable, share the answers and experiences that result from these questions and exercises with colleagues or friends.

NURSING ROLES

1. Several times during a working day stop for a moment and assess the amount of time you have spent both in an instrumental role and in an expressive role. Do this for

several days, keeping track of the approximate percentage of your time in each role and noticing how and why the percentage changed. Review the diagram in Figure 3–1. Do you agree with the role divisions shown there?

VALUES AND ATTITUDES

2. Sometimes we are acutely aware of the problems posed by our own values; sometimes we are less aware of long-standing, deeply buried attitudes. Suppose you are working as a school nurse and Donna, a 16-year-old student, confides in you that a pregnancy test has just confirmed that she is about 5 weeks pregnant. Write down your immediate thoughts and feelings about Donna and her situation. In what ways do these thoughts and feelings reflect your values and attitudes, for example, about abortion, unplanned pregnancy, single parenthood, or teenage relationships? What in your life influenced the development of these attitudes and values? What do you think you should do or say to help Donna? If you are part of a learning group, role play several variations of conversations between Donna and a nurse, noting the expressed and implied attitudes of each person.

3. Suppose you have been assigned to care for Scott, a 20-year-old patient, who has recently been admitted to the hospital after a motorcycle accident. You have been told that he has a fractured pelvis and that a 17-year-old girl who was riding on the back of the bike was killed when the bike left the road. What are your immediate thoughts and feelings about Scott and his situation? In what ways do these reflect your values and attitudes? What kinds of emotional needs do you think Scott might be experiencing? How might you respond to these?

4. You now find out that Scott was being pursued by a police car at the time of the accident because he was riding dangerously. His blood alcohol level was found to be 0.14. Does this information alter your attitudes toward Scott and his needs? In what ways might your approach to him be affected?

5. Each of the patients listed below represents a common stereotype. They are listed this way not to stigmatize them, but to help you identify some patient characteristics toward which you may respond especially positively or negatively. For each patient, ask yourself these two questions: (1) In what ways might my attitudes to life and my values differ from his or hers? (2) How might these differences affect my ability to communicate helpfully with them?

— a frail elderly patient

— a chronic middle-aged male alcoholic patient

— a gay AIDS patient

— an obese female patient

— a very vocal fundamentalist religious patient

— a patient who advocates a Communist revolution

— an anorexic patient

— a cerebral palsy patient who wants to die

— a patient whom you suspect is a hypochondriac

— a patient known to be a child abuser

— a very wealthy female patient

— a young rape victim

Can you see any patterns in your answers? Can you identify influences in your life that might explain this pattern?

NONVERBAL COMMUNICATION

6. This exercise requires that you think of a concern of yours; not a lengthy and involved problem, but one that can be expressed in a few minutes. Tell three persons of this concern in approximately the same way. (Do not tell them until afterward that you are doing an exercise.) In what ways did the specific behavior of your three listeners differ? How did the behavior make you feel? Did any of your listeners exhibit warmth, respect, empathy, or genuineness? In what ways?

7. Choose several exchanges with people and pay attention to your own listening behavior. Are you able to use the attending behaviors of C-A-R-E? Do your facial expressions reflect empathy with the mood of the speaker? Does he or she seem to respond to your effort to hear? What barriers to effective listening did you encounter?

8. For this exercise you will need a cooperative partner. You are to carry on a conversation while in a variety of positions or postures, conversing for 2 to 3 minutes in each position. Mentally note how you feel while doing each of these variations. Start your conversation while sitting back to back. After a short interval turn to face each other, continuing your conversation. Now move your chairs very close together and continue. Have one person stand while the other remains seated, continuing the conversation. Now reverse positions, with the second person standing while the first sits. Talk with each other about how you felt in each of the positions. Did either person show more tension at times? What effect did this have on the conversation? How can your insights be applied to nurse-patient communication?

OPEN RESPONSES

9. *Open* responses focus on feelings as well as facts and invite exploration and clarification of a problem. *Closed* responses focus on factual information and invite short, specific replies. Suppose the following statements are made to you. For each write down both an open and a closed response. For example, a friend says: "My husband's boss is talking about transferring him again. That would mean uprooting the children and everything." An open response might be: "How do you feel about moving?" and a closed response might be: "How long have you lived here?"

PATIENT: My arthritis has really been acting up lately.

FRIEND: Sometimes I wonder whether I did the right thing by going back to work full time.

DOCTOR: I can't help but think that Mrs. Jones just isn't telling the whole story.

PATIENT: The doctor just has to let me go home today.

Compare your responses with those of other nurses. What effect do you think each one would have on communication with the person?

10. Suppose you are interacting with each of the following people. Your objective is to communicate an understanding of the person's feelings. What is the feeling being expressed? What would you say to convey your understanding?

FEMALE PATIENT: I don't know if I can talk about it. Right now my world is just upside-down. I never expected this to happen to me.

MALE PATIENT: I've been trying for three hours now to get somebody to do something about the air conditioning in here! What's the staff do all day, sit in the back room and drink coffee?

WIFE OF PATIENT: Two years ago my son was killed in a car accident. My husband never seemed to get over it. He had his heart attack on exactly the same day as our son died. It's strange. . . .

FRIEND: I can't believe that I got accepted to graduate school! It's frightening in a way, but I'm really excited too.

Compare your responses with those of other nurses. If possible, role play the situations, using a variety of responses, and then talk about the results of each.

PERSONALITY CHARACTERISTICS

11. Answer the following two questions:

I prefer events to happen (a) by careful selection and choice.
(b) spontaneously and by chance.

I admire more the ability to (a) organize and be methodical.
(b) adapt and make do.

What personality characteristic is reflected in your answers? How does this characteristic affect your care of patients?

12. Answer the following two questions:

I would prefer to be known as (a) logical and coolheaded.
(b) sensitive and warmhearted.

In making decisions, I go by (a) standards and procedures.
(b) feelings and needs.

What personality characteristic is reflected in your answers? How does this characteristic affect your care of patients?

4

HOW TO PREPARE FOR TEACHING

In this chapter some of the concepts discussed so far will be drawn together and applied to practical steps for beginning the teaching-learning process. Thorough assessment and planning are perhaps the most important aspects of effective teaching. This chapter presents the Health Balance model for use as a patient assessment tool, some specific methods for collecting assessment data, and a discussion of teaching objectives and plans. For purposes of clarity, this chapter's focus is limited to prepared patient teaching. The variations and abbreviations necessary for spontaneous or informal teaching are discussed in Chapter 7. The main points contained in this chapter are as follows:

- The kinds of responsibilities that must be taken by the patient or his family members are a general guide to the nurse in identifying need for teaching intervention. (Introduction).
- Health can be described as a balance of needs, stressors, strengths, and resources. (Section 4.1)
- The Health Balance model provides the nurse with a broad framework on which to base patient assessment and planning. (Section 4.1)
- Sources of data on which to base an assessment of learning needs include the patient himself, medical observations, written reports, and other people who know the patient well. (Section 4.2)
- A CONE interview is an approach that uses both open and closed questions to gather patient data relevant to particular areas of concern. It can be used in conjunction with the Health Balance model. (Section 4.2)
- The general goals common to all health care situations are treatment, maintenance, primary prevention, and developmental prevention. Although teaching intervention is most closely associated with developmental prevention, it may be appropriate to any of the goals of care. (Section 4.3)
- Clearly stated learning objectives provide the basis for effective teaching. (Section 4.3)

- An important aspect of planning teaching is to decide how the patient's past experiences and present perceptions are to be used to support the learning process. (Section 4.4)
- Use of a written teaching plan helps the nurse organize materials and content and coordinate resources for complex or multiple-session teaching programs. (Section 4.4)

The place of teaching as an integral part of the Nursing Process was discussed in Section 1.2. In this chapter we will look specifically at the assessment and planning phases of that process and the ways in which they provide a basis for effective teaching intervention. Detailed information on general assessment approaches, writing a nursing diagnosis, planning patient care, and the use of a Nursing Care Plan is available from many sources, ranging from basic nursing practice texts, such as that of Sorensen and Luckmann (1986), to texts dedicated specifically to the Nursing Process, such as that of Yura and Walsh (1983). Rather than repeat this extensive material, we will review some major principles. As in Chapter 3 some additional considerations, methods, and approaches are suggested that can be helpful to the nurse as she plans patient care that includes teaching intervention. The basic premises from which we begin our discussion are as follows:

> The Nursing Process provides a framework for organizing comprehensive patient care to meet patient needs and reach health goals. Teaching is one of several intervention strategies used by the nurse in giving excellent patient care. Teaching, like counseling, coordination, and physical care, is not a separate process but an integral part of the Nursing Process.

Teaching is a future-oriented activity. Its purpose is to prepare a person to take action that will help him recover from ill health, maintain his present level of health functioning, or improve his state of wellness.

> Whenever responsibility for future action is to be taken by the patient himself or a member of his support group, helping him prepare for this responsibility through learning is an essential part of his care.

The goal of patient responsibility is a key concept in helping the nurse identify who would benefit from teaching intervention, how teaching might be approached, and when it should start. With the probable future responsibilities of the patient or his family members in mind, the nurse has some focal points for more detailed assessment and planning of teaching. Some examples of patient responsibilities that would alert the nurse to learning needs are that he:

— report medication effects and side-effects to caregivers;
— tolerate discomfort during certain procedures in order to experience their longer-term benefits;
— decide whether to proceed with suggested treatment or surgery;
— take medications at home as prescribed;
— master the skills necessary for carrying out treatment procedures at home;

— plan and carry out changes in life-style, such as diet or exercise, which will improve health; and

— accept limitations in physical abilities.

As demonstrated in these examples, patient responsibilities may involve learning new knowledge or new skills, adopting new attitudes, or a combination of these.

This chapter begins by presenting a broad-based model for gathering and interpreting patient data that will lead to the identification of learning as well as other kinds of patient care needs. The practical aspects of using this model as a basis for assessment and the definition of learning goals and objectives will be followed by notes on how to plan teaching intervention.

4.1 HOW TO ASSESS A PATIENT'S HEALTH BALANCE

A number of assessment tools for obtaining data relevant to patient care have recently been suggested for use by nurses. The nature of these models has changed somewhat as nurses themselves have increasingly used this data to formulate a Nursing Diagnosis. The nursing assessment has come to include information not only about the patient's illness and present condition, but also concerning his emotional and social health. Stressful situations and limited time often prevent the nurse from obtaining complete data within this broad context at the time of a patient's first contact with a health service. It is therefore useful to have an organizational tool that allows the nurse to collect information over a period of time without losing track of what still is needed and to be able to evaluate the importance of data even while she is collecting it. The Health Balance model has these advantages. By classifying information into four broad areas of concern, it helps the nurse establish priorities for nursing intervention.

The basis for this model is a concept of health that includes the notion of "positive" health as being more than the absence of illness. Just as the World Health Organization did in 1947, it recognizes health as complex in nature and dependent on social and community factors as well as individual mental and physical well-being. The term *wellness* conveys the positive aspects of this concept.

One important criterion for a useful assessment tool is that it take individual variation into account. Health is, after all, relative and personally defined. When a person enjoys bounding enthusiasm for life and seemingly limitless energy, we would agree that he is "healthy." At the other extreme, a person's experience of acute physical pain and bodily dysfunction qualifies as obvious illness. It is between these extremes of obvious health and dramatic illness that definitions become blurred, personal, and subjective. Various studies have shown that a large percentage of people suffer from bad backs, arthritis, indigestion, sore throats, and difficulty sleeping but still regard themselves as basically healthy.

The Health Balance model defines health as a state of *dynamic balance*, a constantly changing relationship between the factors that influence one's personal well-being. A child's seesaw illustrates this concept. The children (representing

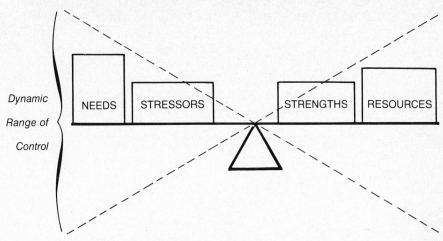

Figure 4–1. The health balance model.

influential factors) must be in balance in order to maintain their game. Once balance is established, they move up and down within a limited range, just as a basically healthy person can adjust to a range of changes and challenges. Illness or distress occurs when one or more of the factors overwhelm the adaptive powers of the balance by becoming too "heavy" or too "light." Assessment, using this model, is a process of identifying how the four basic factors are influencing the health balance. A diagrammatic representation of the model is shown in Figure 4–1.

Factors That Influence the Health Balance

Unmet Needs or Deficits. This factor includes basic human needs that all people share (see Section 2.3) as well as those individual and personal needs perceived by the person as deficits. They may be either acute, demanding prompt attention by caregivers, or chronic, requiring continued work over a longer time. For example, a patient may *need* immediate information and reassurance about his survival and safety. His health balance may also be affected by what he sees as a *deficit* of close and loving relationships or the need for a greater sense of fulfillment in his job.

Demands or Stressors. This factor is made up of the demands placed on a person from a variety of sources and stressors in his environment. They may be physical, emotional, or social. (See Section 2.4 for a discussion of the effects of social and cultural demands and Section 2.5 for a description of the positive and the negative aspects of environmental stressors.) For example, a patient who has been injured in a traffic accident away from home may experience *stress* owing to physical impairment, emotional distress owing to inability to contact and receive support from his family, and concern about being absent from work. Other stressors and demands on his time and energy that could affect his ability to regain his health balance may include financial responsibility for a young family, less-than-adequate housing, or marital discord.

Strengths. A person's strengths include physical, intellectual, motor, and affective or emotional abilities. The knowledge, attitudes, and skills gained through previous experience make a major contribution to a person's present strengths (see Section 2.2). If, for example, the accident victim is in good physical condition as a result of regular exercise, has previously had experience walking with crutches, has good problem-solving ability, and is even-tempered and emotionally stable, the accident will have less negative impact on him than it would if he did not have these internal strengths.

Resources. Another factor whose presence positively influences health is the external resources to which a person has access. These may include material resources, access to health care, and the emotional support of other people. A hospitalized patient, for example, who has good medical insurance coverage and sick leave benefits and whose church membership provides strong personal support and emotional care may well regain his health balance after an illness more quickly than someone without these resources. The improvement of health resources and community services such as paramedic teams, trauma centers, special medical equipment, and public health screening programs positively affects the health balance of all community members.

Using the Health Balance Model

Assessment of these four factors gives the nurse a broad-based picture of a person's present condition and provides the basis for identifying problems and goals.

> The nurse, by analyzing how she might improve the patient's health balance through helping to eliminate or neutralize negative factors and strengthen positive ones, has a starting point for planning patient care.

Awareness of a person's strengths and resources as well as needs and stressors helps the nurse anticipate the impact that an episode of illness is likely to have on the individual in emotional and social as well as physical terms. The Health Balance model helps the nurse organize information about the patient and begin to set priorities for nursing intervention. The following case study illustrates use of this model.

Example 4.1   THE HEALTH BALANCE OF A POSTPARTUM PATIENT

Leslie Peters, aged 27, had just given birth to a 5-pound premature boy by cesarean section. A surgical delivery had been performed because of placenta previa, diagnosed by ultrasound studies when Leslie began to bleed heavily during early labor. Leslie's primary care nurse, Pat Irvine, had admitted her to the unit and had the opportunity to gather information for the following summary of Leslie's Health Balance. Items are not necessarily listed in order of importance or priority. The majority of data included here are subjective, that is, they reflect statements made by the patient and not directly observed by the nurse. This summary is included in the Data Base section of the patient record, along with complete physical assessment data.

Needs and Deficits

— Recover physically from surgery
— Recover emotionally from disappointment of not delivering naturally at the birth center
— Receive reassurance of baby's survival and safety
— Develop self-confidence in handling premature infant
— Successfully breast-feed infant (bottle-fed other son, now 2 years old)
— Regain self-image by losing 40 pounds gained during pregnancy.

Stressors and Demands

— Sibling rivalry already evident in 2-year-old
— Husband disappointed that baby is not a girl
— Mixed feelings about having mother-in-law helping at home

Strengths

— Previous experience with infant care
— Attended prenatal exercise classes with husband
— Good general health: no history of hypertension, heart disease, severe infectious diseases, or mental illness
— Planned pregnancy

Resources

— Husband actively supportive; present during delivery
— Has medical insurance coverage for complications of pregnancy
— Own three-bedroom home; husband steadily employed as engineer
— Mother-in-law in home caring for 2 year old

This Health Balance summary provides a broad picture of some of the positive and negative factors influencing the health of Leslie Peters at this time. The record form used in the hospital in this example allows the nurse to add to this summary as other factors come to light.

Each of the Health Balance factors listed for this patient give additional insight into how best to organize and plan care. Many suggest responsibilities that must be undertaken by the patient and her family over a period of time. The patient's *needs* are the focus of nursing care. They represent goals that caregivers and patient will be working toward. The listing of *stressors* provides a broader view of the patient's world, including environmental and social demands on her time and energy. This patient's *strengths* and the *resources* she has available to her are balancing factors. By collecting this information, the nurse gains an impression about the possible longer-term impact the present episode will have on the patient's health. It alerts her to ways in which previously gained knowledge and experience can be used to more effectively and efficiently prepare Leslie for such responsibilities as breast-feeding, handling sibling rivalry, and maintaining good nutrition while losing weight. Social and cultural factors can be more easily considered with information about resources at hand.

In summary, the Health Balance model has been presented in this section. It offers a framework for assessing a person's present level of adaptation to his health situation and makes clear those areas in which intervention can contribute to restoration of the balance and future wellness.

We will return to the Health Balance model in subsequent sections as we discuss how to gather data for patient assessment, how to identify patient health goals and prioritize nursing interventions, and how to plan for teaching.

4.2 HOW TO GATHER ASSESSMENT DATA

The gathering of data about the patient's present condition and the factors contributing to it is the key to being able to provide care that meets patient needs and helps to restore his health balance.

> Patient care is only as good as the quality of the information on which patient assessment is based.

Because this step is so important to the nurse's ability to teach effectively, an entire section has been devoted to the "hows" and "whys" of this activity. The section begins with some general comments about data collection, proceeds to a discussion of sources of data, and then explores a specific method for obtaining broad-based data from the patient or other people significant to him, using an interview procedure. Useful and more extensive information about data collection and assessment as the first phase of the Nursing Process can be found in basic nursing texts or specialized texts, such as that of Yura and Walsh (1983).

In times past the nurse's role in assessment was largely a matter of collecting and recording patient data for the doctor to use in diagnosing patient problems and needs. The nurse was careful not to obviously interpret the data she collected and certainly not to diagnose. While these attitudes prevailed, data gathering was often seen as an end in itself for the nurse, not as a step toward other nurse-initiated activities. Although still valuable to other members of the patient care team, the data collected by the nurse is now also used by the nurse herself to assess, plan, implement, and evaluate nursing care. She has increasingly taken her place beside the doctor, working with him in a collaborative relationship.

Avoiding Data Collection "Traps"

There are three kinds of "traps" for the unwary nurse in gathering data for the patient assessment. One of these is the historical trap just mentioned: that of regarding the collection of *data as an end in itself*. For the person who falls into this trap, the next logical step in the process, that of interpretation of the data, is avoided or delayed. Delay is especially destructive to effective teaching, which must be started early in order to ensure that patients and family members actually learn.

Some people find it difficult to commit their identification of patient needs to writing in a legal record; they never seem to have quite enough information to make them feel confident and invulnerable to criticism. Reality is, of course, that exhaustive data, especially concerning attitudes, behavior, and feelings, are seldom available in a short time span. The nurse must strive to gather the best-quality information she can, make an educated estimate of need, and, especially where teaching is concerned, check out any assumptions she makes with the patient.

A second trap is the opposite extreme of that just described; it is *rushing to interpretation* before available data has been collected. This is particularly a trap for strongly closure nurses, in Jungian terms (see Section 3.4). They become anxious to have this first phase of the Nursing Process completed and make the mistake of jumping to conclusions. The ancient tale of the blind Indian gentleman who feels the elephant's leg and imagines it to be a tree is an illustration of how judgments based on insufficient data can be very wrong!

In fact, the collection of patient data is not limited to an initial "fact-finding mission." If the quality of nurse-patient interaction is high, then every contact with the patient or his family members, every step in his progress can and should contribute additional data. On this basis the nurse can continue to monitor progress toward goals, modify her approaches, and refine her plans for care. The kind of flexibility that results from continuing assessment is especially important for teaching and counseling interventions.

Finally, there is the trap of *special interest*: that of assigning importance only to data that falls within one's own knowledge area or field of specialization. One of the reasons for the emphasis in these pages on a broad basis for assessment such as the Health Balance model is that nurses are increasingly specializing in clinical areas, and therefore are especially vulnerable to falling into this trap. Strong beliefs or firmly held attitudes can also narrow one's vision when gathering data. Unless the nurse is able to assess the full range of patient needs, she will miss opportunities to help with learning.

Any of these three errors in gathering assessment data results in failure to fully plan patient care. Without a plan that responds to the wide range of patient needs, the nurse can only react to what seems the most important at the moment. Reactive care may meet the patient's basic physical needs but tends to be inconsistent, task rather than goal oriented, and limits the contribution of nurses to physical care interventions.

Kinds and Sources of Assessment Data

There are two basic kinds of information to be gathered from or about the patient and a number of potential sources for obtaining it. A broad-based assessment such as that needed to plan teaching intervention requires both objective and subjective kinds of data and is best collected from several sources.

Objective information is that which can be directly observed and, preferably, quantified by the caregiver. Clinical findings, such as temperature or hemoglobin level, and observable behavior, such as crying or requesting pain medication, are examples of objective data. *Subjective* information is the patient's statements about his thoughts, feelings, and experiences.

Although it is often possible to use objective data to verify subjective statements, and vice versa, subjective information, by nature, is not quantifiable. For

TABLE 4–1. Sources of Patient Data

Source	Methods of Collection
Patient	Interview Physical examination Observation of behavior Questionnaire
Other people significant to the patient (family members, special friends)	Interview Observation of behavior in relation to the patient Questionnaire
Medical records (past and present)	Review Use as basis of consultation with other team members
Other health team members	Consultation regarding knowledge of patient Consultation regarding information about patient's condition
Medical and nursing literature	Review for guidance regarding patient's condition

this reason the subjective has often been regarded as relatively unimportant in planning patient care. Because it is much less "scientific," it continues to be ignored by many caregivers. Yet subjective information is important for a number of reasons: it helps the caregiver understand the experience of medical care from the patient's point of view, gives some insight into his frame of reference, and indicates the degree to which he is motivated to participate in his care. The understanding that results from subjective data allows the nurse to perform her expressive role effectively (see Introduction to Chapter 3).

In Chapter 2 the factors that influence learning were discussed in detail; information about each of them is subjective and personal.

> Assessment of a patient's readiness to learn depends on subjective data concerning his previous experiences, his present perceptions of need, the influence his social group and culture have on him, and his present experience of stress. Obtaining these kinds of subjective data demands a high-quality nurse-patient relationship based on trust.

Of all the relevant subjective data that might be recorded on the patient's chart, the statement: "The patient states that right now he is most concerned about . . ." is one of the most valuable for understanding the subject and complexity of appropriate communication with him. Whatever it is that concerns him is the starting point for teaching, a clue to his motivation, and a guide to building a trusting relationship.

The patient is the first and foremost source of information. For a complete and broad-based assessment, however, secondary sources of information should also be used. When the patient's medical condition or mental state prevents him from being a source of subjective data, one is reliant on his medical record and on other people who know him. Table 4–1 outlines the major sources available in most patient care situations and lists some methods by which relevant data may be collected.

The most common method of data collection is an interview with the patient or about the patient with another person who knows him well. The interview lends itself especially well to collecting the subjective information so important to effective teaching. In the following paragraphs we will look at interview procedures generally and then discuss one particular interview format in detail.

Conducting an Assessment Interview

Because an assessment interview is likely to occur soon after a patient is admitted for health services, it sets some important precedents for the nurse-patient relationship. An old saying applies here: "You only have one chance to make a good first impression." The first moments of the nurse-patient relationship teach the patient what to expect from the nurse. If she immediately begins a staccato series of closed questions, the patient "learns" that he is expected to passively supply information while his caregivers take control. Although this approach may be reassuring to an anxious patient, the pattern of passivity, once established, is difficult to break.

When faced with having to quickly collect data for an initial assessment, the nurse can soften the impact of a "checklist" interview by explaining to the patient *why* she needs information quickly and asking his cooperation. She can also use some of the communication skills usually associated with open questions by *listening* attentively to an extended answer to a question and by *exploring* a hesitant response. These techniques provide the nurse with more complete information and give the patient the message that the nurse is willing to hear both his words and their meaning.

> Skillful interviewing is a conversation with a purpose. Careful preparation is essential to the fulfillment of that purpose.

Although additional useful information is often revealed in unplanned conversation, the initial assessment interview must provide enough detailed information on which to base the Nursing Diagnosis.

The CONE Interview Approach

The CONE interview approach combines open and closed questions within specific, preselected areas of content. Nurses readily grasp the main concept of this approach and appreciate the structure it provides. This is not to suggest that it is the only way to usefully conduct an interview or that it is appropriate for all situations.

This approach is so named because the focus of questions begins broadly and becomes increasingly narrow as the interview progresses, suggesting a conical shape. Each cone has four distinct steps, shown in Figure 4–2.

A reasonably broad-based interview usually consists of four or five CONEs. Without serious distractions or interruptions, each CONE normally takes 5 to 10 minutes. The nurse can therefore plan on such an interview taking between 30 and 45 minutes, including an explanation of just what she will be doing and why. The end of a CONE is a natural breaking point if an interruption makes continuing impossible.

Preparation for this kind of interview consists of identifying *broad subjects* of concern and, within each, *specific kinds of information* for which the nurse is looking.

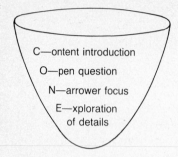

C—ontent introduction

O—pen question

N—arrower focus

E—xploration
of details

Figure 4–2. Steps in the "CONE" interview.

This planning may well serve, with few modifications, for all assessment interviews on a particular unit, whether they are with patients or with significant persons giving information about patients. For example, on a surgical unit, subjects chosen for exploration may include "previous experience and present knowledge about surgical procedures" and "the patient's experience with medications of various types." On an obstetrical unit, subjects of concern may include "preparation for parenting."

The success of the CONE interview as a method of patient data collection depends on the patient's cooperation. Those who are physically able to express themselves usually welcome the opportunity to allow the nurse to get to know them better and appreciate having their thoughts and concerns heard. It is wise and tactful to advise the patient of the confidentiality of the information he shares with the nurse. An example of a statement by the nurse to introduce the interview to the patient might be: "Mr. Jones, I'd like to talk with you for a little while so I can get to know you better. There are some things I especially want to find out from you, so that we can give you the best possible care. Of course any information that you share with me will be used only by the professional staff immediately involved in your care." It is important that this introductory statement be warm, genuine, and respectful, whatever words are used. The nurse is attempting to give the patient the message that she is willing to really listen to him. She also needs to be physically relaxed, unhurried, and willing to sit down. Once the nurse is assured that both of them are comfortable, she may proceed to the first CONE.

Step 1: Content Introduction. The purpose of a short introductory statement for each CONE of the interview is to help the patient understand *what* the nurse is concerned about and *why*. For example, Mr. Jones' nurse might say: "I'm interested in the medications you have taken in the past and how they affected you so that we can better monitor the effects of those you are now taking." Such an introduction helps to direct the patient's attention to the the subject of concern.

Step 2: Open Question. The characteristics of open (as differing from closed) questions were discussed in Section 3.3. They invite the patient to talk freely about a subject, sharing what *he* thinks is important about it. What he chooses to relate gives the nurse valuable clues to his concerns and priorities. An open question for Mr. Jones might be: "Can you tell me about your experience with medications before you became ill this time?" The nurse must then listen CARE-fully (see

Section 3.2) so that she really hears the patient's response. She may want to follow up on some parts of the response later.

Step 3: Narrower Focus. After a full response to a broad open question, the nurse will need to *summarize, clarify,* and ask more narrowly focused open questions. These bits of communication follow directly from what the patient has said and help the nurse more clearly understand the meaning of his words. For example: "So you've been taking Lanoxin, Diuril and Slow-K for two years now without any side effects. Is that right? (Waits for response.) Is there anything else you've taken on a regular basis? (When the patient shakes his head no, the nurse follows with a related open question.) You mentioned that you occasionally take aspirin for a headache. What has your experience been with other non-prescription medications or vitamins?" As in the example, narrower focus questions often take the form of "You said. . . . Can you tell me a bit more about. . . ." This step may be repeated several times as the nurse follows up and clarifies information given in response to the initial open question.

Step 4: Exploration of Details. During this last step the nurse seeks specific information identified during the preparation for the interview as being important but not yet discussed. Mr. Jones' nurse might ask such closed questions as: "Did you take your morning medication before coming to the hospital?" and "Do you have your medications with you?" (If he has, she can objectively verify part of what the patient has told her.)

The cone is brought to a conclusion by briefly summarizing the information shared by the patient during this segment and then proceeding with the introduction to the next cone. For example: "You've given me a lot of useful information about your medication history. I'm also interested in finding out about. . . ."

The Health Balance Model as a Basis of a Cone Interview

An example of a fully planned CONE assessment interview based on the Health Balance model is shown in Table 4–2. Some simple modifications would make the interview useful for obtaining information about the patient from another person. By using this kind of interview format, the nurse is able to gather a wide range of subjective information pertinent to planning patient care. She uses largely open questions that invite the patient to fully express himself but that are relatively nonthreatening to answer because the patient can choose the information he is comfortable sharing. The interview is guided in specific directions without the nurse having to take an aggressively controlling or directive approach. The overall message presented to the patient is that the nurse is genuinely attempting to hear and understand him as a person so that she can work *with* him in overcoming his present difficulty. This kind of message presented by the nurse's verbal and nonverbal behavior is a major step in encouraging the patient's trust and participation in care.

As was pointed out, this is not the only source of valuable data, but it is the most effective way to gather the subjective information that is so important to patient teaching. Guidance for the use of medical record review and consultation with other health team members as sources of data are to be found in such basic nursing texts as Sorensen and Luckmann (1986).

TABLE 4–2. Notes for Health Balance Assessment Interview

Purpose of Interview—to help nurse assess patient's overall health as well as present illness.

Topic of Cone A—*Strengths* of patient
  Introduction: Interest in overall health background
  Initial open question: "Can you tell me about your health before this illness/accident?"
  Looking for: Background experiences and health knowledge
            Perception of prior physical health
            Attitude toward present situation
            Familiarity with hospital/clinical procedures
            Ability to express self verbally

Topic for Cone B—*Needs* of patient
  Introduction: Interest in what is presently going on
  Initial open question: "What sorts of things most concern you right now?"
  Looking for: Unmet basic needs
            Present anxiety level
            Present/future orientation
            Areas of needed information/reassurance
            Willingness to discuss feelings
            Motivation to learn

Topic for Cone C—*Stressors* affecting the patient
  Introduction: Interest in how patient sees his future
  Initial open question: "What kind of changes do you think will be occurring in your life now?" or
      alternatively, "Can you tell me about other things that are going on in your life that might affect
      your recovery?"
  Looking for: Sociocultural context of illness
            Level of awareness of consequences of illness
            Life-style changes foreseen by patient
            Present or impending crises
            Attitude of patient toward changes
            Apparent ability to cope with change
            Motivation to participate in decisions and care
            Areas of knowledge, attitude, or skills deficits

Topic for Cone D—*Resources* available to the patient
  Introduction: Interest in other people in patient's life
  Initial open question: "How are your family and friends affected by your illness/accident?"
  Looking for: Extent of social resources and support
            Strength of bonds with others
            Self-image in relation to others
            Importance of social roles
            Identification of people who are most significant to patient

Questionnaires are most commonly used to gather data on the patient's medical history. They are also useful in certain patient teaching situations in which they may be used to assess knowledge or attitudes or as an adjunct to other written material to stimulate the patient's interest in a subject and involve him in active participation. The use of written materials in patient teaching is discussed in Section 6.2 and the use of questionnaires for the purpose of assessment or evaluation, in Section 9.3.

Writing the Nursing Diagnosis

The Nursing Diagnosis is the summary statement that results from the analysis and interpretation of assessment data. It concisely identifies patient problems and deficits and their causes or contributing factors. Unlike the medical diagnosis, which focuses on disease entities, the Nursing Diagnosis focuses on the patient's level of adaptation to his present circumstances. It acts as a guide for nursing intervention, including patient teaching.

> By reflecting the broad-based interest of the nurse, the Nursing Diagnosis points the way to teaching opportunities that lead the patient to better adaptation in his present situation and better health in the future.

The Nursing Diagnosis will undoubtedly have a number of parts. Those related to responsibilities that must be undertaken by the patient or his family members now or later will require teaching intervention. For example, the Nursing Diagnosis for Leslie Peters, the postpartum patient discussed in Example 4.1, might read in part:

— Lack of self-confidence in breast feeding infant related to inexperience
— Deficit in knowledge about nutritionally adequate postpartum diet owing to lack of previous learning in areas of nutrition and dietary weight control
— Anxiety about sibling relationship related to observed jealous behavior in 2-year-old

These diagnostic statements suggest that teaching intervention would be appropriate to help the patient gain the new knowledge, attitudes, and skills she needs to resolve these issues.

In summary, this section has focused on the importance of comprehensive patient assessment in ensuring broad-based care. After a discussion of some common traps that may limit the scope of data gathering and the necessity for subjective as well as objective data to guide nursing interventions, particularly those with a high component of the expressive role, a particular type of patient interview was suggested. The CONE interview was described in detail and then applied to gathering data about a patient's Health Balance. Finally, the role of the Nursing Diagnosis in summarizing the interpretation of patient data and guiding the nurse in planning patient care was briefly described.

4.3 HOW TO IDENTIFY LEARNING GOALS AND STATE OBJECTIVES

The transition from discovering what needs to be done and deciding what can and should actually be done to taking constructive action is sometimes more difficult than it appears on the surface. A clear statement of goals and objectives provides the link between these steps in the problem-solving process.

The Health Balance model has been suggested as a starting point for organizing patient data and discovering what *needs* to be done. This organization is readily done even as the nurse collects the data thereby simplifying interpretation and the writing of a Nursing Diagnosis.

In working with community health nurses whose major area of intervention is teaching, Waring and McLennan (1979) found that dividing general "goals of care" into four major groupings helped nurses more clearly construct patient objectives and come to terms with what *could* and *should* be done. The four categories of goals acted as a kind of checklist so that problems that were important but not urgent were not forgotten in the rush to help with more immediate needs. More recently this division of goals has been adapted to nursing intervention in clinical settings as well. It has been found useful for clarifying the whole range of patient objectives, not just those involving learning.

> The establishment of clear goals and objectives ensures that nursing intervention remains practical and relevant to the patient's Health Balance.

Goals of Care

The goals that are common to all health care situations are *treatment, maintenance, primary prevention,* and *developmental prevention.*

Treatment

For the identified patient in a medical care setting, the goal of treatment is an obvious starting point. The activities of caregivers with this goal in mind seek to eliminate or reduce the impact of factors that are currently having a negative effect on the patient's Health Balance.

For example, the positive result of treatment for a diabetic patient would be to control his blood sugar levels, thereby minimizing the effects of too little natural insulin on his body's metabolism. Treatment for the person with a broken femur might include removing bone fragments that are impinging on nerves and blood vessels, stabilizing the limb, and giving analgesics.

> Specific patient objectives with *treatment* as their goal may be identified by answering the question:
>
> "How can this patient's Health Balance be restored by reducing or eliminating the negative factors that are upsetting it?"

Nursing interventions that may be involved in this goal of care are physical nursing care, coordination with other members of the medical team, supervision of the patient's self-care, and teaching the patient or a family member how to continue treatment at home.

Because of the priority necessarily given treatment activities and the strong medical care orientation of many caregivers, sometimes these are the only goals identified and knowingly acted on. It may be up to the nurse, with a broader *health* focus, to go on to identify other goals of care.

Maintenance

Concern over iatrogenesis, or treatment-caused disorder, is very real in today's complex medical practice. The goal of maintenance is devoted to, at the least, not doing harm to the patients we care for. Besides giving the patient effective treatment, we would like to help maintain those strengths and resources that positively support the Health Balance.

For example, specific nursing activities that help the patient keep up the good nutrition and muscle tone he had before his illness have a general goal of maintenance. Encouraging those who are part of the patient's primary social group to continue their emotionally supportive roles is a way of helping the patient maintain the personal relationships that affect his general health.

Specific patient objectives with *maintenance* as their goal may be identified by answering the question:

"What strengths and resources does this patient have that should be maintained?"

Primary Prevention

Because the general goal of prevention includes so many kinds of activities, this goal has been divided into two types of prevention. (See Table 4–3 for a comparison of the goals of care presented here with Caplan's [1964] definitions of "prevention.") The first type is primary prevention, the major goal of which is to avoid a stressor entirely, eliminate it from the environment, or create a barrier between the stressor and a vulnerable individual. Attainment of this goal usually involves environmental manipulation.

Examples of large-scale primary prevention are the installation of equipment that prevents toxic industrial wastes from entering the domestic water supply, reforestation projects that prevent soil erosion after a fire, and laws requiring motorcyclists to wear helmets to reduce the likelihood of head injuries. On a smaller scale, examples of primary prevention include using side rails on the bed of a sedated patient to prevent a fall, using a lambskin on the bed of an elderly person whose skin might be irritated by rough sheets, using masks and gloves during surgery to protect the patient from infection-causing organisms, and using condoms as a birth control method. Primary prevention activities require knowledge of a likely stressor in the environment, thorough planning, and careful attention to the motivation required to use the changed environment appropriately.

Specific patient objectives with *primary prevention* as their goal can be identified by answering the question:

"From what negative factors in the environment should this person be protected?"

Developmental Prevention

The goal of developmental prevention is similar to that of primary prevention: to protect the individual from harmful stressors. The approach in this case, however, is to help make the person less vulnerable through improving his personal strengths and resources. Even if the stressor is unavoidable, its impact is reduced.

Specific patient objectives with *developmental prevention* as their goal may be identified by answering the question:

"How can this person be helped to be less vulnerable to physical, emotional, and social factors that could adversely affect his health?"

Education is the principal method by which developmental prevention is

TABLE 4–3. Comparison of Goals of Care Terminology

Goal of Care	Definition	Preventative Activity Level*
Treatment	Overcoming present disruption in the Health Balance by reducing or eliminating negative factors	Secondary and tertiary
Maintenance	Protecting and maintaining factors that positively affect the Health Balance	Secondary and tertiary
Primary prevention	Eliminating negative factors from the environment or creating barrier to protect the individual from disruption of the Health Balance	Primary
Developmental prevention	Helping an individual become less vulnerable to the impact of negative factors on his Health Balance	Primary and secondary

*Caplan, 1964.

accomplished. Examples of developmental prevention include helping a person learn how to include daily vitamin C in his diet, how to begin an exercise program, why it is important to stop smoking, or how to develop constructive communication patterns with his spouse. Sometimes developmental prevention takes the form of helping other people learn how to better protect the patient. Examples of this kind of developmental prevention include helping a mother learn why it's important to immunize her child, helping a patient's wife learn how to reduce cholesterol in his diet, or helping the family of a handicapped person learn how to include him in social activities and daily tasks.

Although developmental prevention usually involves patient teaching, other nursing interventions may also be appropriate. The nurse may, for example, meet developmental prevention goals by massaging pressure areas to increase circulation and prevent skin breakdown or by helping a patient develop positive self-esteem through counseling, thereby making him less vulnerable to depression.

> The four general goals of care help the nurse identify specific, realistic patient objectives. The clear statement of objectives (a) focuses nursing care on the patient rather than on the disorder or the nurse, (b) helps to coordinate the efforts of all caregivers working with the patient by promoting more complete communication, and (c) facilitates evaluation of the effectiveness of care.

The reader may well be familiar with Caplan's (1964) division of prevention into primary, secondary, and tertiary levels. In Table 4–3 these are compared with the four goals of care presented here. The nurse who considers how she can help the patient with each of these four goals of care will find not only that construction of patient objectives is simplified, but also that the whole range of activities that will improve the patient's Health Balance are considered.

Stating Patient Objectives

Nurses have become increasingly aware of the contribution that nursing assessment and nurse-planned intervention make to patient care. At the same time the need for legal accountability has dominated many aspects of practice. As a result, various formats for record keeping have been instituted that seek to clarify the activities of nurses in relation to a patient, set expectations for patient progress, and simplify nursing audit and other evaluation procedures. The Nursing Care Plan is part of all these formats. Older-style Nursing Care Plans have the nurse identify patient "problems" and related nursing actions. More recent plans have used the phrase "Expected Patient Outcomes" or "Patient Objectives" instead of problems, signifying an important evolution in the concept of what nursing care attempts to accomplish. Emphasis has shifted away from the nurse as a fixer of problems to the nurse as a facilitator and expert clinician who works with the patient to resolve difficulties the responsibility for which he has not relinquished.

Although the word *objectives* has been associated especially with learning activities, many nurses have mastered the skill of writing patient objectives that reflect a full range of health needs. The objectives are phrased to show what the *patient* will be able to do, encouraging the inclusion of the patient and his family members in mutual goal-setting activities. This kind of orientation makes it much easier for the nurse to include patient teaching as an integral part of nursing care.

The well-stated learning objective performs the same function for the learner that a detailed road map does for the traveler: it tells you how to proceed toward your goal, how far it is, and how you will know when you arrive. Like the road map, objectives may be used for planning, for teaching or other nursing intervention (traveling), and for evaluation. Robert Mager (1975) identifies three components of a well-stated objective:

Behavior + Conditions + Criteria = Learning objective

Behavior. Learning has taken place if the newly acquired knowledge, attitudes, or skills lead to an ability to take action. The behavioral part of a learning objective states what the learner will be able to do, what action he will take.

Clearly some of the things that are learned by patients are not put to the test of action until well after they have left the clinical setting. A person who has learned to modify his diet, for example, will not fully practice what he has learned until he returns home. Yet it is important that both teacher and student have some means of evaluating whether progress in learning has been made. For this reason the objectives guiding the teaching-learning process must identify behaviors that can realistically be seen and evaluated in the shorter term. An objective for the patient who is learning about his diet may specify that he be able to *name* three ways to reduce his cholesterol intake or *write* a plan for five low-sodium menus. Such short-term objectives function as a road sign along the way to let both teacher and learner know that they are on the right track and making progress. The importance of feedback is discussed in greater detail in Section 9.1.

Conditions. The demonstration that learning has taken place occurs within a given set of circumstances or under certain conditions. These need to be stated specifically to signify what kind and level of learning is involved. (See discussion of levels of learning in Section 4.4.) The statement of condition may reflect the degree of responsibility the learner is to take for the behavior. For example, learning may progress from a condition in which he is coached by the nurse while performing the desired behavior to the ability to initiate the behavior on his own.

Other possible conditions involve the use of particular equipment, supplies, or references. They may specify the position, location, or environmental setting for the desired action.

Criteria. Two commonly used criteria for the performance of an action included in an objective are a target date and a target standard. The former represents a schedule for learning and is especially important when time is limited. A patient who is to be discharged in 2 days needs to be well on his way to performing complex self-care activities without intensive guidance or he will be unable to take full responsibility at home. When several levels of learning are involved, setting target dates helps to focus the attention of both teacher and learner on the tasks required to meet them.

Standards for the performance of learning vary from the absolute (without contaminating sterile field) to the conditional (will succeed in three out of five trials). The statement of standard must include how "success" is to be measured or whose authority is to be used (according to Dr. Blogg's instruction sheet).

Let us look at some patient objectives that might have been listed for Leslie Peters, the mother of a premature infant, described in Example 4.1. Each of these reflect a general goal of care. Notice that they are not limited to teaching intervention.

- By ———, the patient will be able to sit in chair at bedside for 30 minutes. (Goal of care is treatment.)
- By ———, the patient will have resumed normal voiding of at least ...ml per 8 hours. (maintenance)
- By ———, the patient will be able to demonstrate cleansing procedure for preparing breasts before nursing. (developmental prevention)

Each of these meet the following test for useful and realistic objectives:

> Patient objectives should clearly specify patient *behavior* that can be observed and evaluated by the nurse herself, along with the *conditions* under which the behavior will occur and the *criteria* that apply to its performance.

Both patient and caregivers are rewarded when an objective has been attained. Helping patients and their family members participate in the formulating as well as the meeting of objectives, particularly learning objectives, promotes this sense of accomplishment. It also enables the nurse to fully use the patient's previous experiences and present perceptions in her teaching (see Sections 2.2 and 2.3). Mutual objective setting encourages mutual trust. In Section 9.3 the use of patient-kept records and patient contracts are discussed in more detail.

Assigning Priority to Objectives

The next step in planning patient care is to assign priority to the stated objectives. Theoretically, the more basic the need to be fulfilled by an objective, the higher priority it will be given. One has to ask, however, whose perception is going to influence this determination. Outside of needs that are clearly urgent,

TABLE 4–4. The Care Planning Process

Identify Goal of Care	→ State Patient Objective	→ List Nursing Intervention/Orders
Treatment	To state apply perform name describe verbalize	Physical care Coordination Supervision Counseling Teaching
Maintenance	To resume practice recognize demonstrate recall	Physical care Coordination Supervision Teaching
Primary prevention	To remove avoid use ensure plan	Physical care Supervision Teaching
Developmental prevention	To develop describe choose identify distinguish compare	Teaching Counseling Coordination Supervision

the perception of the patient represented by his immediate concerns and anxieties should be considered. Effective teaching must start with these.

Generally, treatment and primary prevention goals receive the first attention of caregivers. Maintenance objectives are important throughout care, but unless the objectives of maintenance are carefully included in the Nursing Care Plan, they can be overlooked.

The objectives of developmental prevention are often relegated to the if-we-have-time category. This is unfortunate because, as was discussed in Section 2.5, there is an opportunity for learning and a willingness to change behavior patterns at a time of stress that may be lost by placing priority only on acute care.

> Helping a patient learn how to become less vulnerable to illness is a responsibility of all health professionals and deserves high priority when planning care.

Because it often takes longer to meet learning objectives than it does to complete other forms of care, teaching intervention should be started early. If the nurse has assessed the patient's learning needs and planned her intervention at the time of admission, she can then proceed to teaching as soon as the patient is physically and mentally able to begin the learning process.

The steps for planning nursing care using the framework of goals of care are summarized in Table 4–4. For each of the general goals, some verbs that are useful in stating objectives are listed and commonly identified nursing interventions shown.

In summary, four general goals of care have been described and a format for specifying patient objectives suggested. A Nursing Care Plan based on these concepts can be expected to clarify the direction and purposes of care for all caregivers involved with the patient, encourage patient participation in goal setting, attainment, and evaluation, and help the nurse identify a full range of nursing interventions based on patient needs.

4.4 HOW TO PLAN TEACHING INTERVENTION

As discussed at the beginning of this chapter, teaching intervention by the nurse is appropriate whenever a patient objective involves responsibility for future action by the patient or his family. Such responsibility for decisions or action may be part of any of the four goals of care (see Appendix A for an extended example of goals of care applied to common patient teaching situations). In this section the preparations necessary for effectively initiating teaching intervention are outlined in the form of a series of four questions that the nurse might ask herself.

What Shall I Teach?

The first guide for planning teaching is the specific patient objectives. They point to subjects within which the patient may need to develop knowledge, attitudes, or skills and may suggest the content areas to be included. For example, a common objective related to the patient's responsibility for continuing treatment at home states:

- By ———, the patient will be able to identify the medications he will be taking at home by their pharmaceutical names.

The subject in this case is "take-home medications." The more specific content of teaching is indicated by the verb used, in this case *to identify*.

> The key to deciding what to teach lies in determining the level of complexity at which learning must occur. Patient objectives may need to be refined to reflect this level.

The levels of learning complexity were described in Section 2.2 (Table 2–3). For ease of reference, the table outlining these levels is repeated (Table 4–5).

In the example given above, the patient objective indicated that the patient should be able to "identify" his medications by name. It probably is sufficient, in this case, that the patient simply be able to *remember* the name and appearance of the medication. This is the least complex level of knowledge to learn and, providing the patient is mentally alert and not under undue stress at the time of teaching, helping him meet this part of the objective should be straightforward.

A second objective that might apply to this patient would be that he be able to *state* how and when the medication is to be taken. While this verb suggests only a recall level of learning, he actually needs to learn at the application level if he is going to be able to take his medication correctly at home. Because the nurse will not be able to observe his at-home behavior herself, she does not include it in the objective statement. There are, however, other behaviors she could observe that would allow her to refine the objective statement to more nearly reflect the

TABLE 4–5. Levels of Learning

Knowledge

1. Remember	To recall information
2. Understand	To grasp the meaning
3. Apply	To use the information
4. Analyze	To understand the underlying principle
5. Evaluate	To judge value and compare with other known information

Attitudes

1. Recognize	To be aware and give attention
2. Respond	To react and give feedback
3. Verbalize	To be able to explain attitude
4. Utilize	To take action demonstrating attitude
5. Conceptualize	To make attitude part of one's larger value system

Skills

1. Perceive	To be aware of component parts and their relationship to one another
2. Manipulate	To be able to handle parts appropriately but separately
3. Combine	To put parts together for coordinated action
4. Perform	To carry out sequenced actions and complete total task procedure
5. Adapt	To modify procedures to fit circumstances

optimum level of learning. For example, the clinical situation may permit the patient to take the medication himself at the prescribed times under the supervision of the nurse. Alternatively, he might come to the nurses' station at the prescribed times and request the medication by name. His wife might be included in the teaching by the nurse so that she can remind and support her husband in taking the medication.

> Effective teaching begins with careful thought about the level of complexity at which learning needs to occur and creative planning so that successful learning can be demonstrated in the clinical environment.

Who Should Be Included in the Teaching?

In Section 2.4, the social and cultural context of learning was discussed. There are three major reasons for including family members or those who form part of the patient's support system in the teaching-learning process. The first reason for including others is that they will be *affected by a change* in the patient's behavior. Unless they understand the need and nature of the change, they cannot be expected to support it. For example, had Mr. Innes' wife (Example 2.6) been included in the explanation of why it was important for her husband to exercise regularly, she might have cooperated and supported Mr. Innes' attempt to jog every day rather than complain about the change.

A second reason for including others is that, although they may not be directly affected by a change in the patient's behavior, they are in a position to *actively lend support* to it. For example, a close friend with whom the patient works may actively support the patient's resolve to stick to a low-calorie lunch.

Finally, others should be included in teaching when they share responsibility for actions affecting the patient. It is important that the person caring for a stroke patient at home be included in learning why it is important for the patient to turn frequently and breathe deeply.

> Other people should be included in the teaching-learning process when (a) they will be affected by the patient's change in behavior, (b) they can lend support to a change, or (c) they share responsibility with the patient for a behavior change.

Including others in a teaching session means that the nurse must plan ahead in order to coordinate attendance and adjust her teaching methods and materials accordingly. (See Chapter 8 on teaching groups of three or more persons.)

When Should I Initiate Teaching?

The short answer to this question is "As soon as possible!" There are a number of factors to be considered, however, that define "possible." One major factor is the patient's and the family member's state of mind. In order to be able to learn, the learner must be able to concentrate attention and respond. Aside from obvious physical limitations owing to medical condition, disturbed concentration and response are most likely to be caused by pain or high anxiety levels. The nurse may need to give pain medication or reduce the level of anxious concern before attempting to teach.

Moderate levels of stress actually help the learning process but only within subject areas directly related to the cause of the stress. For example, a patient anxiously awaiting an x-ray report can be expected to willingly learn what the results mean to him and why, but he cannot be expected to even hear an explanation about the long-term benefits of reducing his cholesterol level.

The amount of time that will probably be required to meet the patient objective is also a factor to be considered when planning teaching. The longer learning takes, the earlier one must begin.

> Generally, the length of time needed for learning increases with (a) the complexity of the new knowledge, attitude or skill, (b) the number of people involved in a change of behavior and (c) the degree of impact the changed behavior will have on the patient's life-style.

Teaching related to continued treatment after discharge is often left until shortly before the patient's discharge. Such teaching is uniformly ineffective for two basic reasons. One reason is that the patient's attention span and concentration ability will probably be limited because of natural anxiety about a transition to home care. Another reason is that teaching done under the pressure of a deadline is seldom well presented and may sound to the patient like a tape recording played on fast forward. He may be unable to make sense of a tangle of admonitions even when offered with well-intentioned concern.

When Should I Write a Teaching Outline or Lesson Plan?

A Teaching Outline is appropriately used whenever teaching intervention would benefit from improved organization or communication with other caregivers.

> As a general rule, a Teaching Outline should be completed whenever teaching is to extend over several related sessions, whenever more than one teacher is involved with the subject matter, or whenever the targeted level of learning is complex.

Because the teaching outline contains all information relevant to a specific learning objective, it serves as a reference for the nurse teacher and as a method of coordinating the efforts of the care team.

There are numerous variations of the Teaching Outline form, sometimes called a Lesson Plan. One is shown in Table 4–6 as an example in an abbreviated version.

The Teaching Outline provides the nurse with a valuable tool for organizing teaching intervention. By summarizing relevant information, it saves time by preventing needless duplication of effort while reminding the nurse teacher of preparation that must be made before beginning teaching.

In summary, some of the practical aspects of planning teaching intervention related to teaching content, timing, and organization have been discussed in this section. As with any nursing intervention, planning is an essential ingredient in effective care.

TABLE 4–6. A Teaching Outline*

Assessment Information
Indicate learner's prior level of knowledge or experience in the subject area:
Describe the learner's perceptions of his learning needs and relevant attitudes toward learning:
List social and cultural factors that may influence learning:

Planning Information
State patient objective(s), including level of learning complexity required and resulting behavior of learner:
List major subject area(s) to be included in teaching:
Indicate planned number of sessions and anticipated length:
Identify learner(s) and indicate reason for their inclusion if other than patient:
Identify teacher(s) and indicate division of responsibilities:
Indicate time and place of planned session(s) and note any preparations that must be made ahead:

Session 1:

Content (List in order of presentation, noting points to be emphasized):	**Methods and Materials** (Note resources or additional equipment needed):
1.	1.
2.	2.
3.	3.
4.	4.
5.	5.

(Actual form includes space to list content and methods/materials for two additional sessions.)

Evaluation Methods: (Note when each is to be used.)

Notes and Comments of Nurse Teacher: (Comment on positive and negative aspects of each session.)

*Identifying patient information and space for answers have been omitted from this example form.

SUMMARY

In this chapter, theory and practical considerations have been combined in a discussion of the assessment and planning phases of the Nursing Process as they lead to teaching intervention. The Health Balance model was presented as an approach to a broad-based patient assessment. After a review of some general aspects of gathering assessment data, the CONE interview was suggested as a useful method for determining a patient's need for and readiness to learn. An example showed how this interview structure could be used in combination with the Health Balance model.

The interpretation of assessment data was discussed in terms of four general goals of care leading to a statement of specific patient objectives. The clear statement of objectives lends direction and purpose to all nursing intervention and is especially important for effective teaching. In the final section of this chapter we have considered some of the practical concerns of the nurse as she plans her teaching approach.

The reader is referred to Appendix A, in which details of needed assessment information and sample teaching plans using goals of care as the basis are shown for some commonly occurring patient teaching situations. In the next two chapters we will look at the teaching strategies and materials that might be used to help patients learn.

Study Questions and Exercises

1. For two patients in your care, list his or her responsibilities for decisions or actions. Include both large and small responsibilities: those that require immediate attention and those that are longer term but related to the patient's present illness. Discuss your lists with classmates or colleagues. Can you identify several categories of responsibilities? What implications do these have for nursing intervention?

2. Ask three or four persons for their definition of health. Find out whether they regard themselves as healthy and what factors they consider important to this state. Ask what they typically do when they do not feel well, but not ill enough to seek medical help. Share the answers you receive with your classmates or colleagues and discuss what implications the answers have for health care workers.

3. Review the assessment format currently used in your hospital or clinic. Compare and contrast it with the Health Balance model outlined in Section 4.1.

4. Make a survey of at least six nurses, asking them how they gather data for a patient assessment, what they find most useful, and why. Summarize these findings and discuss them with classmates or colleagues.

5. Construct an interview CONE, as described in Section 4.2, for a topic of special importance to a unit with which you are familiar. Role play, using this CONE, with a classmate or colleague. Evaluate the information this technique provided and note changes you might make in it for next use.

6. Using the notes shown in Table 4–2, conduct a Health Balance assessment interview, first with a classmate and then with a patient. Evaluate the information you receive and discuss with classmates or colleagues how this information might be used to plan teaching.

7. Write at least three patient objectives in each of the four goals of care discussed in Section 4.3 for each of two patients in your care. Be sure to include behavior, conditions, and criteria in each objective. Discuss how these objectives fit in with the present record-keeping format and how they might be used in planning comprehensive patient care.

8. Choose an objective from exercise 7 for which teaching intervention is appropriate. For that situation, note answers to each of the questions posed in Section 4.4.

9. Compare and contrast the Teaching Outline used on your unit with that shown in Table 4–6.

5

HOW TO
CHOOSE AND
USE TEACHING
STRATEGIES

The preceding four chapters have presented theoretical and practical material that help the nurse understand and prepare for teaching. This chapter begins a series of four chapters devoted to practical guidance for the nurse as she carries out a teaching intervention. It focuses on teaching strategies for use with one or two learners. First some general considerations in selecting and combining teaching strategies are discussed and then each major group of strategies is explored in detail. (Strategies for use with groups of three or more are considered in Chapter 8.) The main points included in this chapter are as follows:

- Whether the style of teaching is formal or informal, structured or open, prior organization and patient participation are important to learning. (Introduction)
- In choosing teaching strategies the nurse should consider her own knowledge base, interpersonal relationship with the patient, and the environment in which learning will take place. (Section 5.1)
- Giving attention to the sequence of a lesson and planning ways in which the learner will be able to give the nurse feedback during the lesson improve the efficiency and effectiveness of learning. (Section 5.1)
- Explanation and lecture are efficient means of transmitting information from teacher to learner. Used properly, they are especially effective in helping a person acquire new knowledge. (Section 5.2)
- Discussion promotes an open exchange between learner and teacher. It is especially effective for helping with attitude change. (Section 5.3)
- Demonstration-coaching strategies, in which the learner tries out procedures under the guidance of the teacher, are particularly effective for the development of motor skills. (Section 5.4)
- Role play, behavior rehearsal, and experiential exercises are based on the

principle that people learn best that which they actually experience first-hand. They are emotionally powerful techniques that promote complex learning. (Section 5.5)

Throughout this book the interactional nature of teaching and learning has been emphasized. In this chapter we will explore strategies of teaching in detail and examine what the teacher does in order to teach and what she asks the learner to do to participate in learning. Because we are focusing specifically on the teaching of only one or two learners, the quality of interaction between teacher and learner is emphasized.

Because of childhood experiences, most people have some preconceived notions about what teaching-learning situations ought to be like. There are two basic elements to these notions: one is the relative *formality* in which teaching-learning ought to be conducted; the second is the relative *structure* that ought to guide the interaction of teacher and learner. While notions of what "ought to be" derive from past experiences, they reflect preferences and comfort with particular teaching and learning styles in adulthood.

In a large group peer pressure usually results in tolerance of, if not individual adjustment to, the teacher's preferred style. A class member might "escape" an uncomfortable style of teaching by withdrawing attention or participation. In a one-to-one situation there is no comparable escape. In individual patient teaching the preferred styles of both learner and teacher are important and may need to be negotiated. Presumably, the nurse as teacher has the major responsibility to adapt to the preferences of the learner. Her flexibility will increase as she gains experience with a patient teaching role.

In choosing a teaching style that is acceptable to the patient, the nurse can be guided by the tone and nature of interactions that precede planned teaching and by the patient's verbal and nonverbal responses as teaching begins.

Formality denotes the psychosocial distance between teacher and learner. This element of the teaching-learning situation may be regarded as a continuum, with strict formality at one extreme and casual informality at the other. The more formal the situation, the more obvious the role of the teacher as "expert" and the greater her sense of control. Teachers who are relatively inexperienced or lack some confidence in presenting the material selected generally prefer a more formal role. As Rankin and Duffy (1983) point out, some potential for conflict exists between a nurse who prefers to present herself as an expert and a patient who especially wants to feel in control of his environment. (See Section 3.4 for a discussion of personality factors and their relevance to teaching and learning.)

The degree to which the learner actively participates in learning is a dimension of formality; in very formal situations the teacher expects to speak while the student listens passively. While a formal style allows less freedom for give and take, opportunities for participation by the learner can, and should, still be included. There is good reason to believe, as discussed in Section 2.2, that active participation is an important aspect of learning. It helps the learner make sense of new knowledge, attitudes, and skills and apply them to his personal situation.

At the same time learner participation helps the teacher follow the learner's progress and respond more fully to his needs.

> Whether teaching is conducted in a formal or informal style, learner participation is an important part of effective teaching.

A second element of teaching style is the amount of structure that is included. This, too, might be regarded as a continuum, with carefully detailed structure at one extreme and an open, free-flowing approach at the other. Highly structured learning situations may include the use of written notes or an outline that the student can follow during discussion or explanation. A more open style might appear more conversational. Many counseling situations are conducted in an open style, with the counselor following the lead of the client in discussing topics of concern. The CONE interview approach to assessment, described in Section 4.2, is an example of a structured format, with topics carefully selected before the interview.

A concept often associated with structure is organization. In order for a lesson to be organized, the teacher needs to have carefully considered the objectives to be achieved and the probable means of achieving them. The organizational aspect of effective lesson planning has little to do with the style of presentation, although it is usually more apparent in a structured style.

> Whether a structured or open style of teaching is used, organization is essential to the achievement of patient objectives.

The nurse teacher's preferred style of teaching, in terms of relative formality and structure, reflects her personality. As teaching skills develop the nurse will become more flexible in varying her style to match the preferences and comfort of the patient. Keeping in mind that the overall goal of teaching is to help the patient learn, she will ensure that patient participation and basic organization are included, whatever style is used.

5.1 WHAT TO CONSIDER WHEN CHOOSING A TEACHING STRATEGY

Before examining specific teaching strategies, we will explore some of the general considerations that will help the nurse plan the activities that make up the learning experience. These considerations include the nurse's own knowledge in the subject area, her interpersonal relationship and level of communication with the patient, the environment and time available for teaching, and, perhaps most important, how teaching can be sequenced to promote maximum learning.

The Knowledge Base for Teaching

Clearly one must know something before being able to teach it. If the nurse who has done the patient assessment and nursing care plan has an adequate knowledge base in identified areas of learning need, she may go ahead and select a teaching strategy with which she is comfortable and to which she anticipates the learner will respond positively. If she does not feel confidently knowledgeable in an area of need, she has two basic options: she can learn enough to be able to teach, or she can delegate the teaching responsibility in that area to someone who is more knowledgeable. A careful analysis of the level of complexity at which the patient needs to learn may guide the nurse in this decision.

Example 5.1   PATIENT PREPARATION FOR A CARDIAC PROCEDURE

Mr. Quinn had been admitted to the medical unit after an episode of chest pain. He was scheduled for a cardiac catheterization procedure in the morning. His primary nurse, Julie Johnson, was an experienced nurse but had only recently joined the staff at this hospital. Because she had previously worked in orthopedic and neurological units, she was unfamiliar with the newest advances in the cardiac catheterization procedure as well as with the protocol at this hospital. However, Mr. Quinn and his wife needed to learn what to expect tomorrow and have an opportunity to ask questions of someone who was knowledgeable in this area.

Ms. Johnson's first thought was to contact the catheterization laboratory and ask for help. Unfortunately, the nurse who often did patient preparation was unavailable. Her next resource was her nursing colleagues on the unit. By asking others, Ms. Johnson soon located Sandra Holt, a nurse who had worked in the catheterization laboratory up until a few months ago. Ms. Holt was happy to talk with Mr. and Mrs. Quinn. Ms. Johnson planned a convenient time with the nurse, asking whether she might join in the session in order to learn about the procedures herself.

In this case example, the nurse met her obligation to provide for the patient's learning need through coordination with a more knowledgeable colleague. She also took the opportunity to join in the session herself, so that she could progress in her own learning. If she were able to accompany Mr. Quinn to the catheterization laboratory and observe the procedure, she would be well on her way to being able to handle patient teaching in this area.

Levels of Communication and Rapport

The nurse who has had an opportunity to get to know both the patient and the people who are important to him has the best chance of being able to clearly and specifically identify learning needs and choose the most effective strategies for teaching. A basis of rapport and background of communication with the patient will enable the nurse to initiate teaching easily and naturally as part of her nursing care.

Sometimes a learning need must be met immediately, even though the nurse has not had an opportunity to develop communication or rapport. Ms. Holt, in the example above, was in such a position. Because she knew the content of the lesson well, she might just have proceeded with an explanation of the material to the Quinns. In this instance she had an opportunity to find out a little more about the patient from his nurse so that her teaching could be more effective. She might have assessed the patient's readiness to learn by inquiring whether the patient had ever had similar tests, what his major concerns were about the procedure, what his knowledge about cardiac anatomy and physiology was likely to be, and what level of detail was likely to interest him. Such information would have vastly improved the nurse's ability to relate to Mr. Quinn and more fully meet his learning needs.

Many hospitals and other medical facilities employ nurse teachers, whose job it is to provide learning opportunities for patients, usually concerning specific subjects, such as home care or stoma care. Such nurse teachers are at a distinct disadvantage in their ability to relate to individual patients, since they are seldom able to get to know a patient before beginning to teach. In addition, many of the subjects that are taught by the special nurse teachers produce stress or carry high emotional impact for the patient. Before she initates teaching, a nurse in this kind of position must use whatever formal and informal channels are open to her to discover something of the patient's relevant previous experiences and present perceptions of need. She is also well advised to select interactive strategies for teaching that will help her build a trusting relationship with the patient and provide her with the feedback necessary to modify the content and direction of teaching to meet individual learning needs.

Limitations of Time and Environment

In Chapter 3 a number of aspects of environment, such as lack of privacy, distractions, and interruptions, were mentioned as being hindrances to patient-nurse communication. Keeping in mind that the goal of teaching is to help the patient learn, careful assessment of the learning environment must be made before teaching. If the environment cannot be freed of negative factors, then the teaching strategy may need to be altered to accommodate the situation. For example, if the patient cannot be moved from a noisy area that is also full of visual distractions, the nurse might pull the curtains, adjust the light, and provide written materials to the patient to supplement a brief explanation or discussion, or perhaps she could plan teaching for a less noisy time of day. As Cunningham and Baker (1986) point out, it is appropriate for the nurse to take control of the learning environment, trying to make it as conducive to effective learning as possible.

Likewise, time limits imposed by the situation can alter choice of teaching strategy. The nurse may have only a few minutes to help the patient prepare for a procedure that will begin immediately. The nurse herself may feel pressured by other demands and activities and not be able to sit down at the patient's bedside for prepared patient teaching, even though she recognizes the importance and need for this. Early identification of learning needs, as discussed in Chapter 4, will help to alleviate some time complications. By anticipating how much time will need to be spent helping a patient learn, the nurse is in a better position to plan her own time. In those situations where a time limit is imposed, a careful selection of teaching strategy may help. For example, a videotape of a self-care procedure may partially substitute for a personal explanation by the nurse. Discussion, role play, and other highly interactive methods predictably take longer initially, but the quality of learning may be such that time is actually saved later by using them (Bruner, 1961).

Because patient teaching often takes place in a stressful environment, a person's involvement through participation in discussion or other activities not only improves the quality of the learning, but also helps the person focus his attention on a future-oriented objective, and thereby may help to reduce his stress level.

The Sequence of Learning

A final, and important, consideration in selecting teaching strategies is the order, or sequence, of steps in the lesson being planned. Although the sequence may differ from time to time and from subject to subject, a typical pattern is shown in Table 5–1.

TABLE 5–1. Sequence of Steps in a Lesson

Beginning	1. Confirm knowledge base and motivation 2. Get learner's attention 3. Clarify objectives/present "organizer"
Middle	4. Present content of lesson and get feedback 5. Provide an example
End	6. Reinforce learning 7. Summarize and evaluate learning

A lesson may be only 5 minutes long or nearly an hour; it may be one of a series of lessons on a particular subject, or it may be a lesson planned as an isolated, individual response to a patient's question or concern. In each of these circumstances the pattern of beginning, middle, and end steps in the lesson will apply. The meshing of two gears illustrates this phenomenon: the gears are moved together and begin to engage their cogs; they are then able to run smoothly together. Finally, they disengage and move apart.

> The use of several teaching strategies as nurse and patient progress through a lesson sequence reinforces learning and keeps the interest of the learner.

Even short lessons may combine teaching strategies, such as explanation and discussion or demonstration and role play. Chapter 6 includes guidance on using teaching materials to vary lessons and reinforce learning.

Steps in a Lesson Sequence

Step 1: Confirm Knowledge Base and Motivation. This step may either precede the lesson or be part of the beginning phase. It is essential that the teacher know the learner's present knowledge level for a particular subject so that she knows how and where to start. Making assumptions about this without checking with the patient puts the nurse at risk of wasting time by trying to teach irrelevant material, thereby reducing the learner's motivation and interest. The nurse teacher's goals in confirming the learner's present knowledge and concerns are to link teaching to something already known and to guide the progression of the lesson. As discussed in Section 4.4, the nurse may simply ask the patient what he knows or what his experience has been, or she may give him a questionnaire or pretest. When complex concepts or skills are involved, the nurse may want to review previously learned material with the patient as part of this step before proceeding to new content.

Step 2: Get the Learner's Attention. Certain college lecturers have been known to go to the extremes of explosions and the staging of dramatic incidents to gain the attention of their students. Although these kinds of ploys will not be necessary for the nurse teacher, it is important that the full attention of both learner and teacher be focused on the subject at hand. This focusing may be accomplished by telling an appropriate story or anecdote, advising the patient ahead of time to anticipate a lesson on a particular subject, having the learner perform an activity related to the subject before the lesson begins, or arranging the environment so that he is aware that something requiring his attention is about to begin.

Step 3: Clarify Objectives/Present "Organizer." Of major importance at the beginning of a lesson is letting the learner know what he can expect. One of the best ways of doing this is to clarify what behavior is expected as a result of learning, i.e., the learning objectives. This may be done verbally through explanation or discussion, nonverbally through use of a written version of the objectives and perhaps content of the lesson, or through a combination of these approaches. The teacher may present the learning objective as she sees it and invite feedback from the learner, or teacher and learner may decide on specific objectives together.

An "organizer" is material that is relevant to the subject of the lesson; it provides the learner with a context within which to understand the new learning (Ausubel and Robinson, 1969, p. 145). Organizers are especially useful when the content of teaching is novel to the learner or when connections with past experiences are not clear. Teaching patients about clinical procedures is often in this category.

A statement of objectives can serve as an organizer, as can a lesson outline. For example, the listing of major points at the beginning of each chapter in this text is a form of organizer, as is Table 5–1 which summarizes the material covered subsequently in more detail. By using an organizer, the nurse can emphasize points of special importance while showing how other material relates to these points. The following case example demonstrates how and why an organizer might be used in patient teaching.

Example 5.2   USE OF AN ORGANIZER IN TEACHING

While in the hospital Mr. Quinn was started on atenolol, a beta-blocking agent. Because he would be continuing this medication at home, his nurse, Julie Johnson, planned a lesson devoted to helping him learn about the medication and how to take it. Mr. Quinn had never taken a beta blocker and, in fact, had not been on regular medication before this hospitalization. As Ms. Johnson prepared the lesson, she jotted down notes to herself about what she would like to include. Her list was as follows:

Take with meals.

Check pulse regularly.

May cause tiredness.

Must be taken regularly to prevent angina.

Nightmares and nausea sometimes are side effects.

Do not discontinue med suddenly.

On collecting these notes, the nurse decided that Mr. Quinn would probably not remember all these points, since this medication was different from any he had taken before. She constructed the following teaching aid to be used as a lesson organizer. Under each title she left space so that Mr. Quinn could write his own notes.

_____ is a medication you will be continuing to take at home.

This medication is a "beta blocker."

You should take this medication as follows:

Some effects that may be caused by the medication are:

You should notify your doctor if:

IT IS DANGEROUS TO STOP THIS MEDICATION SUDDENLY. BE SURE TO TAKE IT REGULARLY AS PRESCRIBED.

After introducing the subject generally to Mr. Quinn and his wife, Ms. Johnson handed each of them a copy of the teaching aid, explaining that it was an outline for what they would be discussing. She gave them time to read through it and made sure they had pencils so they could write their own notes on the sheet.

In this case example the nurse presented a written list of topics as an organizer. Another approach would have been to ask the Quinns what they wanted to know about the medication and start the lesson with these topics. Their limited experience, however, could have made it difficult for them to appreciate the complexity of the material they needed to learn for safety's sake. The organizer introduced the couple to the scope of the lesson and established the lesson's structure. The written outline had the added advantage of allowing the Quinns to participate in the lesson by writing notes as well as interacting verbally. By printing the caution on the sheet in large type, the nurse emphasized this point visually as well as verbally.

Step 4: Present Content and Get Feedback. This step is the lesson's "main course." The teaching strategies described later in this chapter relate specifically to the presentation of content and reception of feedback. This step is not complete unless it has both components—content and feedback.

Step 5: Provide an Example. In Section 3.4 Jung's theory of personality dimensions is presented, along with its implications for teaching. According to this theory most people learn specific material initially, generalizing it to concept level later. Examples and illustrations are therefore important adjuncts to teaching. Examples not only help the learner see how facts and ideas can be applied in a practical way, but also stimulate interest by helping the learner identify with the person in the case study or the problem solved in the example. This is why so many case examples and illustrations have been included in this text.

Step 6: Reinforce Learning. Just as it is important to follow through with a tennis or golf swing so that the ball gets to its destination, it is essential that the nurse follow through on teaching to ensure that the objective will be reached. Reinforcing learning is more than just repeating important points; it is helping the learner make the new knowledge, attitude, or skill his own. The best reinforcement is the practical application of the learned material to the learner's situation under the nurse's guidance. When skill learning is involved, this may mean a return demonstration by the patient. In the case of Mr. Quinn, had his wife not been present during the initial lesson, the patient might have "taught" the lesson to his wife under the supervision of the nurse as reinforcement of his new knowledge.

The reinforcement step gives the opportunity to not only repeat material, but also involve the learner emotionally—and perhaps physically—as well as intellectually with learning. In most cases the nurse will want to select a strategy for reinforcement that is different from that used for initial presentation of content. To the extent possible, she will want to involve the learner in an activity related to the material.

> Learning is aided by involving as many of the learner's senses as possible in the learning experience: sight, hearing, touch, smell, and taste.

For this reason, it was important to Mr. Quinn's learning that he not only hear the nurse describing his medication and how it should be taken, but also write down the information himself and see it on paper. Repeating the information in his own words would have reinforced this lesson.

Step 7: Summarize and Evaluate. In this final step in the lesson sequence both teacher and learner have the chance to look back over the lesson, summarize what was learned, and decide to what extent objectives were met. In briefly reviewing the content of the lesson, the major and most important points can again be emphasized. Evaluating the lesson may be as informal as a brief discussion with the learner about his progress, or as formal as a written evaluation stating planned objectives in full and asking the learner to identify specific ways in which they were met or not met.

Both teacher and learner are, of course, evaluating the learning situation throughout the lesson. In one-to-one teaching the nurse can receive constant feedback by carefully noting the learner's nonverbal behavior as well as his willingness to participate and respond verbally. This ongoing evaluation allows the nurse to alter the pace, strategy, or even content of a lesson to match the learner's needs. At the same time the learner continuously evaluates the credibility of the teacher and the usefulness of the material being presented. One of the advantages of developing a trusting relationship between teacher and learner before teaching begins is that, during the lesson, the learner spends less time evaluating the teacher and more time learning. In Chapter 9 the process of evaluation is considered in a broader and more formal sense.

In summary, in this section we have discussed some of the considerations that influence the nurse teacher's choice of teaching strategy. These include the nurse's own background knowledge of the subject to be taught, the nature of her relationship with the learner, the environment and time available for teaching, and the specific demands of each step in the lesson sequence. In individual teaching the nurse has the opportunity to use continuous feedback from the learner to adapt teaching to the learner's concerns, interests, and needs.

The remainder of this chapter focuses on a variety of teaching strategies and offers specific guidance for their use. Each section includes a definition of the strategy under discussion, some reasons for selecting the strategy, how to prepare for its use, some guidelines for the conduct of a lesson using the strategy, and some hints about how to handle a situation in which the strategy does not meet patient needs.

5.2 USING EXPLANATION OR LECTURE AS A TEACHING STRATEGY

The traditional and most common method of instruction is for the teacher, the expert, to "tell" the student what she thinks he needs to know. Most of us have recollections from our school days of ineffective lectures: boring hours in a classroom during which the instructor droned on in a monotone or, worse yet, read from a text while students tried to figure out what might appear on the inevitable test. As Gayles (1966) so succinctly put it: "The lecture at its worst consists of transferring the notes of the teacher to the notebooks of the students without passing through the minds of either."

The term *explanation* is generally used when describing the strategy of "telling" only one or two individuals; *lecture* implies that a larger group of learners are present. In either case, verbal messages are transmitted in only one direction: from teacher to learner.

Advantages of Explanation

The major advantage of this teaching strategy is that it is an efficient way to transfer information to the learner. Because the teacher is in control, facts can be carefully organized and presented with attention to emphasis and important detail. Most older learners *expect* that teaching will be done using a strategy of explanation. Meeting this expectation establishes the credibility of a younger nurse teacher as an expert.

Explanation is a useful method of introducing a lesson and may be used for the clarification and organization step of the lesson sequence. It is otherwise limited to helping with the learning of *knowledge*, rather than with the learning of attitudes or skills. Health educators often make the mistake of thinking that the learner's attitudes will be greatly influenced by an explanation of ideas and facts without further reinforcement or experience, or that skills can be developed through simple explanation of their principles.

> Explanation is effective as a patient teaching strategy only when it is used in combination with other, more learner-participative strategies such as discussion.

Preparing for an Explanation

Every teacher expects to prepare for a formal lecture or speech by organizing material, making notes to ensure a logical progression of ideas, and perhaps preparing handouts or written outlines for students to follow. When the strategy of telling is used with an individual learner, the presentation is seldom lengthy but preparation is just as important to its success. For example, Ms. Johnson in Example 5.2 carefully prepared the explanation she gave Mr. Quinn about his medication. At the very least, preparation for an explanation should include the basic organization of material and notes as to important points to be emphasized.

In some cases it will be necessary for the nurse to prepare for an explanation by delaying it. This is preferable to risking the pitfalls of an incomplete, unorganized, off-the-top-of-the-head explanation that is isolated from other prepared teaching. It may be better to acknowledge that the subject is a valid concern and return to it later, when the nurse is prepared and organized to teach and the learner is expecting to learn.

There are three general situations in which explanation is useful as a teaching strategy. Each of these require special attention to an aspect of preparation.

1. When an explanation is given because of an *anticipated patient need*, the nurse must be sure to link the explanation to something that is already known to the patient. For example, anticipating the patient's need to know about the cardiac catheterization procedure, the nurse might start her explanation by linking it to other kinds of diagnostic tests already completed.

2. When an explanation is given in response to a *known patient need*, the nurse must be sure to include how the information can be used by the patient to meet that need. For example, if Mr. Quinn had been apprehensive about going home, fearing the possibility of another angina attack, his nurse might have begun her explanation about his medication by pointing out that this information would enable him to correctly take medication that would make another attack much less likely. With a little planning the nurse can, in this way, make use of existing patient motivation to promote learning.

3. When an explanation is given in response to a *patient's question*, it is wise to first find out what kind of need triggered the question. Because it is socially acceptable to ask factual questions, people sometimes disguise an emotional need in this way. There are few situations in which an explanation cannot be delayed at least long enough to clarify its intent by asking, "What is it that is concerning you?" and paying close attention to the patient's nonverbal communication. The patient may in fact not want information, but rather reassurance, a kind touch, or a chance to describe his feelings to a concerned listener.

Guidelines for Using Explanation

In using an explanation strategy to help others learn, some points should be kept in mind.

• Advice and threats are ineffective and send to the listener the message that the teacher is interested only in her own powerful position as an expert. If the teacher needs to encourage or discourage a particular behavior, the "who, what, when, why, and how" (4W-H) of that behavior should be included in the explanation so that the learner is helped to understand why the teacher is making this point.

- The use of humor, stories, anecdotes, and examples helps to enliven an explanation, allows the listener time to mentally sort through the points being made, and involves the listener emotionally as well as intellectually. The nurse must take some care in using such material, however, because unless it is well planned to supplement the lesson, it is simply a distraction.

- When an explanation includes instruction on patient responsibility that will be taken outside the clinical setting, it is wise to include a family member in the session. This reduces the possibility of error in the recollection of important details, such as what to do if medication side effects are experienced. If there is a discrepancy in recall between the two persons present at an explanation, it is likely that they will consult a caregiver for clarification rather than proceed with an erroneous assumption.

- In order for learning to result from an explanation, teacher and listener must use the same language. Although superficially this point seems self-evident, in practice, language is a real concern. The more obvious version of this problem occurs when teacher and learner are from different cultures. A person may understand elementary English and yet be unable to translate a lengthy or rapidly spoken explanation by the nurse into anything understandable. In working with many people of non-English-speaking background, I have found that a useful tactic is to interact with the person in conversation or discussion before attempting to teach. This helps to establish rapport, clarifies the nurse's intentions, helps the person become accustomed to the nurse's voice, and alerts the nurse to cultural differences that will pose problems of meaning. (See Section 2.4 for a discussion of the many ways in which a person's social and cultural group influence learning.)

- A subtler version of the language problem occurs when the nurse inadvertently uses in her explanation medical terminology that is unknown to the patient. Although television has certainly contributed to some terms, such as "malignancy" and "cholesterol," being widely recognized as familiar, the nurse should not take for granted that such terms and their implications are understood by patients in the same way that she understands them. Nor should the nurse expect that a patient receiving an explanation will be brave enough to stop the nurse and ask for clarification. Stephany (1986) tells of a patient who became hysterical when an explanation about the presence of a hydatidiform mole aroused fears of a brown, furry animal growing inside her. This kind of problem is compounded when the nurse and the patient are not from the same socioeconomic background. In effect, this kind of discrepancy poses the same problems as differences in culture in terms of word knowledge and usage.

- As mentioned previously, the major disadvantage to the explanation strategy is that the teacher has no automatic way of knowing whether the listener is also becoming a learner. This means that the nurse must periodically stop speaking and reverse the flow of communication to get feedback. The most frequently used, but largely ineffective, questions for this purpose are "Do you have any questions?" and "Do you understand?" Because these are often asked abruptly, the listener is taken by surprise by the change of roles and seldom can do more than respond no and yes, respectively. A more effective way of obtaining feedback is to shift to discussion about a particular point. For example: "I've told you that you will need to take this medication three times a day. How do you see that fitting in with your schedule?" Here the nurse gives the patient a specific topic on which to focus and then asks an open question. His response will give her information about his level of understanding.

Another way of checking out the listener's learning is to pose a problem to which the new information can be applied, such as: "Suppose you forgot your noon pill and only discover it at 3 P.M. What would you do?" The nurse might also introduce an activity, such as a worksheet, a game, or a role play, that would use the information covered in the explanation.

- As a general rule, the fewer the number of learners participating in the lesson, the shorter an uninterrupted explanation should be. For example, 5 minutes without verbal feedback for a single learner is maximum. Beyond this time, information is poorly assimilated, if indeed it is heard at all.

What If . . . ?

Most teachers, especially those who are relatively inexperienced, have fantasies about all the things that can go wrong during a lesson. The explanation strategy is usually not chosen unless there is important information that needs to be communicated to the patient in a time-efficient way. The worst that can happen, therefore, is that nothing happens; the listener does not understand, remember, or use the information offered. In the following case example the nurse was confronted by such a fear.

Example 5.3   AN UNCOMMUNICATIVE LEARNER

Pam Kepler, a public health nurse, had been referred to Terry Reynolds, a 16-year-old now in her eighth month of pregnancy, for prenatal teaching. Ms. Kepler had visited Terry several times to try to find out what she knew and needed to learn about pregnancy, delivery, and child care.

So far, the nurse had been unsuccessful in having any kind of conversation with Terry, whose demeanor was pleasant but passive. No matter how she phrased her questions, Terry's answer was always one or two words or a shrug. Not knowing quite how to handle such an unresponsive learner, and having no clues about Terry's knowledge background, Ms. Kepler decided to launch a formal teaching approach based on her previous experience with pregnant teenagers. She told Terry that on her next visit, she would bring some pictures of what the baby looked like at various stages of development and discuss with her what would happen when she went into labor.

Several days later, armed with a birth atlas, the nurse settled down on the couch with Terry. She hoped that Terry would be sufficiently interested that she would participate, but her real expectation was that she would have to give a lecture. Once again Terry was silent for most of the lesson, but seemed nonverbally more involved than previously, looking at the pictures with apparent interest. The nurse kept her explanations brief and repeatedly invited discussion, but got little verbal response. She even attempted a form of confrontation by saying: "It's hard for me to know whether these things are interesting to you and are things you want to know when there's no feedback." Terry's response was to frown and shrug.

Feeling frustrated about the session, the nurse packed up her books to leave. As she stepped out the door, Terry said, "Thank you, I learned a lot."

Although such a situation is, fortunately, uncommon, teachers frequently suffer the frustration of wondering whether learning has actually taken place. Terry's passivity may have been the result of her view of the nurse as being relatively powerful, older than Terry, and an expert. These perceptions carried with them an injunction to "be quiet and listen." In the circumstances Ms. Kepler probably did the best she could by first trying to find out what was of interest and concern to Terry and then sharing lesson objectives with her, stopping repeatedly to attempt discussion, using visual support for her explanation, and being overt about how Terry's behavior made her feel. She could have just given up, but as it turned out, she did make a contribution to Terry's knowledge. Faced with an unresponsive listener, the teacher can but do the kinds of things Ms. Kepler tried. Sometimes the introduction of a second learner can be helpful for modeling more interactive responses for the quiet participant.

In summary, the teaching strategy of explanation or lecture has been explained in this section. Its usefulness for communicating information has been emphasized and its major disadvantage, that communication is limited to one way, has been discussed. Some authors list "lecture-discussion" as a separate teaching strategy. This is usually defined as short periods of explanation followed by discussion of the points made.

> Whether the strategy is called lecture, explanation, or lecture-discussion, only short intervals of one-way communication flowing from teacher to learner are appropriate when teaching involves only one or two students.

5.3 USING DISCUSSION AS A TEACHING STRATEGY

A discussion can be defined as a verbal exchange between two or more persons. Discussions, even those that occur in a social context, allow those involved to share knowledge, attitudes, and opinions, and therefore contribute to learning. Unlike the explanation, a discussion is two-way communication between participants of equal "power," with no one having "all the answers."

The discussion strategy is used in two basic ways: either as an adjunct to an explanation strategy, with the intent of helping learners individualize information and apply it to their own needs, or as a method of learning by itself. When people are able to hear themselves working through a problem, receiving feedback and contributions of information from other people, they generally learn at a level of complexity not possible from explanations or lectures.

The discussion strategy is based on the belief that the people involved in the interaction have within them all of the pieces of knowledge, attitudes, and skills that will be necessary to "discover" the solution to a problem or meet a need. The discovery is made through sharing of individual resources, and, because interaction often inspires creative thinking, the resulting solution often surpasses that which an individual might find alone. In Chapter 8 the use of group process in nurse-patient teaching is explored in detail.

The oral "quizzes" given learners at the end of an explanation are not discussions; they are "return" explanations. Asking the patient to repeat what he thinks were the major points of the nurse's explanation, or having him summarize what he learned, results in one-way communication from learner to teacher. This may be useful feedback, but it is not a discussion.

Advantages of a Discussion Strategy

The advantages of discussion have to do with the fact that a two-way exchange makes it possible to use information in small pieces, making sense of each and applying it to one's own situation as one sees it. If explanation is like being presented with a whole meal, discussion is like being handed small bites when one is ready to eat and digest them. Because the learner is involved in progressively acquiring and using increasingly complex information, the result is greater depth of understanding than can be expected of explanation methods. Discussion is especially appropriate when patient objectives require learning at one of the more complex levels, such as analysis (for knowledge) or verbalization (for attitudes). Because of the involvement implicit in discussion, it is an ideal method for stimulating attitude examination and change.

An additional advantage of a discussion strategy is that the nurse need not be an expert in anticipating the best solutions to particular patient problems. Instead, she contributes her knowledge and support while the patient works on the problem himself. The nurse may *lead* a discussion, but she does not dominate it. She expends her effort in listening to and interacting with the patient rather than in talking to him. To this extent, discussion makes serious demands on the communication skills of the nurse and requires her to be patient with the learner's own pace.

Preparing for a Discussion

Although discussion is a much less formal teaching strategy than explanation, preparation is just as important for its success. Particular attention must be given to the clear definition of learning objectives, to the questions that will be used to initiate a discussion and guide it toward the objectives, and to the environment in which discussion takes place.

Clear patient learning objectives are especially important to a discussion strategy because they provide not only a goal but also guidance for helping the patient through increasing levels of learning complexity. For example, an objective that states "by (date) the patient *verbalize* at least three ways in which he will reduce stress in his life" suggests that he must first become *aware* of stress and its affect on him and he then must *respond* to this awareness by identifying ways in which he can actively take control of his stress level. (See Table 4–5 for a listing of levels of learning complexity.) Clearly defining objectives before a discussion begins also prevents the discussion from being sidetracked into other issues or dissolving into social conversation, the two principal dangers of discussion methods.

Discussions are usually initiated by a question, or a statement of a problem. The kinds of broad, open questions discussed in Section 4.2 as being appropriate for the "top" of a CONE interview are also suitable for launching a discussion. Such questions should be framed before a discussion begins so that they reflect, as nearly as possible, the objective to be met.

> The major difference between an interview and a discussion is that the purpose of an interview is to help the nurse learn about the patient, whereas the purpose of a discussion is to help the patient learn about himself.

Through use of the relationship skills described in Chapter 3, the nurse forms a partnership with the patient, encouraging him to talk about feelings as well as facts and guiding him to discover solutions to the problems he faces.

An attitude of equality is vital to an effective discussion strategy. The environment is an important factor in reinforcing that attitude. Discussion participants should be at or near the same physical level. The nurse should be sitting—a signal that she will not be acting as expert or judge during the exchange. Because learning through discussion often takes longer than an explanation strategy, reflecting the more complex learning that is taking place, it is important that the nurse plan some protection against distractions and interruptions. Many modern hospital units now have staff-patient conference rooms available for this purpose.

Guidelines for Using Discussion

In using discussion as a strategy for helping others learn, some points should be kept in mind.

- The goal of discussion is to help the learner reach his own conclusions and discover his own solutions to his problems. These conclusions and solutions may be vastly different from those that the nurse might choose for herself. The nurse's role in a discussion is to guide, facilitate, and contribute useful information, not to advise, dictate, or demand. Until they gain a fair amount of experience, most discussion leaders find themselves getting impatient with apparently slow progress or becoming fearful that the learner will not choose to do what is "right." The nurse must avoid offering her own opinions or launching an explanation in an effort to direct the patient's thinking. When the nurse does gain experience with discussion, she will have learned to trust the process of patient self-responsibility.

• One way to avoid the temptation to take control of a discussion and give advice inappropriately is to start a discussion with a question to which the nurse does not have an answer. Although this approach might seem risky to a strongly closure nurse, it is one way of ensuring that she begins a discussion with the intent to work *with* the patient as an equal.

• Learning that involves putting facts together with feelings generally takes some time and is not necessarily a totally verbal process. People need "thinking time" to consult their emotions or phrase their thoughts before they are able to articulate them. Discussions frequently contain relatively long silences. The nurse must control her impatience and allow these to occur without breaking in or permitting her own thoughts to wander too far afield.

What If . . . ?

The fantasies usually related to a discussion strategy involve having the discussion get out of control or take too long. The real advantage of a discussion is that the nurse has a partner in it. When a discussion seems not to be going anywhere or gets off the track, she can consult with her patient-partner to determine what is happening and how it can be fixed. Some examples of statements that might be used to confront such difficulties are:

— "We seem to have drifted away from the subject we started with. I'd like to go back to talking about . . . "

— "It seems to be difficult for you to talk about . . . . Can you tell me how you're feeling?"

— "I'm not sure just how far we've gotten toward our goal. Maybe we ought to stop and summarize."

Such statements are evaluative; they are expressed from the point of view of one of the discussion participants, inviting a similar evaluation by the learner. Clearly they can be made only if a goal or objective has been previously stated and agreed on.

Another fear commonly associated with the discussion strategy is that the patient, invited to share his feelings, will express anger or begin to cry. Many caregivers find it difficult to deal with these emotions. It is generally helpful for the nurse to "listen through" such an expression of emotion. She must avoid trying to talk the person out of feeling that way or offering platitudes such as, "I'm sure things will be better soon." Because strong emotions sometimes get in the way of confronting issues and discovering solutions that are important to the patient, their expression can be a positive step in the learning process. By staying with the learner through the feelings, this kind of barrier can be overcome.

In summary, discussion as a strategy for teaching has been described in this section. Its success depends on the communication skills of the nurse and the willingness of the patient to work toward an objective. This strategy is especially suited to helping with attitude change and complex levels of knowledge.

> In using a discussion strategy the nurse is a facilitator rather than an expert; she works *with* the learner in reaching objectives and solving problems.

5.4 USING DEMONSTRATION-COACHING AS A TEACHING STRATEGY

Demonstration-coaching is a multiple-step strategy used to teach a desirable behavior involving motor skills. It is based on the educational principle of modeling or imitation (see Section 2.1). Initially, the demonstration-coaching strategy uses one-way communication from teacher to learner, but as learning progresses, the learner is more involved, both verbally and physically. The nurse teacher's major use of the demonstration-coaching strategy is to help patients and family members learn care procedures. Modeling in other forms may also be used to teach interpersonal skills; the use of role play and behavior rehearsal are discussed in the next section.

Demonstration-coaching requires sequential steps in learning, progressing through a number of skill levels. The learning sequence allows the learner to develop increasing familiarity with the procedure and improved motor skills. Teaching within several of the following levels of demonstration and coaching are chosen to reflect the present knowledge and skills of the learner, the complexity of the procedure being learned, and the learning objectives.

Level 1. The nurse explains the procedure and then demonstrates it completely as an introduction to or overview of what is to be learned.

Level 2. The nurse slowly demonstrates each part of the skill to be learned, describing each and pointing out *why* it is done that way, *what* is being done, and *when* that part is to be done in relation to other parts of the procedure.

Level 3. The nurse performs the procedure while the learner describes each part and "coaches" the nurse on what to do next.

Level 4. The learner handles the equipment, tries out the parts of the procedure that require development of new skills, and practices these under the nurse's guidance.

Level 5. The learner slowly performs each part of the procedure under nurse's guidance and coaching.

Level 6. The learner performs the complete procedure, explaining what he is doing and why.

Level 7. The learner demonstrates what to do if something goes wrong during procedure, while the nurse coaches.

Keeping in mind a desirable sequence of learning events, several of these variations are chosen to correspond to organizing, presenting, and reinforcing the skill to be learned.

> Reinforcement through practice is the most important aspect of learning a motor skill.

One of the levels, or a variation of it, may need to be repeated many times in order for the learner to develop the skill at a "performance" or "adaptation" level of learning complexity.

Advantages of Demonstration-Coaching

The clear advantage of the demonstration-coaching strategy is that it helps patients learn concrete, practical skills that lead to self-responsibility and a sense of control over their situations. When learning involves motor skills, knowledge about what has to be done, or even an attitude of willingness to carry out a procedure, is not enough. Learners must have the opportunity to manipulate equipment and develop motor skills to the level at which they can perform a procedure competently without coaching. The demonstration-coaching strategy is especially useful for patients who need to learn self-care procedures, such as injecting insulin, walking with crutches, using a hemodialysis machine, or bandaging an injury. This strategy may be used to demonstrate the multiple skills of a complex procedure or the simple application of familiar equipment.

Preparing for Demonstration and Coaching

As with other teaching strategies, the clear definition of patient learning objectives is the first step in preparing to use demonstration-coaching. In this case, however, thorough analysis of the behavior that will be the result of learning is essential. The various parameters of the analysis can be explored through use of the following questions:

- Can this task or procedure be logically divided into several components to make learning easier?
- Is there only one right way to perform this task? If so, what are the rules of performance, what standards are used to measure success, and what must be emphasized in teaching?
- If there is more than one acceptable way to complete the task, is the person to learn several alternatives or should he be able to modify a model procedure to fit his preferences and needs?
- What knowledge, attitudes, and skills does the learner already have that might be applied to this task?

After thoroughly analyzing the task or behavior to be learned, the nurse can turn her attention to two other aspects of preparing for a demonstration. One is to plan enough *time for practice*. The more complex the learning, the more variable the procedure, and the less the learner already knows that can be applied to the task, the longer will be the time needed for practice.

Another important aspect of preparation is *checking out the equipment* to be used, the environment in which the demonstration is to be given, and the skills of the demonstrator. The assembly of needed equipment is necessary before a demonstration begins. Surprisingly often, teachers are in a hurry and fail to check the equipment before they begin. Equipment failures are at least embarrassing, are potentially dangerous in some cases, are certainly a waste of time, and fail to instill confidence in the would-be learner.

Likewise, a failure of the nurse teacher's own skills are upsetting to all concerned. The nurse preparing a demonstration must be able not only to perform the task or procedure, but to do so with a *minimum of concentration*. During the demonstration she will be busy explaining the steps and paying attention to the learner and not be able to fully concentrate on what she is doing. Finally, in order for a demonstration to be successful, it must, as nearly as possible, approximate reality and the learner must be able to see and hear it adequately, ideally from the same perspective he will have when he performs the task. For example, he may need to watch the demonstration from over the nurse's shoulder as she manipulates the equipment.

In helping others learn new skills, thorough preparation and sufficient time for practice are essential.

Guidelines for Using Demonstration-Coaching

In using a demonstration-coaching strategy to help others develop skills, some points should be kept in mind.

- The demonstration is only the first step in helping a person master a skill. Effective coaching demands that the nurse help the person, first, overcome any barriers to learning, such as fear, embarrassment, or anxiety, and, second, take increasing responsibility for carrying out the procedure himself. These goals can be accomplished through a combination of organization, encouragement, verbal reinforcement and praise, gentle guidance, and patience. As any parent can attest, sometimes it is difficult, yet necessary, to stand by and watch the first fumbling attempts to do a new task. In a clinical setting the environment, medications, and emotional content of the situation all erode mental concentration and manual dexterity, necessitating more time for learning. The investment in the patient's future well-being and independence is, however, well worth the effort.

- It is important that the nurse clearly identify the criteria for success in performing a task or procedure and share these with the learner during the demonstration. In this way the learner will be able to help evaluate both his progress and his failures, relieving the nurse of the need to criticize. For example, a patient learning to apply a sterile dressing needs to know, before attempting the procedure himself, what contamination is, how it occurs, and how it should be avoided. During practice he then can say, "Oops, I touched it," rather than having to wait for the nurse to say, "No, no, don't do it that way!"

- Most procedures that the patient or a family member will carry out at home will benefit from including practice in how to recover from an error. The time spent in rehearsing the "what would you do if..." scenarios will save anxiety, frustration, and perhaps urgent telephone calls later.

- Remember that it takes time to acquire speed in doing a task. When speed or complex set-up procedures are required, it may be possible for the patient to practice on his own once he has mastered basic competence, with the nurse consulting from time to time.
- As with the explanation strategy, it is advisable to include another person in addition to the patient in demonstration-coaching sessions. The other person need not learn the skills to the same degree as the patient, but he or she does need to be able to evaluate performance and reinforce success. Once the patient is at home, the person can then take the role of coach.

What If . . . ?

Most of the concerns of nurse teachers in relation to this strategy have to do with the demonstration going wrong. Such a fear is usually fueled by vivid memories of a demonstration mishap during nursing education. I clearly recall one incident in which the instructor, who was demonstrating intramuscular injection technique, hit her finger instead of the student-patient. One would like for the learner to remember the demonstration, but it is not necessary for it to be that memorable!

The best insurance against the demonstration going wrong is to practice and carefully examine the equipment before beginning. Other than that, a sense of humor will make it possible to salvage some perspective even from a misfired demonstration.

Another area of valid concern for the nurse is "What if the patient won't, or can't, cope with the procedure?" Some patients who are faced with the reality of handling the colostomy irrigation equipment or the insulin syringe cannot bring themselves to proceed. This kind of barrier to learning can be dealt with more successfully by changing to a counseling intervention, in which the person is encouraged to talk about the disabling feelings, than by persistent urging to continue the procedure. To feel as though he has failed both himself and the nurse is not helpful to the patient's acceptance of his physical condition.

In some instances the nurse may find that the patient is much more awkward than she anticipated. Again, rather than proceeding, it is useful to stop and discuss how the procedure can be made easier for the learner. Sometimes innovative modifications can be developed together.

In summary, in this section the demonstration-coaching strategy has been described. Emphasis has been placed on preparation and on providing adequate opportunity for the learner to develop skills through practice. This strategy uses the learning principle of modeling or imitation to help people learn motor skills. Chapter 6 includes notes on using films or television programs as adjuncts to live demonstrations.

5.5 USING EXPERIENTIAL STRATEGIES: ROLE PLAY, BEHAVIOR REHEARSAL, AND EXERCISES

The experiential strategies are similar to demonstration-coaching in that they provide an opportunity to the learner to experience a situation as nearly like reality as possible and practice his behavioral responses. Whereas the demonstration-coaching strategy focuses on the learning of motor skills, the experiential strategies discussed here focus on the learning of interpersonal skills. Because behavior toward other people engenders feelings, attitudes, and values, the experiential strategies are ways of clarifying, illuminating, and practicing the emotional components of behavior as well as the behavior itself.

Some authors have used other schemes for categorizing teaching strategies. Redman (1984), for example, includes the teaching of intellectual skills and attitudes, as well as motor skills, under "Demonstration and Practice" but places role play in a separate section. I have chosen to separate motor and interpersonal skills learning because the manipulation of equipment and the teaching of procedures present a much different challenge to the nurse teacher than does the guidance and interpretation of interpersonal behaviors.

Each experiential strategy presents a situation, problem, or decision-making opportunity to the learner that may be a simulation of reality or an extension into the future of the present situation. The strategies are often initiated with words like "Let's pretend that . . ." or "Suppose . . . ." They are effective in both one-to-one teaching and group teaching.

Advantages of the Experiential Strategies

Throughout these pages the role of experience in learning has been emphasized. A person's experiences in the past form the basis for present learning (see Section 2.2). The experiential strategies provide controlled experiences in a supportive atmosphere. In this way the learner does not have to wait for a "real" situation in which he can try out a behavior and experience the consequences of it. Instead, he can practice, explore alternative behaviors, and see consequences in anticipation of reality.

> Planned experiences that anticipate reality allow the learner to develop mental connections between principles, concepts, or theories and actual behavior. They stimulate complex, multidimensional learning in which knowledge, attitudes, and skills come together.

Because the experiential strategies anticipate real situations, they are emotionally, as well as intellectually, involving. Although this combination may stimulate complex learning in a powerful way, the learning experience may be emotionally unsettling. Care must be taken to make the experiential strategies "safe" for the learner; he must feel that the risks he takes by acting out the future in the present will contribute positively to his ability to cope with reality and that he will be protected from serious negative consequences while he is taking these risks. A trusting and supportive relationship with the nurse is essential to this "safety" requirement.

Preparing to Use the Experiential Strategies

As with the demonstration-coaching strategy, the majority of learning takes place after the initial role play, rehearsal, or game. It is not the experience itself which teaches, but the meaning that is later attached to the experience in discussion and introspection. For this reason the nurse teacher needs to have developed skills in leading discussion, attentive listening, and sensitive exploration of the feelings of others in preparation for using experiential strategies.

The first specific step in preparation for using role play, behavior rehearsal, or experiential exercises is to identify an appropriate situation in which they can facilitate learning. The psychosocial and medical realities faced by the patient must be taken into account. Generally, the experiential strategies might be considered when the learner expresses anxiety about anticipated interactions with other people, when it seems to the nurse that the learner is compartmentalizing knowledge and feelings, or when, in the nurse's estimation, the learner has an unrealistic view of the consequences of planned future behavior and its impact on other people. The following patient statements are examples of these three conditions that might lead to the nurse's choice of experiential strategies for further learning.

Example 5.4   STATEMENTS SUGGESTING EXPERIENTIAL STRATEGIES

- "My wife is just going have to stop this emotional nonsense. So what if they found a growth in my colon. Lots of people have had that sort of thing."
- "I'm so worried about how I'm going to handle the questions that I know the women in my church group will ask me about my condition."
- "I'm planning to go back to work next week [despite a cast that confines him to a wheelchair]. I'll get Fred to pick me up in the morning and then Janet can take me to physiotherapy at noon, and George can drop me home in the evening."

For the nurse, in addition to identifying appropriate situations for the use of experiential strategies and being secure in her own interactional skills, the major factor in planning is time. Using any of these strategies requires time to carry it out and at least double that amount of time afterward to help the person make sense of the experience and learn from it.

Unless there is adequate time to follow experiential learning with thorough discussion, these strategies should not be attempted.

To some extent, experiential strategies are difficult to plan in detail. Because they are interactive, the nurse has only a general idea of what will happen and what will be learned from the experience. The challenge of using these powerful tools for learning is that the self-awareness, sensitivity, and communication skills of the nurse literally create a learning opportunity out of present events. Thus, the learning experience has an immediacy and relevance that not many other teaching strategies can duplicate.

Guidelines for the use of role play, behavior rehearsal, and experiential exercises will be discussed separately.

Guidelines for Using Role Play

In role play a "part" is assigned to the learner, but it is not rehearsed. The players do not play themselves as they do in behavior rehearsal, but someone else with whom they are familiar or about whom they are given information. In one-to-one teaching the nurse teacher will also be taking a role and interacting as a participant as well as the leader of the learning experience. Some points to keep in mind when using role play are as follows:

- Make clear at the outset what role is being played by each participant. Allow some time to adjust to the idea; it takes most people a few minutes to "get into" a role.
- Allow the interaction within the role play to go on long enough for there to have been significant communication between "characters" but not so long that communication reaches an impasse or gets bogged down. When used in an individual teaching context, 2 or 3 minutes is usually adequate to expose enough material to facilitate learning.
- Expect to spend a few minutes as participants "de-role" talking about how they felt while playing the character. During this phase the nurse should continue to refer to the person by his role name. For example, the nurse might say to Mr. Smith, "Alice, how did you feel when you were talking about what's worrying you?" The nurse should then make clear the distinction between the role and reality by saying, "And Mr. Smith, how did you feel about playing Alice?"
- Feelings and their relationship to facts are the content of role play. Learning takes place when the person is able to bridge the gap between them and feel the support of the nurse's acceptance, attention, and trust.

In the following case we will see what happened when the patient who made the first statement in Example 5–4 was encouraged to role play.

Example 5.5   APPRECIATING ANOTHER'S FEELINGS

Mr. Smith had commented to the nurse that his wife's emotional response to his diagnosis of a mass in the colon was "nonsense."

Nurse: Let's try out something. Suppose you pretend that you're Alice, your wife. I'll pretend I'm you and we'll see what happens when I tell you that you shouldn't be so upset.

Patient: Hmm. Well, okay, I guess we can do that.

Nurse: All right, now you're Alice. How do you feel Alice?

Patient: Well, I don't know. Let's see . . . I feel worried about my husband, like maybe he won't be able to go back to work or maybe he'll have to have more surgery.

Nurse: (Seeing that Mr. Smith is getting into the role) Okay, and I'm Clarence. I feel pretty annoyed that my wife is so upset. Let's try it. I'll start: Look, Alice, I can't understand why you're so upset about this situation.

Patient: Well, you know, I'm worried about what's going to happen in the future . . .

Nurse: I'm not sure what you mean, Alice.

Patient: Well, I mean . . . what if you can't go back to work? What about the house payments?

Nurse: Are you mostly worried about finances?

PATIENT: Well, not only that . . .

The patient, playing the role of his wife, Alice, now begins to think about how she feels. His speech slows down and the nurse models good listening behavior, helping him to clarify these feelings as he names them. In another few minutes he has talked about Alice's worries concerning her ability to care for him, her fear about his continued disability, and her anxiety about the tumor "coming back."

NURSE: (At a convenient pause the nurse breaks in.) Okay, let's stop there. (She then proceeds to the de-roling, as described earlier.)

The patient talked through his feelings as he played the role of his wife with new awareness of what she is experiencing. He still thinks that her fears are unfounded, but now he is less likely to dismiss them. He has learned to be aware of Alice's feelings, he has had the opportunity to get his own feelings together with the facts of his situation, and he has learned, through the model presented by the nurse, how to have a positive and supportive discussion with his wife about her concerns.

One aspect of experiential strategies in general, and of role play in particular, is that they often lead to long-term learning as well as immediate progress. Because the "pretend" experience above, for example, was an emotional one, it has the potential to color in a positive way the interaction between Mr. Smith and his wife for some time to come.

Guidelines for Using Behavior Rehearsal

Behavior rehearsal is much like role play except that the learner plays himself in an altered situation. The scenarios for behavior rehearsal are often worst-case circumstances; acting these out relieves some of the anticipated anxiety. The patient who made the second statement in Example 5.4—the woman who was concerned about handling the questions she would be asked by her friends—is a good candidate for behavior rehearsal. The nurse would first have asked the patient to explain what kinds of questions she anticipated with anxiety. The nurse would then play the role of a friend asking questions, while the patient would try out some responses. After each trial the patient would be helped to discuss how she felt about that version and why and the nurse would contribute how she, as the friend, reacted. Some points to keep in mind when using behavior rehearsal are as follows.

- Unlike role play, which loses some of its impact if not initiated right away, when the opportunity presents, behavior rehearsal can be returned to later. The decision to use this teaching strategy might be made after several widely separated clues have been given by the patient about a particular anxiety. The nurse in our example might say in introduction: "You've said a couple of times now that you're feeling anxious about confronting the women in your church group. I wonder if it would help if we tried out some of the conversations you anticipate."

- Be sure that there is a clear beginning and end for the rehearsal segment. The nurse can offer to start the interaction and should declare a stop after a short interval: "Let's stop there." The discussion that follows is the most important part of behavior rehearsal.

- There are three parallel learning dimensions of behavior rehearsal, any of which may be talked about during the discussion. One is the communication skills that the learner is developing by trying out ways of interacting. A second dimension is the insight into the consequences of the learner's behavior that is developing. Concurrent with these two important dimensions of behavior rehearsal is an increased awareness of one's own and other people's feelings.

It is usually relatively easy for the nurse to identify situations in which behavior rehearsal might be an effective teaching strategy, since there is less time pressure to act on her awareness. Because behavior rehearsal requires skills that are similar to those needed for role play, the nurse teacher is encouraged to practice using behavior rehearsal and become comfortable with it before attempting role play.

Guidelines for Using Experiential Exercises

Experiential exercises may be as simple as a suggested activity, as elaborate as a carefully planned "game" that is symbolic of a real situation, or anything between these extremes. The exercises described at the end of each chapter of this book are examples of activities designed to give the reader experience with some aspect of patient teaching. In patient care situations the nurse teacher might make use of already prepared exercises, such as crossword puzzles or video games, or she might design her own simple exercises to meet the patient's learning need.

Some guidelines to keep in mind when using experiential exercises are as follows:

- The nurse should be straightforward about her objectives in presenting an exercise. If she has hidden motivations for doing so, the patient can feel like a victim rather than a learner.
- Once again, the discussion that follows an activity is more important than the activity itself.
- As with behavior rehearsal, experiential exercises allow a person to try out ways of doing things and permit him to gain some insight into the consequences of his behavior.

While working on a rehabilitation unit, a nurse devised a game she called "Murphy's Time Machine." To a piece of cardboard she had affixed a spinning dial (a tongue depressor with a large straight pin through the center). When a patient started making plans to go home, the nurse would give him a piece of paper on which had been drawn a large circle divided into 24 segments. Each segment represented an hour of a "typical" day after the patient went home. The patient was to fill in what he expected to happen during that hour on such a typical day. When it was completed the paper was taped to the cardboard and the dial positioned in its center. The game consisted of the patient spinning the dial and the nurse making up a "what if" scenario related to the activity shown. The patient's part was to think up how he might handle such an event. Sometimes the nurse would follow his response with "How does that make you feel?"

The patient described in Example 5.4 who had made detailed plans for how he was going to return to work with the help of several friends would have been a prime candidate for "Murphy's Time Machine." He might have been asked, "What if Janet calls at 11:30 and says she can't take you to physio today?" or "The dog gets out while Fred is helping you out to his car and you're already late for work. What do you do?" or, when the pointer lands at 2 P.M., "You're so tired this afternoon and your leg hurts and you figure you are just going to have to go home. How do you get there?"

The point of the game is to inspire the patient to plan realistically for his discharge from the unit. But since it is a game and is presented with good humor, it's also fun. Games and other experiential exercises take some creative thinking on the part of the nurse, but they are a valuable teaching strategy.

A special category of experiential exercises is patient activities, such as field trips or visits with other patients. The family of a patient who is now confined to a wheelchair may find that a visit to the home of a former patient to view the modifications necessary for wheelchair access may be much more valuable than any number of books and pamphlets or verbal descriptions. Similarly, a patient may be helped to develop a more positive attitude toward his condition and have many of his questions answered by talking with a former patient with that condition. Mastectomy, ostomy, and diabetic patients are often especially helped by this approach.

Thorough preparation is most important when using these special kinds of learning experiences. Not only should learning objectives be clear to all participants and the resource environment, equipment, or person "reviewed" before teaching by the nurse, but the patient should also be helped to prepare for the experience by making a list of what he wants to know, questions he wants to ask, or problems he wants to discuss. As with all experiential methods, the follow-up discussion with the learner, in which he is helped to put the experience in perspective and apply new insight to his own situation, is all important to real learning.

What If . . . ?

The fantasies and fears of nurses surrounding the use of the experiential strategies usually concern (a) refusal of the patient to participate or (b) inadvertently stumbling into emotional territory that would be better handled by a therapist. The experiential strategies should not be presented in such a way that the patient feels that he has no choice or that he has been trapped in an uncomfortable situation. Having taken the precaution of being sure that the patient has an "out," the nurse should respect his decision as to whether or not to participate. This will take care of most instances of the second problem as well as the first, since those who are on unstable emotional ground will generally not expose themselves to introspective situations.

The purpose of the experiential strategies is to stimulate thinking. As emphasized earlier, it is the discussion following a brief learning experience that is really important. The nurse who chooses one of these strategies must be alert to nonverbal clues of discomfort or distress. When such clues are given it is best to stop and discuss what has happened so far. If the nurse still feels uncomfortable about the incident after the discussion, she should discuss it with a staff psychologist, therapist, or others who have experience in working with people's emotions. She can learn a great deal by doing this.

In summary, three experiential strategies for learning have been described. Although their use requires a commitment of time and a high level of interpersonal skills in the nurse, they can effectively be used to facilitate complex learning.

> Experiential learning strategies allow the learner to take action and see the consequences of it in a condensed time span. For this reason they are effective in facilitating problem solving, attitude change, and preparation for anticipated events.

An especially important aspect of the experiential strategies is the quality of the nurse-patient relationship that precedes their use. Only within a relationship of trust is the nurse able to evaluate the potential benefit of using these methods, and only within such a relationship is the exploration of feelings and thoughts at this depth emotionally "safe" for the patient. Experience is a fine teacher, but it is to be arranged for others with caution.

SUMMARY

In this chapter the practicalities of using a variety of teaching strategies have been discussed in detail. Attention has been focused on individual teaching situations in which only one or two learners are involved. In Chapter 8 we will again discuss a number of teaching strategies as they can be used for group teaching. This chapter has emphasized the need for thorough planning of teaching strategies and the importance of involving the learner as a participant, whatever strategy is chosen. Appendix A contains notes about the choice of teaching strategies relevant to some commonly occurring patient teaching situations.

Study Questions and Exercises

1. For three lessons in which you have recently participated, rank the style of the teacher on the following continuum:

Formal 5 ——— 4 ——— 3 ——— 2 ——— 1 Informal

Structured 5 ——— 4 ——— 3 ——— 2 ——— 1 Open

Were the lessons organized? In what ways? Was active learner participation included? What teaching strategies were used?

2. Using the same continuum scale as in Exercise 1, what style of teaching do you prefer when you are a class participant? What style do you prefer as a teacher? How do you decide what style to use? Discuss your answers with classmates or colleagues.

3. List the topics that you would feel comfortable helping patients learn. Referring to the "Levels of Learning" in Table 4–5, indicate next to each topic the level of complexity at which you feel you could teach. Compare your list with that of classmates, adding to it as others suggest topics that you may not have included. Make notes for yourself about what you need to learn about common patient-teaching topics in order to teach.

4. Analyze a lesson in which you have recently participated, identifying the steps in the lesson sequence and the strategies used by the teacher for each.

5. Plan a patient-teaching session using a plan outline such as that shown in Table 4–6. For each item of content to be included, indicate your planned teaching strategy and the reason for your choice. Present this plan to classmates, describing the session's organization, sequence, and plans for learner participation.

Microteaching. Microteaching is a valuable technique for helping nurses learn how to use teaching strategies. It involves planning and actually teaching a 5- to 10-minute lesson to a classmate or a small demonstration group. The "learners" then analyze the lesson presented, helping the "teacher" modify and improve it. If videotaping facilities are available, viewing oneself teaching is an invaluable, and usually supportive, learning experience. Nurse teachers involved in a teacher education program usually need at least three demonstration sessions using each of the major teaching strategies in order to feel comfortable with everyday patient teaching.

6

HOW TO CHOOSE AND USE TEACHING MATERIALS

Teaching materials and audiovisual media are important adjuncts to effective teaching. In this chapter we will continue to explore the practical aspects of conducting patient teaching by reviewing a variety of visual and audiovisual aids. (See Appendix B for information on how to obtain materials from various organizations and agencies.) For each of the materials discussed, the advantages, guidelines for their use, and hints for the nurse in preparing her own materials are included. The focus is again on prepared patient teaching in which only one or two learners are involved. Notes on the modification and use of teaching materials for larger groups can be found in Chapter 8. The main points contained in this chapter are as follows.

- Teaching materials aid memory by stimulating interest and involvement and by helping the learner focus his attention. (Introduction)
- Teaching materials are most effective when they are used in conjunction with teaching strategies as part of a planned program of learning. (Section 6.1)
- Any teaching materials chosen should be reviewed for accuracy, content, organization, and specific objectives. (Section 6.1)
- Written materials are extremely flexible tools for helping to organize, facilitate, summarize, or reinforce learning. The learner's visual acuity and reading comprehension must be assessed before their use. (Section 6.2)
- Pictures and other visual aids provoke emotional responses in the learner and are important aids to memory. (Section 6.3)
- In order to derive maximum learning benefit from films and programs using electronic media, the learner must be helped to prepare for them and apply their content to his individual needs. (Section 6.4)

- Self-paced learning materials allow the learner to take responsibility for his own learning. They can be a valuable aid to complex learning. (Section 6.5)

In Section 5.1, in discussing the sequence of steps in a lesson, it was suggested that the use of several teaching strategies during the course of a lesson helped to stimulate the learner's interest and reinforce learning. The use of media or materials other than the nurse's voice similarly increases teaching effectiveness.

Teaching materials serve the important functions of focusing the learner's attention, involving him emotionally in the learning process, and aiding his memory.

Attention, involvement, and memory are critical links in the chain of learning. Attention and memory deserve special consideration by the nurse teacher.

Gaining and Maintaining Attention

Attention to a subject is a kind of open door through which new knowledge, attitudes, and skills can enter. Without the attention of the would-be learner, teaching is futile. Not only is it important to gain the learner's attention initially, but it is also essential that it be maintained throughout a lesson. The skillful use of teaching materials does this by involving visual as well as auditory senses and providing interesting variety.

A patient in a clinical setting is likely to experience a range of physical and psychological factors that compete with the nurse teacher for his attention. A major barrier for the nurse to overcome is a *lack of expectation* that learning is to take place. Students in a classroom expect to be taught, if not to learn. Patients are unlikely to have the same level of expectation. Unless they are carefully prepared for the learning experience, the nurse cannot assume that they will be in a state of mental arousal that will permit attention and foster concentration at the time the nurse chooses to teach. Presentation of a short film or written material can help to break through this barrier by promoting interest in a subject.

Another significant barrier to attention is *high stress levels*. When the learner is anxious or in an emotional crisis, he will give his attention to teaching only if he perceives it as helping to reduce his stress level. Teaching materials that demonstrate the successful result of learning and highlight the solution of problems will increase this positive perception. Those that show the patient how new learning is linked to what he already knows will further reduce stress.

Even under the most advantageous conditions, *attention span* is limited. Research has shown that attention span not only varies with interest in a subject but also with time of day, body temperature, and fatigue (Wingfield and Byrnes, 1981). Even under the most advantageous conditions, 45 minutes is about the maximum that can be expected in concentrated attention from an adult. The results of my own studies with nurse teachers in a community health setting suggest that active learning occurs for a maximum of 20 minutes during planned individual teaching sessions, with a reduced level for an additional 10 minutes as measured by recall the next day. In a clinical setting the effects of medications and pain and an environment that is noisy and distracting further erode the length of time a patient can reasonably be expected to pay attention. Short, relevant teaching sessions are a necessity. Audiovisual materials can significantly increase the impact of teaching on the patient by showing the relevance and making it easier for him to concentrate by providing a visual focus for his attention.

In choosing teaching materials that will be effective in overcoming barriers to attention, the nurse considers their *appropriateness* for the subject of concern and their *availability*. She also needs to consider their *acceptability* to the learner.

> Teaching materials will stimulate the attention of the learner if they are neither too simple nor too complex for him. They must interest without overwhelming and provoke involvement but not distress.

Although most people are able to accept a range of materials and approaches when they are motivated to meet learning objectives, this motivation can be quickly undermined by poor choices of material. Presentations that are too simple may be regarded as silly or, worse yet, condescending, inspiring the learner's anger or boredom or his discreditation of the teacher. For example, cute cartoons about serious subjects might be poorly accepted by a middle aged executive or a medical professional, who may regard this approach as too simplistic.

At the other end of the spectrum, material that is too complex for the learner's present level of understanding will probably be ignored or tolerated with boredom. Teaching materials are intended to stimulate interest and attention; boredom is the exact opposite of the intended reaction. When the first nonverbal signal of lagging attention and boredom is noted, the nurse must be prepared to shift gears and introduce material that will regain interest. In some instances materials that are too complex can cause fear or anxiety. For example, television programs showing the details of open heart surgery may be overwhelming to someone about to undergo such surgery.

Remembering What Is Learned

The human memory is fascinating and complex. It is only beginning to be fully appreciated and is not yet completely understood by scientists (Tulving, 1983).

> Gaining a learner's attention is prerequisite to his remembering what is taught. Unless he can remember and use the knowledge, attitudes, and skills offered, teaching has been ineffective.

To define memory as simply as possible, it is a mental process that results in the storage of ideas, thoughts, facts, feelings, and skills for later use. Remembering, and the retrieval of what is stored, is helped through establishing connections between what is already known and what is being learned (Wingfield and Byrnes, 1981). Communication experts report that visual perceptions and ideas associated with feelings are easier to remember than verbal learning (Bailey, 1976). For example, most people soon forget the details of words spoken or written during even important events in their lives but remember for years the feelings inspired by them and visual "pictures" of the scenes. The brain has several avenues by which to code information for the storage system. The most powerful memories are those involving several code systems (Wittig, 1981). For this reason, teaching materials that stimulate emotional involvement and present visual images are especially helpful in promoting memory.

The ability of well-chosen teaching materials to stimulate attention and aid memory is central to our consideration of various materials in this chapter.

6.1 CHOOSING EFFECTIVE TEACHING MATERIALS

In this section, three important considerations in choosing teaching materials are discussed. Special attention is given to a procedure for reviewing materials to estimate their appropriateness, availability, and acceptability.

The Importance of Combining Teaching Strategies and Materials

Teaching materials can contribute interest, emphasis, and reinforcement to a lesson. Their potential is seldom realized, however, when they are used alone.

Teaching materials are most effectively used in combination with teaching strategies.

There are instances in which posters, pamphlets, and television programs teach effectively even when isolated from other learning experiences. This happens when the reader or viewer already has a concern or interest that these materials build on. They then act as simple reinforcement, validation of already suspected truths, or examples of a known theory. (See Chapter 2 for discussion of factors that influence readiness to learn.) Teaching materials presented by themselves are too inefficient and too unpredictable to be useful for planned teaching.

For the nurse who is preparing patient teaching, a wide variety of materials and audiovisual aids can contribute positively to learning goals. They may be as simple as a sketch of an organ drawn by the nurse as she describes it, or as complex as a computer-assisted learning "game." Anatomical models, written instructions, pictures, or pieces of equipment are all valid teaching materials. Such supplements to explanation, discussion, or demonstration can be used in any part of the lesson sequence (see Table 5–1) but are most frequently used in the presentation of content or in reinforcement of learning.

A critical aspect of their effectiveness is that teaching materials must actually further learning progress, rather than just entertain. They do this best when the learner is prepared to use the teaching material and then has the opportunity to discuss his reactions to it. This kind of verbalization allows the patient to apply the messages contained in the teaching material to his own reality and the larger picture of his health and well-being. The following example describes a study that illustrates this principle.

Example 6.1 APPOINTMENT CARDS AS A TEACHING MATERIAL

Brownbury Hospital is a 350-bed acute care facility in the suburbs of a large city. Its discharge planning unit was primarily concerned with nursing home placements and arrangements for visiting nurse services and was staffed by social service workers. If a patient needed extensive instruction in self-care procedures, responsibility for this was taken by his primary care nurse, who usually included information on follow-up in her teaching by instructing the patient to contact his doctor's office for an appointment. Patients who did not need extensive teaching were simply given an instruction sheet on which the nurse had filled in medication orders and a time interval in which the doctor was to be contacted.

An informal study was initiated in 1982 when medical staff members complained that a large proportion of their patients were not returning to them for outpatient care after discharge. The study excluded those who received extensive discharge teaching and those referred to other care services. Of the remaining discharged patients who were interviewed by telephone, 90 per cent recalled the doctor or a nurse telling them that they ought to see their doctor again, although in many cases a specific instruction was not remembered. Only 55 per cent of the patients contacted had, however, made an appointment with their doctors within six weeks of discharge.

A nurse, Wanda Lyons, was subsequently appointed to a position in the discharge planning unit. Her job was to be sure that every patient discharged from the hospital received instruction on home care and follow-up medical care. In most cases she was able to prearrange an appointment with the patient's doctor so that her instructions about follow-up could be specific.

After meeting with the nursing staff of each patient unit to clarify her role and gain their cooperation in letting her know as early as possible of a patient's impending discharge, the nurse developed a plan for teaching that would take approximately 30 minutes. When an appointment had already been made, she gave the patient an appointment card to supplement her explanation of the importance of having follow-up care.

The nurse kept a summary record of items included in teaching, together with a note as to the time and place of the appointment. Between 4 and 6 weeks after discharge she either contacted the doctor's office or telephoned the patient to check on whether the planned visit had been kept. Over a period of 6 months, 86 per cent of those given specific appointments kept them, whereas only 62 per cent of those given more general instructions to make an appointment for themselves had actually done so.

Although many variables in this study make the results less than conclusive, the findings suggest that the nurse's intervention had a positive effect on patient cooperation with the instruction to return to the doctor for follow-up care. When her teaching could be specific, it also was more successful. The teaching material in the form of an appointment card or other written instruction was more effective when it was included as part of a larger teaching program than it was previously, when it had just been handed to a patient leaving the hospital.

Teaching materials are like a racquet connecting with a tennis ball: the potential for useful impact is great and just connecting may push the ball over the net. The best use of the potential power is realized, however, when the racquet is prepared for the impact and a follow-through helps the ball reach its target.

The Importance of Using Relevant and Individualized Materials

Most people can recall instances from their educational experiences in which they were left wondering why a particular film had been shown or why they had received a handout that seemed to have no relevance to the topic of a lecture. These misused teaching materials may have been interesting or entertaining in their own right, but if the student was unclear about their intention, they probably contributed nothing to meeting learning objectives. Sometimes teachers become so fond of an audiovisual program, pamphlet, or picture that they use it regardless of learning objective and then wonder why learners fail to share their enthusiasm.

In patient teaching the nurse has the opportunity to demonstrate her grasp of the patient's learning needs by choosing relevant materials that clearly help with the learning process.

> The most effective teaching materials are those which are immediately relevant to learning objectives and individualized to meet unique patient needs.

Individual teaching gives the nurse an opportunity to individualize materials so that they make the most of the interactive aspects of this kind of teaching. The combination of relevant and individualized teaching materials is especially powerful in helping with behavior and attitude changes.

There are two paths the nurse can follow in choosing teaching aids that are relevant and individualized. She can *prepare her own materials*, which are designed with a particularly common problem or a special patient in mind. In the remaining sections of this chapter a segment on preparation of one's own teaching materials is included. Alternatively, she can carefully select materials appropriate to particular learning objectives and then *prepare the patient* to individualize the messages contained in it. Thoughtful patient preparation and follow-up permit the nurse teacher to make use of a wide range of prepared films, games, video programs, and worksheets. (See Appendix B for information about locating such materials.)

The Importance of Reviewing Patient Teaching Materials

An appreciation of the importance of relevance and the individualization of teaching leads the nurse to review all materials before use. There are four major elements in the review of teaching materials that help the nurse judge their relevance and usefulness in stimulating attention and memory.

> A careful review of teaching materials includes an assessment of their accuracy, content, organization, and specific objectives.

Notes entered on file cards or in a notebook when a material is reviewed remind the nurse of important details and guide her in planning its use.

Accuracy. A primary consideration when choosing teaching materials is whether the information they contain is *correct, complete,* and *current.* The publication date is not always a reliable indication of how up-to-date the content is. Sometimes companies who sponsor a publication, film, or other teaching material fail to include information about recent advances in treatment or technology made by competing companies.

Clearly, if the information included is simply wrong in the light of current knowledge, the teaching material is useless and possibly even dangerous. Sometimes, however, it is possible to salvage materials, even though they are incomplete or out of date, by carefully planning their use in a teaching session. Supplemental material might be used or only a portion of a film or handout shown. For example, I used a book published by a maker of oral contraceptives as a teaching material for several years after its information was outdated because it included anatomical drawings that were easy for patients to understand. I simply stopped using some of the other diagrams and drawings that were product specific.

The nurse has a legal as well as professional obligation to see that information given patients is correct. Carefully assessing teaching materials for their accuracy is therefore important.

Content. In reviewing the content of teaching materials the nurse is especially interested in discovering its contribution to learning and its use in relation to other planned content. Some of the aspects of content that she might look for include the following:

- *Breadth* of content: How extensively is the subject covered?
- *Depth* of content: What level of complexity is the material designed to teach?
- *Clarity* of content: Are audio and visual components clear and easy to understand?
- *Objectivity* of content: Is content well balanced, or slanted in its point of view? Is it intended to sell a product?
- *Appropriateness* of content: With what audience would the nurse feel comfortable using the material?
- *Topics* covered by content: What specific topics are included and in what detail?
- *Special features* offered: Is the content especially interesting, involving, detailed, or comprehensive?

Teaching materials, other than those constructed by the nurse herself, are seldom ideal for specific instances of teaching. Notes as to strengths and weaknesses of prepared teaching materials are helpful when planning teaching. For example, a diagram or picture might be attractive and interesting but poorly labeled; or a film might emphasize a particular point that is not appropriate for all patients. On the basis of the evaluation of relative strengths and weaknesses of any material, the nurse can decide whether or not to use it in a given situation. The time taken to write thorough notes about content when first reviewing a teaching material is well spent, since it saves so much time later.

Organization. As discussed within the context of planning teaching, the organization of presentation either makes material accessible to the learner or confuses him and undermines his motivation to learn. Basic questions about organization to be asked by the nurse as she reviews teaching materials are as follows:

- What is the learner expected to know before using this teaching aid, i.e., what are its *prerequisites*?
- What kind of *organizer* is used to orient the learner to the content covered? (See Section 5.1 for definition and discussion of organizers.)

- Does it proceed from simpler to more complex content in an organized, *logical* way?
- With what specific content does it *begin* and *end*?

By analyzing the organizational framework used in a teaching material the nurse can decide whether or not it fits well with her planned approach and whether or not it is useful as a logical extension of her teaching.

Objectives. All teaching materials have a purpose or an objective. A diagram or picture might simply be intended to represent or illustrate a part of the body, a piece of equipment, or a relationship. A film or videotape program might intend to demonstrate a skill, increase awareness of an issue, or inform the viewer of recent developments in research. In reviewing teaching materials the nurse needs to assess how and what the material was intended to teach, whether these objectives are clearly stated or just implied, and to what degree they are consistent with learning objectives in the immediate situation. If the objectives of a material are simple or general, they can often be individualized by the nurse with little effort. She can time the presentation of the material or emphasize particular aspects of it to meet the patient's unique needs. It is more difficult to individualize more complex materials, however, and therefore more important that the objectives of material and learner match.

No matter how well a nurse knows a particular teaching material, its objectives should be reviewed before every use. This will allow her to make the most of the opportunity for individual and personal teaching that is present in one-to-one patient education.

In addition to reviewing teaching materials for accuracy, content, organization, and objectives, there are two other important pieces of information the nurse needs. One has to do with the *availability* of the material. Many a teaching plan has foundered because a film had not been booked the necessary 2 weeks in advance.

A second piece of important information is whether *special guides* are available for the teacher, such as manuals, evaluation data, suggestions for use, or references. The nurse will want to note the author or sponsor of any teaching material she uses. Special guides do not replace the nurse's own critical review of materials, but some do contain valuable information and suggestions.

In summary, three basic considerations in the choice and use of teaching materials have been discussed. Whether a simple drawing or a complex program, teaching materials are important additions to teaching strategies. Used wisely, they stimulate interest and involvement that lead to attention and retention of learning. If carefully reviewed and sensitively chosen for relevance and contribution to learning objectives, they make the teaching-learning process more interesting, fun, and challenging for both teacher and learner.

6.2 USING WRITTEN MATERIALS

Written teaching materials are, by far, the most flexible of the aids available to the nurse teacher. They must, however, be used with caution. Because written materials are so concrete and can be so comprehensive, they give the illusion of being more effective than they often are. In order to actually be effective, they must be read and comprehended by the reader; only then do they fulfill their potential for helping him learn. As all of us know from our school days, simply being given something to read does not guarantee that we will learn from it what is hoped and expected by the teacher.

Written teaching materials range from a few notes on a page that outline a lesson, to lengthy books. They include pamphlets, lesson notes, bibliographies, labels, newspapers, magazines, and package inserts for prescription medication. Some of these intend to be instructive, while others have no specific learning objective. In this section we will explore some advantages and guidelines for using written materials to supplement individual teaching. The nurse is also offered some notes on preparing her own written teaching materials.

Advantages of Written Materials

The written word is probably the largest single contributor to learning. Because written instructions, labels, letters, and newspapers are all around us, we often learn informally, even unknowingly, from them. As supplements to verbal teaching, written notes, outlines, pamphlets, and articles offer a method by which information can be made visual and relatively permanent. Seeing an appointment date and time helps to fix it in memory; a card with this information helps to reinforce the learning by acting as a reference.

Written materials can be used in several ways to assist with learning. Outlines, notes, and "pre-reading," such as articles or pamphlets, help to organize a lesson, giving both teacher and learner a head start on the content to be covered. These kinds of materials are especially effective if they are accompanied by a statement of learning objectives. The nurse might give a patient an article to read from a health-related magazine telling him: "Before you go home I want to help you learn about how diet can help prevent another heart attack. Here is an article that gives some general information about diet. I'd like you to read this and jot down the questions that occur to you. Then this afternoon, when your wife is here, I'll spend some time with both of you helping you learn why decreasing your salt and cholesterol is important and discussing ways you might do that at home." This kind of verbal and written organizer helps the patient focus on the learning task ahead and begin to actively think through his own personal objectives.

Written materials are also used to supplement the content of teaching. An example of this kind of use is described in Example 5.2. An outline, initially presented as an organizer for a patient learning about taking beta-blocking medication, became an aid to the lesson content when the patient wrote down information on the sheet as it was explained. The visual stimulation of the written outline could be expected to assist his memory. Even more useful to memory was the mental processing required to write down what he heard.

Much of the supplemental written material used as part of the content of a lesson or used to summarize and reinforce material already presented, in effect, is a lecture on paper. Like a lecture, it is an efficient way of transmitting information but communication is similarly one way and nonparticipative (see Section 5.2). Unless materials have been prepared or modified by the nurse with a particular patient in mind, they may be impersonal or general. For these reasons it is important to include an introduction to written materials in the lesson and, if possible, provide for discussion of them later.

Like explanations or lectures, written materials are most effective in teaching new *knowledge* or giving information. Chosen carefully, however, they may also stimulate awareness of an attitude or value and even begin the learning that will result in development of a skill. In order to help the reader alter an *attitude*, the material must provoke a positive emotional response, and in order to teach a *skill*, it must provide clear, step-by-step instructions and simple descriptions of why the procedure should be done as shown. The pamphlet reproduced in Figure 6–1 does all of these things effectively. When used as a teaching material to supplement a nurse's individual explanation and discussion or demonstration, it could be useful in facilitating, reinforcing, and summarizing learning. The pamphlet initially attracts attention and invites identification with the picture of a well-groomed young woman. Inside, the question-and-answer format, bold headings, clear diagrams, and simple explanations make the content easy to read and understand. The reader does not have to start at the beginning and read sequentially through the material in order to have it be meaningful. Because people often glance at a pamphlet, reading paragraphs in random order, this is an important aspect of teaching through this medium.

> Written materials provide a varied and flexible aid to verbal teaching. They are efficient ways to transmit information and, because they are visual, stimulate memory. Wisely used to supplement teaching strategies, they can help to organize, facilitate, summarize, and reinforce learning.

Written materials that can be used as teaching materials are available from a wide range of sources. Most medical facilities have education departments that keep stores of pamphlets and articles. Appendix B lists a number of sources from which one can obtain patient-teaching materials and information about what is currently available.

Guidelines for Choosing Written Materials

In choosing materials to supplement teaching, both the patient or learner and the material need to be carefully assessed so that an effective match can be made. The following guidelines will help the nurse make this assessment.

Mental and Visual Acuity. It is essential to assess a person's mental and visual acuity before giving him reading material. Medications, stress, advanced age, and a wide range of physical disorders can act to disrupt a patient's normal ability to concentrate, his interest, and his visual focus. He may be able to carry on a conversation with a nurse or answer questions but be unable to see or clearly comprehend written materials. Sometimes finding his reading glasses is all that is required. Asking a patient the straightforward question "Are you able to read this?" is reasonable if the nurse is unsure about his visual acuity.

Mental acuity can best be assessed by a nurse who knows the patient and has interacted with him over a period of time. The reading material, such as books, magazines, or newspapers, in evidence at his bedside gives some indication of his interest and ability. Sometimes relatives and friends who come to visit can offer helpful guidance to the nurse as to whether a patient is ready to read, listen, or comprehend.

Reading Ability. An assessment of the learner's reading ability helps the nurse choose appropriate written teaching materials. Knowing the grade level achievement of a person does not help one accurately predict their reading ability. For example, it cannot be assumed that because a person has completed high school, his reading comprehension level is grade 12. The number of people in the United States who are functionally illiterate has increased markedly in recent years. Conversely, a person with minimal education but an interest in reading may have developed his skills far beyond his grade level accomplishment. Likewise, a person for whom English is a second language may have much better reading skills than verbal skills.

Many people with poor reading skills are defensive about this deficiency. They cover up the fact by pretending that they are reading and understanding materials presented to them. In order to avoid this situation or the learner's acute embarrassment, the nurse must approach an assessment of reading ability with sensitivity. One method is to ask the patient "Do you like to read?" If the response is positive, it can be followed by a second question: "What kinds of things do you read regularly?" These questions can be asked in the course of general conversation so that the person does not feel that the nurse wants a particular answer. The first question provides useful insight into the person's motivation to learn through reading, an important factor in the use of written teaching materials. The second question gives some indication of preferred reading level. For example, most newspapers are written at an average reading level of grades 7 through 9. *Time* and *Newsweek* are somewhat more difficult, at grade 10 or 11. The pamphlet shown in Figure 6–1 is easy to read and represents a grade level of 5 or 6.

Reading difficulty is usually assessed by counting the number of sentences and syllables in several 100-word samples of a document. (See Redman [1984], Chapter 7, for details of several readability formulas.) For example, a sample from an average newspaper is likely to have five to six sentences and 140 to 150 syllables.

One of the best ways to assess a person's interest and skill in reading is to observe him reading. For anyone with the reading skills to make reading pleasurable and a developed habit of obtaining information through the written word, the long hours of boredom in a hospital bed are likely to prompt interest in reading as soon as mental concentration is equal to it. If the patient is reading his own materials, it is likely that he can be interested in reading those of the nurse teacher.

Readability of Materials. Teaching materials must be assessed for the level

GOT A FEW MINUTES?

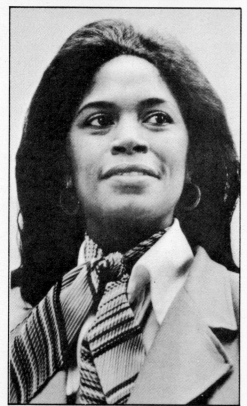

Do what I do. Use them to check your breasts every month to help protect yourself against breast cancer. It's a lifetime habit that could add some time to your life.

Who needs to do a breast check?

Every woman—

from early teens on. It's a good habit to get into and stay with for the rest of your life.

Why do it yourself?

Most lumps are found by women . . . by chance. Most lumps are not cancer though. But the quicker you see a doctor, the quicker you'll get peace of mind if you've found a lump. Or if it does turn out to be cancer, get it taken care of. Early breast cancer is easiest to cure.

Why every month?

You check on a regular basis for two reasons: (1) to find things early and (2) to get to know what is normal for *you*.

How do you check yourself?

It's two basic steps. The easiest step is *The Mirror Check.* Just look at your breasts in the mirror with your arms at your side. Raise your arms over your head to see if either breast shows any unusual

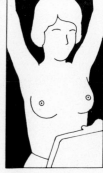

Figure 6–1. Pamphlet on breast self-examination. (Source: American Cancer Society pamphlet No 2078–LE. Used with permission.)

Illustration continued on opposite page

change in size or shape. Also put your hands on your hips, press down and see if you notice anything different. Look to see if there are changes in the skin—any redness, a swelling, or a scaly area or sore on the nipple.

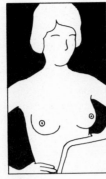

The Clock Exam

This second step takes longer to explain than to do. Lie down on your back on a bed or flat surface. Pull a small pillow or folded towel under your right shoulder and put right arm behind head. Use your left hand to check the right breast. Keep fingers flat and together. Think of your breast as the face of a clock. Start at 12:00 and gently press around till you're back up to 12 again. You must cover every part of each breast. When you've finished, put the pillow under the left shoulder, left arm behind head and use your right hand to check your left breast. Simple. Then squeeze each nipple to see if you have a discharge.

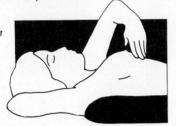

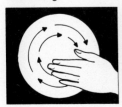
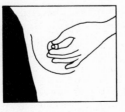

What time of the month should you check yourself?

One week after your period is the best time. Your breasts are softer and easier to examine. If you've stopped having periods, do it on the same date each month. (A lot of women pick the first because it's easy to remember.)

What if you find something?

It's important to see a doctor right away. Most lumps are not cancer, but only a doctor can find out for sure.

How do you know what is normal?

By checking your breasts every month you can learn what is normal for *you*. Ask about BSE when you see the doctor next for any reason. And you and your doctor or the nurse can go over the BSE check together.

Spend a few minutes a month. It might save your life.

Figure 6–1. *Continued.*

of demand that they place on the reader, or their readability. Some medical units that have a store of pamphlets and patient-teaching materials label them easy, average, or difficult to read, thereby saving the nurse from having to do a detailed assessment each time she plans patient teaching using them. Materials in languages other than English also need to be assessed for readability and accuracy. When written materials have been previously rated and labeled, the nurse's normal review of materials should be sufficient to confirm its readability level.

Environment and Timing of Presentation. A well-lighted, relatively quiet environment is necessary for learning through use of written materials. Although this point is obvious, it is included because it is easy to forget to first instruct the patient in turning on the lights before expecting him to read the material he has been given.

Written materials should be presented when you want the learner to read them. The written word is powerful in diverting attention from a verbal exchange. Presented with something to read, most people will immediately begin to do so, surreptitiously if necessary. A material given a patient to "read later" may well be lost or forgotten.

Preparing Your Own Written Materials

Written materials are the easiest of all the teaching aids for the nurse to prepare herself. In individual teaching the relevance of materials to the personal goals of the learner is especially important for meeting learning objectives. The fact that the nurse teacher takes the time and makes the effort to make teaching materials herself contributes greatly to her rapport with the learner. For patients, it is more important to be given personalized teaching materials, even if they are crudely lettered, than it is to be given beautiful, professionally formatted, but not really relevant teaching materials. Handwritten *notes* or *outlines*, for example, can be valuable aids to learning because they are so immediately relevant and personal.

Flip charts with large sheets of newsprint or butcher paper attached to a board and often on a tripod stand are easy to construct and to see. Using the flip chart like a blackboard, the nurse can use a marking pen to write key words or phrases as they are discussed, to aid memory. Similarly, she can prepare a number of sheets before the lesson, noting important points or major sections of content. These might then be added to or modified during the session as appropriate.

Overhead projectors, which project what is written on a transparent sheet onto a screen or wall, can be used in the same way. The transparencies are easy to prepare ahead of time and transport to the bedside; the projector itself may be somewhat more awkward. The nurse can then add to the visual aid as she teaches. Transparent sheets can be photocopied, and the patient can be given a copy as a reminder after the lesson.

A common form of personalized teaching materials involves the writing of *instructions*. Instructions are deceptively difficult to write well. It is easy to forget that the reader does not have the same acquaintance with the problem as has the writer. Jargon can sometimes complicate the simplest set of rules.

I recently encountered a photocopier with the following instruction taped to it: "Insert cassette carefully. Raise top first." Although this note probably made sense to the writer, it was not helpful to a first-time user. After some investigation it became apparent that the "cassette" was the plastic drawer that held the paper. This basic information, along with where the cassette could be found, and instructions which reflected the appropriate sequence of actions would have improved the written instructions. When motor skills and the manipulation of objects are involved, it is helpful to include diagrams in the instructions.

A list of instructions should be reviewed by a colleague or someone who is not included in the teaching before it is given to the learner. After the learner receives the list, he should read through each instruction, reinterpreting it verbally for the nurse, so that they can agree on the meaning. In some instances the nurse might help the patient make his own list of instructions for a procedure he is learning.

Nurses who have developed an awareness of the need to help their patients and others learn are often creative in making teaching materials to aid them. A major source of ideas on how to make teaching more effective through the use of teaching materials is a nurse's colleagues. Some staff development or nursing education departments collect and coordinate the use of teaching materials developed by nurses to solve particular learning problems creatively. Workshops or seminars on the use of teaching materials are especially helpful to those who are just beginning to develop teaching skills.

In summary, in this section attention has been focused on the use of written teaching materials. Because they are so varied and flexible, they can aid teaching in many ways. In order for them to be used effectively, however, the abilities of the learner must be carefully assessed and the readability of the material matched to the situation. Written materials are easy to construct and can often be designed to meet specific learning needs by creative nurse teachers.

6.3 USING PICTURES AND DIAGRAMS

As the old saying goes, a picture is worth a thousand words. When choosing teaching materials and aids for a learner's memory, this truth should be firmly kept in mind. Pictures and diagrams represent an alternative to words in communication. Not only does an alternative method act to reinforce spoken or written messages, but it also has an emotional impact of its own. Visual memory uses a "channel" of mental process that is different from the one used for words (Wingfield and Byrnes, 1981). Pictures are more readily recalled than specific words. Therefore, pictures and diagrams are ideally suited to communicating concepts and complex relationships. For example, the visual images that accompanied news coverage of the devastating earthquake in Mexico in September 1985 surpassed the thousands of words devoted to the story in communicating the complex combination of despair, fear, pride, and grim determination experienced by the people of Mexico City.

The visual representations of ideas that might be used by the nurse in individual patient teaching range from color photographs to rough handdrawn illustrations. They may include anatomical diagrams, charts, puzzles, or meta-phorical pictures, such as gears to indicate the interaction of factors affecting a problem.

Pictures are especially useful for focusing attention, showing detail, and representing values; diagrams are useful for simplifying concepts and representing complex relationships.

Guidelines for Using Pictures and Diagrams

Once a nurse starts looking for pictures and diagrams which could assist her in teaching, she will find them in widely scattered, but readily accessible places such as magazines, books, pamphlets, posters, and newspapers. Combined with her own creativity, these teaching materials can be extremely effective. The following are a few guidelines for their use.

- Pictures and diagrams communicate most effectively when they are used as the *focus of interaction* between learner and teacher. Visual images, like written teaching materials, transmit their message in only one direction. Their effective use, therefore, requires the teacher's help to prepare the learner for their visual impact. After their introduction the learner will also usually need help in applying the message to his own situation. The photos from the Mexican earthquake would not have been as memorable had they not been surrounded by words that contributed meaning to the images.

- The most effective pictures and diagrams are *simple and uncluttered*. Both of the charts in Figure 6–2 present information about the health risks of smoking. The learning objective in both cases is for the patient to develop a positive attitude toward stopping smoking. Because the drawing on the right presents information in a dramatic way, it is likely to be the more effective of the two in stimulating an emotional as well as intellectual response, thus helping to alter attitudes. The chart on the left would be improved by simplifying the information it presents and adding a heading that attracts attention to the subject of concern.

The effectiveness of pictures and diagrams is enhanced by simplicity of format and complete, legible labels. Because pictures and diagrams can evoke an emotional response in the viewer, they are especially useful when learning objectives involve attitude change.

- The use of *color* increases the impact of pictures and diagrams on the viewer's attention and memory. While simplicity of design and clarity of the message are the most important aspects of pictures and diagrams used as teaching materials, color should be included when possible. A simple underline in a contrasting color or a colorful border can help to focus attention.

- Finally, whenever *actual equipment* is available to be used as a teaching material, use it rather than a picture or diagram of it. This principle especially applies to the teaching of skills. Showing a mother how to strap

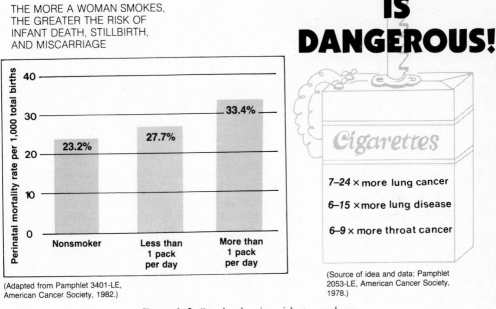

THE MORE A WOMAN SMOKES,
THE GREATER THE RISK OF
INFANT DEATH, STILLBIRTH,
AND MISCARRIAGE

(Adapted from Pamphlet 3401-LE,
American Cancer Society, 1982.)

SMOKING IS DANGEROUS!

Cigarettes

7–24 × more lung cancer

6–15 × more lung disease

6–9 × more throat cancer

(Source of idea and data: Pamphlet
2053-LE, American Cancer Society,
1978.)

Figure 6–2. Graphs showing risks to smokers.

a doll into a real infant safety seat is much more likely to result in learning than showing her a diagram of how this is to be done. The use of a diagram, however, is more effective than words alone.

Preparing Your Own Pictures and Diagrams

Pictures and diagrams that give visual impact to individual teaching are easy to prepare and fun to use. They can easily be personalized. Diagrams quickly sketched by the nurse while teaching progresses have an immediacy and relevance that more than compensate for their lack of professional design. Those that are made before teaching begins can be constructed from readily available supplies, such as butcher paper and marking pens. Accuracy, simplicity, legibility, and color are the key factors in making your own effective teaching materials.

Once the nurse directs her attention to possible sources of ideas and pictures which might be incorporated into her teaching, she will find them all around her. Professional magazines are an excellent source of anatomical diagrams, for example. When photocopied and legibly labeled, they can be effective teaching materials. The graphic arts section of a large stationery store or an art supply store are good places to begin to learn about the variety of supplies available to help the nurse prepare interesting and effective visual aids.

> The preparation of effective visual teaching materials does not require extensive artistic skills; it does require imagination and a firm grasp of the subject of concern.

In summary, the use of pictures and diagrams as teaching materials to supplement verbal teaching has been explored in this section. Such visual aids can easily be made by the nurse teacher using available materials. Pictures are especially likely to arouse an emotional response in the learner and are therefore useful for helping with attitude change, while diagrams help to make concepts and complex relationships clear. Adding a visual component to verbal teaching stimulates interest and aids memory.

6.4 USING AUDIOVISUAL PROGRAMS

Films and electronic media programs that are suitable for use in individual patient teaching come in many sizes and shapes. Included are 8mm and 16mm films, filmstrips with audiotapes or records, slides with or without recorded audio, videotapes, and television programs. They may offer explanations of detailed or broadly comprehensive topics or demonstrations of procedures. The best of these present interesting, involving programs that are useful in introducing information, clarifying concepts, showing relationships, influencing attitudes, and beginning skill development. They add a dimension of entertainment to instruction.

The major disadvantage of audiovisual programs is that they are necessarily one-way communication usually designed for diverse audiences. The material presented is often general and not individualized. Like books and pamphlets, films and television can potentially teach even in the absence of a teacher; they do so when the reader or viewer has interests or learning needs that happen to be met by the material presented. This hit-or-miss method of learning is inappropriate when important learning objectives need to be met in order to prepare a patient to better care for himself and his health. The nurse can help the learner benefit fully from audiovisual materials by integrating them into her teaching plan with careful preparation and follow-up.

> Audiovisual programs teach most effectively when they are combined with discussion and other interactive teaching strategies.

The challenge for the nurse teacher is to choose programs that are as relevant to the learner's needs as possible.

Guidelines for Using Audiovisual Programs

Television holds a central place in the lives of a majority of Americans. Most people expect to be entertained when they watch an audiovisual presentation. A number of steps can be taken by the nurse to ensure that the patient will be helped to learn from the experience as well as enjoy it.

Previewing. Previewing audiovisual programs before attempting to use them in patient teaching is essential. This means that the nurse must take the time to watch the program all the way through. If she writes detailed notes or uses an evaluation system such as that suggested in Section 6.1, she will not have to review the program again in this detail. By referring to her notes she will refresh her memory of what the program offers a learner.

> Without seeing for herself how material is presented in audiovisual programs, what visual images are used, and what points are overtly and subtly made, the nurse is unable to plan associated interactive teaching that stimulates and reinforces learning.

Embedding Audiovisuals in Interactive Teaching. Films and electronic media programs promote learning most effectively when they are surrounded by interactive teaching that helps the learner see the relevance of the program's messages and apply them in a personal way to his own needs. The first step in preparing the learner to view the program is to clarify his learning objectives. This can be done by presenting an organizer in the form of a written outline of points emphasized in the program, discussing the major points, or explaining what the nurse anticipates that the learner will derive from watching it. The nurse may also alert the viewer to particular points of interest or value.

The learner may be asked to jot down notes or questions while he views the program. When videotapes are used, which can be stopped at the will of the viewer, response forms can be used such as that used for Mr. Quinn by the nurse in Example 5.2, in which the patient wrote down in his own words his interpretation of what he heard. Such techniques make audiovisual programs as interactive as possible and provide relevant material for postviewing discussion between nurse and patient.

The period immediately after a program is when real individual learning takes place. The nurse's objectives during this time might include reviewing with the patient what he saw and heard during the program, helping him "make sense" of the information and apply it to his own needs, supplementing the program with additional information or emphasis, and reinforcing learning. When attitude change is part of learning objectives, discussion might include the learner's attitudes or values in comparison with those presented in the program and his feelings about the program's images and information. When skill development is part of learning objectives, follow-up teaching should include practice and coaching.

Choosing Appropriate Materials. As with printed materials and verbal explanations, audiovisual programs are most effective when they are chosen to match the learner's level of comprehension and attention span. Oversimplified material or humorous portrayals of serious subjects may be seen as condescending by the learner, while complex, detailed scientific analyses of a subject may be boring or overwhelming. It is useful to give audiovisual programs an overall rating of easy, average, or difficult to understand so that the nurse will have a starting point for her investigation of a particular program. Review notes should give specific details of language complexity and patient knowledge required before viewing.

The patient's level of comprehension is most easily evaluated by a nurse who has been caring for him and talking with him. The simple question "What are your favorite television programs?" can yield important information about what kinds of programs the patient chooses to watch. Following up with "What do you like best about those programs?" will give the nurse additional data on which to base her selection of effective audiovisual programs.

If patients and their family members are to learn from an audiovisual program, they must be able to give it their concentrated attention. Stress, medications, and pain all interfere with attention span. Because preprogram and postprogram teaching must be added to the actual running time of a program, relatively short programs of 10 to 15 minutes are most effective. The results of one study show that videotaped programs that extend beyond 20 minutes are substantially less effective than shorter ones.

Checking Equipment. An important aspect of successfully using films and electronic media programs in teaching is checking the equipment before its use. This may mean that the nurse will need to acquire some skills in using a film projector, synchronizing a slide-tape presentation, or adjusting a video display terminal. Instructions and demonstrations are often available from the staff development department or nursing education unit. Once the skills needed to successfully use the equipment have been mastered, it is essential that available instruction manuals accompany machines so that problems can be quickly remedied.

> Equipment for the presentation of audiovisual materials must be checked by the nurse before each use to determine its working order and her own skills. Doing so ensures that neither the nurse's time nor the patient's motivation is wasted.

Finding Resources. Resources for information about audiovisual programs include staff development or nursing education departments in medical facilities and the public library. Libraries have listings of film and video distributors, names of films available, and general subjects offered. A short note containing the nurse's areas of interest will usually bring a free catalog. Nearby colleges and universities may have audiovisual materials that they will make available for patient teaching. In Appendix B there is a listing of sources of information about a range of audiovisual patient-teaching materials.

> When chosen with the learner's attention span, level of comprehension, and specific learning needs in mind, audiovisual programs have an impact on emotions and memory that far surpasses that of other teaching materials.

Although sometimes extra effort is required to arrange access to programs and equipment, the learning that can result may well be worth it. As the availability of electronic media, particularly videotapes and computer-based programs, increases, the nurse will have more and more opportunity to use audiovisual programs for the benefit of her patient's learning.

Preparing Your Own Audiovisual Programs

In recent years the growth area in audiovisuals has been *videotapes*. Many hospitals now have the capability of broadcasting educational tapes through the television set in the patient's room. Nurses who are recent graduates have also experienced the value of individual learning through the use of videotapes in their nursing education programs.

The technology for the widespread use of videotapes in patient education now exists. Nurses have the opportunity to take a lead in promoting, designing, and helping to develop programs that will meet patient learning needs.

The following case example demonstrates what can be done by creative nurses who are sensitive to the educational needs of their patients.

Example 6.2   PREPARATION FOR SURGERY ON VIDEOTAPE

In the past 2 years St. John's Hospital had experienced a marked increase in the number of patients being admitted on the day of their elective surgery, rather than the night before. They also were seeing an increase in the number of in-and-out minor surgeries. Jan Morris, head nurse on the surgical unit, was becoming increasingly concerned about the physical and psychological preparation that patients were able to receive on her unit because of these changes. When a memo was circulated by the new audiovisual department asking for ideas for videotapes, Ms. Morris suddenly realized that this could be a vehicle for solving part of the problem.

At the next staff meeting Ms. Morris and her nurses discussed what the staff saw as gaps in patient knowledge, how these gaps were affecting the patients' experience of surgery, and how a videotape designed as a teaching aid might help. The nurses enthusiastically endorsed the idea and participated in consultations with the nurse and the technician who made up the new department. An in-house, closed-circuit television channel was being developed that would allow all patients to receive broadcasts of videotapes in their rooms.

After several weeks of preparation, filming began on a 15-minute videotape that would show the patient a little about the hospital generally and then specifically what he could expect to happen between his admission and his recovery. A picture of a patient receiving premedication was accompanied by a short explanation of why premed is given and that it would probably make the patient feel sleepy or dizzy. The use of side rails was explained, as was the use of special gowns and caps. Views of a patient being transported to surgery were shown, followed by pictures of operating rooms and the recovery room. The videotape ended with pictures of the whole surgical team and an explanation of how they work together to help the patient regain his health.

Everyone in the surgical department was given the opportunity to view the film and comment on it. After final editing it was time to try out the videotape for patient teaching. Three nurses agreed to help with a trial teaching plan in which the film was broadcast at particular times. The nurses first gave patients a questionnaire about their at-home preparation for surgery, which had been in use for some time. One question asked whether the person had previously had surgery at St. John's. The patients then were told of the videotape and its objective of familiarizing them with the unit and the procedures they would be experiencing. The nurse made sure they knew the time of the next showing and how to receive it. Patients were asked to make a note of any questions that occurred to them. After the videotape was shown, the nurse discussed any variation in the taped procedure that would apply to that patient and answered his questions and those of any family members present. On the second postoperative day elective surgery patients in the trial program were asked to fill out a questionnaire including what they remembered from the videotape and an evaluation of whether it had met the objectives and their needs. Response to the trial teaching by both patients and the nurses was extremely positive. Following the patients' suggestions, the film was slightly modified and then broadcast frequently during the 7 A.M.-to-9:30 A.M. time period, when most of the unit's patients were admitted.

In this case example a nurse's concern for a frequently experienced patient-teaching problem led to the creative use of electronic media.

Although video cameras and recorders are becoming less expensive and easier to handle, *slide programs* are still the most straightforward of audiovisual teaching aids to make or alter according to patients' learning needs. Equipment is usually available in medical facilities and easy to transport to a patient's room for an individual teaching session. Single slides can be replaced, substituted, or skipped at will. Because the nurse usually runs the program herself, she can stop to supplement information or answer questions so that it much more resembles an interactive explanation-discussion strategy with pictures and graphics.

In summary, approaches to using audiovisual programs in patient teaching have been discussed in this section. As the availability of such programs improves, along with the technical capability of medical facilities, nurses will have increasing opportunities to use, design, and help produce these powerful aids to patient learning.

6.5 USING SELF-PACED LEARNING PROGRAMS

Self-paced learning programs are a combination of teaching strategy and teaching material. They present information in small segments, or "frames," allowing the learner to progress at his own rate. They require frequent responses from the learner and give him immediate feedback for self-evaluation of progress. First proposed in 1932 by Sidney Pressey, who invented a teaching machine, self-paced, or "programmed," learning became popular in the 1950s in application of B.F. Skinner's work on operant conditioning (Lefrancois, 1975). Pressey's teaching machine did not catch on, but written versions of teaching programs did. Only since the early 1980s, when computers became increasingly available, have machines been used to do what Pressey had in mind. It is likely that computer-assisted instruction will become a major force in patient education in the near future. The capability of a computer to respond to a learner in a nearly personal way, to store vast quantities of information, and to quickly modify the presentation of material in order to meet specific patient needs makes its development truly exciting. Like television, computers are becoming more common in medical care facilities and in private homes. As a result the public in general and nurses in particular are becoming familiar with computer jargon and the computer's capabilities and seemingly unlimited potential to teach.

Until easily accessible, interactive, computer-assisted patient-teaching modules are available, the nurse may well find that the written variety is effective in helping certain patients learn.

> A major advantage of self-paced learning programs is that they allow the learner to take responsibility for his own learning. He alone controls the speed and extent of his acquisition of new knowledge.

Programmed learning is not difficult to write, but it does take practice to do it well. Johnson and Johnson (1975) have written a useful book of programmed instruction whose objective is to teach the skills of writing programmed instruction. The nurse who is interested in this kind of teaching material or who can visualize something of the potential of computers in this field is encouraged to search out examples of written programmed learning and investigate the structure and possibilities of computer "games."

Self-paced programs are of two basic types: *linear* and *branching*. The linear type follows without diversion from one section of the program to another (usually called a "frame"). The branching program can follow a divergent path, depending on the learner's response. For example, this text is normally linear in format, one page following the last. It would become branching, however, by adding an instruction such as "If the reader is familiar with the construction of programmed learning, proceed directly to page ___."

The frames that make up a program normally contain at least one opportunity for the learner to respond with a word or phrase. These responses are prompted in a number of ways. Some of the different kinds of "prompts" are shown in Figure 6–3.

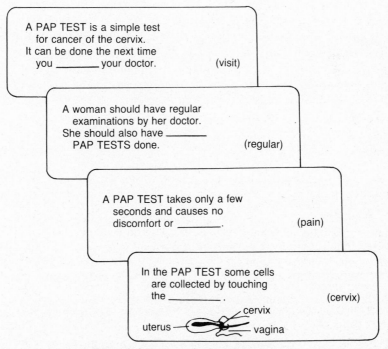

Figure 6–3. Prompts for learner responses.

Well-constructed programs can effectively teach complex levels of knowledge, concepts, and specific problem solving. As with audiovisual programs, they are most effective when the learner is individually prepared for their use and has the opportunity to ask questions, receive further information, or discuss his progress with the nurse teacher after the program.

In summary, self-paced learning programs have been described in this section. They provide the learner with opportunities to take responsibility for his own learning and work at a pace that is comfortable for him. With the increasing use of computer-aided instruction, the potential for such programs in patient teaching seems limitless. Thorough review of self-paced programs by the nurse and careful evaluation of the learner's objectives, motivation, and reading ability help her match patients and self-paced programs most effectively.

SUMMARY

In this chapter the major categories of learning materials have been described, guidelines for their use suggested, and notes on preparing materials offered. Throughout the chapter the importance of thoroughly reviewing materials before using them in patient-teaching sessions has been emphasized. Another point that has been stressed is the importance of using teaching materials within the larger context of interactive teaching so that their relevance to patient learning objectives is ensured. Teaching materials lend interest and enhance attention and memory. They can broaden or deepen learning; they can involve the learner emotionally; and they can demonstrate skills. The challenge for the nurse teacher is to effectively match teaching methods and materials with the needs and abilities of learners.

Chapters 4 through 6 have focused on prepared patient teaching. Many opportunities to teach, however, occur spontaneously. In the next chapter we will look at informal or spontaneous teaching in detail.

Study Questions and Exercises

1.   In order to do this exercise, two groups of ten small objects, such as a key, a needle, the cap from a bottle, or an eraser, are needed. Each group of objects should be arranged on a tray so that they are readily visible. Two or three subjects for the exercise should be chosen from the learning group. Be sure that the subjects have not participated in the gathering of objects. Now ask all but one subject to leave the room and then appoint a timekeeper. Allow the subject to view the first tray of objects for 1 minute. Remove the tray, wait 1 minute, and then have the subject recall as many of the objects as possible. Record her score. Now show her the second tray of objects, allowing her to view it for 3 minutes. Again remove the tray, wait 1 minute, and ask her to recall as many objects as possible. Record her score. Repeat the procedure with each subject in turn, alternating the 1- and 3-minute viewing times in order to partially cancel the effect of familiarity with the

task. Did memory increase consistently with greater viewing time? Were certain objects more memorable to all subjects? Why? What might have happened if the interval between viewing the objects and attempting recall had been increased? What relevance does this exercise have for patient teaching and the use of teaching materials?

2.   Research what is currently known about short-term and long-term memory in your medical facility, college, or public library. Share your findings with classmates or colleagues and discuss practical methods of stimulating memory during patient teaching.

3.   Analyze at least two classes in which you have been a recent participant. What teaching materials were used? How did the teacher prepare for their use and follow-up afterward? In what ways were the materials effective? Ineffective? How could you effectively use similar materials in individual patient teaching?

4.   Select several pamphlets from a health education display. Review them according to the procedure suggested in Section 6.1. Share your reviews with classmates or colleagues.

5.   Begin your own file of patient-teaching materials. A large accordion file labeled according to subject is handy for keeping samples of pamphlets, pictures, diagrams, and the like. Arrange a card file or ring binder in which to keep reviews of films, videotapes, and written teaching materials. Discuss the project with classmates or colleagues, sharing ideas about collecting and reviewing resources for patient teaching.

6.   Make a diagram showing the basic anatomy and blood flow within the human heart. Label it appropriately. Share this teaching material with classmates or colleagues, discussing how it might be used in individual patient teaching.

7.   Review at least two films or videotapes using the procedure outlined in Section 6.1. Add these reviews to your own resource file. Discuss your review with others who have also seen these programs. How would you most effectively use them for patient teaching?

8.   Write a short programmed instruction using material from a pamphlet. Have several classmates or colleagues try it out and comment on what they learned. How could this material be used in patient teaching?

7

HOW TO USE SPONTANEOUS TEACHING OPPORTUNITIES

An opportunity for spontaneous or informal teaching occurs when the nurse is presented with an urgent learning need, one requiring an immediate response. Most such opportunities occur within the context of requests for help with various problems. This chapter begins with a discussion of three kinds of common requests for help that give the nurse the opportunity to assist with learning as part of problem solving. Special attention is given to identifying a person's urgent need to learn. Doing this effectively requires that the nurse use her interpersonal relationship or "expressive" skills to the fullest (see Introduction to Chap. 3). For this reason the discussion of spontaneous teaching will draw on psychological as well as learning principles, and counseling as well as teaching methods. The main points contained in this chapter are as follows:

- The first step toward effective spontaneous teaching is for the nurse to "stop, look, and listen" so that she can begin to identify the person's learning need. (Introduction)
- When people ask for information and advice, they are often in the state of confusion and uncertainty that precedes effective problem solving. (Section 7.1)
- Giving advice is not a useful teaching strategy because it may undermine a person's independence and self-responsibility. (Section 7.1)
- By giving a person "permission" to talk about vague and ill-defined symptoms, the nurse can help him realize the importance of early diagnosis and treatment. (Section 7.2)
- An important aspect of patient teaching is helping a person learn how to appropriately approach and use the community's medical resources. (Section 7.2)

- By actively listening to the message behind the anger and frustration of a complaint, the nurse can reduce the stress of the situation and help the person focus on problem solving. (Section 7.3)
- Two useful criteria in assessing complex problems are their estimated duration and intensity. (Section 7.3)
- Spontaneous teaching is an effective way to help with learning because it is a response to a person's immediate interests and concerns and begins with his involvement and participation. (Section 7.4)
- A thorough initial assessment of a patient's health balance allows the nurse to anticipate learning needs so that she can respond constructively to opportunities for spontaneous teaching. (Section 7.4)

In Section 4.1 health was broadly described as a balance of a person's needs, the stressors acting on him, his internal strengths, and the resources available to him. It was suggested that the Health Balance model helps the nurse to assess areas of need so that she might plan broad-based care and specific nursing interventions. We now return to this model because it provides us with some understanding of how spontaneous teaching situations arise.

When a person experiences needs or an increase in stress, he often speaks of these as "problems" or "concerns." In an effort to reestablish a balance, he is likely to seek out knowledge that will add to his personal strength in dealing with the problem. In order to acquire such knowledge, he will enlist the help of resource people whom he expects to be able to help him and whom he trusts.

Nurses are asked to assist with problem solving because they have access to expert health information and are regarded as personally trustworthy.

As nurses, we expect to help with the problems and concerns related to people's health. We quickly learn that others regard us as a special resource in our families, communities, and work environments. Although we may not always be able to accurately judge what perceptions or previous experiences influence a person's readiness to learn, his questions, requests for advice, and sharing of concerns about his health come as no surprise. (See Section 2.1 for a discussion of factors that influence readiness to learn.) Sometimes we can readily identify major areas of learning need and set about preparing teaching that will help to fulfill it. More frequently we choose to contribute what we can "on the spot" by teaching spontaneously.

Nurses are potential sources of help with more than just a person's immediate medical condition or health concerns. The patient (or people in our social environment) may well imagine that a caring, helping resource in one subject area just might help with other problem areas of his life. Given some reasons to trust the nurse, he may risk asking questions, requesting advice, or sharing concerns about a wide range of subjects. Although the nurse might not have anticipated these requests for help, they nevertheless offer an opportunity to help the patient restore his "health" balance in the broadest sense. She may respond by counseling, teaching, or referring the patient to other sources of help, or by using all of these forms of intervention. Her goal is to assist the person to discover how to take effective action and maintain self-responsibility.

Because interaction concerning problems is often brief, the nurse's helping responses must be sensitive and insightful but also prompt. This chapter focuses on how to quickly assess and respond without delay to learning needs expressed as problems and concerns.

Whenever people are concerned about a problem confronting them and decide to enlist the aid of a possible resource, they make every effort to present their cause in the most favorable light. They intuitively know that first they must interest their resource person in their problem and involve her in their concern. Their appeal must therefore seem plausible and socially acceptable. Nurses are expected to be interested in health care matters. For this reason, whatever the true nature of the concern, an initial request for help may be presented as a health-related problem. Once the interest and attention of the nurse has been secured, the person's perception of the "real" problem may be revealed. The following case is an example of such a socially acceptable request that tested the assessment skills of the nurse.

Example 7.1   GETTING HELP FOR A HIDDEN PROBLEM

Elaine Thomas, an attractive, well-groomed mother of two young sons, was an active participant in school functions. One day she stopped in at the office of Mary Morrison, the school nurse. After a brief social chat, Mrs. Thomas asked Mary about prenatal classes held in the area. The nurse was surprised by the request, since she knew Mrs. Thomas had two children and seemed like such a confident mother. Aware that there might be more to this request for information than was obvious, she invited Mrs. Thomas to sit down while she found the pamphlet describing nearby classes. She spent a few minutes searching through her teaching materials and finally located the pamphlet. Mrs. Thomas seemed anxious and ill at ease while she waited. Mary then sat down and asked gently, "What is it that's concerning you?" There was a long pause before Mrs. Thomas replied, tears welling in her eyes: "Oh, I'm so frightened about this pregnancy! You probably don't know that my last baby was stillborn. We want another baby so much and I'm so scared . . . ."

In this case example, the nurse could have reasonably just given Mrs. Thomas what she requested: information about prenatal classes. Mrs. Thomas may well have attended, and then it would have been up to the instructor to recognize the deep anxiety distressing this woman that no amount of information about child care would have alleviated. Like so many people with concerns they are unable to clearly resolve, Mrs. Thomas approached a known resource person and made what she thought was an acceptable request. At some level she and others like her probably hope that the attention and caring concern they receive will somehow help. In this case an alert and sensitive nurse helped Mrs. Thomas verbalize and begin to explore the real problem.

A simple guideline for the nurse in responding to requests for information, advice, diagnosis, or other forms of immediate help is to first STOP, LOOK, and LISTEN: stop to pay attention to the possible meaning behind the request; look for nonverbal communication that will help clarify the intent; and then listen carefully to the words, asking for further clarification if in doubt.

The easier it is for the nurse to answer the question or respond to the problem posed, the more difficult it is for her to stand back and take the time to find out what the person is really asking for.

In this chapter we will examine a number of ways in which people approach nurses with requests to help them solve a problem. The majority of these requests represent opportunities for the nurse to teach. In the next three sections we will explore how the nurse can identify those opportunities quickly and accurately.

7.1 HANDLING REQUESTS FOR ADVICE AND INFORMATION

Like the problems which are reflected by them, questions come in all shapes and sizes.

> Is it true that . . . ?
>
> What should I do if . . . ?
>
> Are you sure that . . . ?
>
> Can you tell me whether . . . ?

The most important parts of a question are the context in which it is asked and the nonverbal communication that accompanies it. Some questions are phrased in such a way that they seem to plead for an answer, whereas others are rhetorical and require no answer. Some questions flatter the nurse's wisdom and expertise, and others challenge and confront. Generally speaking, questions request either advice and opinions or information. Advice involves the nurse in a personal way; by offering it she is commenting on how she personally would solve a problem and what feelings she has regarding it. Key words in a statement of advice are "should," "must," "always," and "never." In contrast, information usually is presented as a relatively objective statement of fact.

> A request for information or advice indicates that the asker perceives a problem in his life that might be solved by learning facts or finding out how others would approach the problem.

Unfortunately, much of the advice and information people receive does not help them. This gap between asking and using occurs for a number of reasons. One of the most common is that the person's perceptions are incomplete or erroneous; he has not clearly identified the source of his troubles. Like Mrs. Thomas, previous experience may cloud his interpretation of his needs. When a person is primarily concerned about making his request acceptable to the resource person whose attention and interest he hopes to attract, he may well be unable to fully use the information he receives.

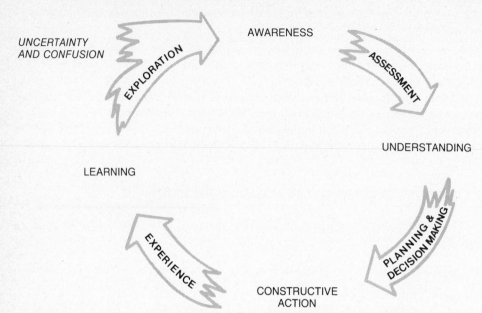

Figure 7–1. Goals of personal problem solving. (Based on the work of R. Carkhuff, 1980.)

Carkhuff's Model of Problem Solving

The work of Robert Carkhuff (1980) is helpful in further understanding the dynamics of asking for and receiving help with problem solving. As a psychologist, Carkhuff is especially interested in how people are helped to solve "personal" problems or those that evoke strong feelings. He suggests that a helper should direct her efforts at helping the troubled person achieve a series of goals related to the problem. These goals are the result of a problem-solving process that parallels that of other authors with one major exception. Carkhuff added the idea that a person confronting a "personal" problem usually experiences a stage of *uncertainty and confusion* before he is able to start on the problem itself. During this stage the facts and the feelings of the situation are unclear, upsetting, and ill-defined.

The role of the helper is, initially, to assist the person who is in a confused and uncertain state to "explore" the problem situation verbally. Doing so gives him the best chance to reach "awareness," the first goal of problem solving. Verbalization is a key concept in Carkhuff's framework, just as it is in Principle of Learning 5 listed in Table 2–1 on page 31 and discussed in Chapter 3. The four goals suggested by Carkhuff, along with the actions that are necessary, are shown in Figure 7–1.

Awareness involves identifying the nature of the problem and looking realistically at how the facts and feelings surrounding the problem affect the person.

This goal is reached through exploration, which may consist of "talking through" the troubling situation with a trusted friend or with a nurse or other helping professional.

Having reached awareness, the next goal is *understanding*. This step involves assessing the problem within a larger context: knowing why this is an important problem to solve, what the consequences of the problem and its solution might be, and perhaps how the situation developed. Understanding is followed by planning and decision making, which results in *constructive action*, or implementation. The problem-solving cycle does not stop here, however; the learning that results from the experience of problem solving gives a person skills and self-understanding that provide extra personal strength for resisting future health imbalances.

Carkhuff's work makes it clear that there are no shortcuts in the problem-solving cycle. One cannot proceed directly from uncertainty to constructive action without going through awareness and understanding. No matter how much we as helpers may want to see a person reach a satisfactory solution to his problem, we can but patiently help him learn to deal with it step by step and then help him learn through the experience. Assessment of the person's real need and his progress in meeting it so far is an important first step in responding helpfully to a question.

> By pausing to find out what is behind a question she has been asked, the nurse can accomplish three things: she can assess the person's stage in the problem-solving process, she can help him feel that he is valued and his concern justified, and, if he is still in a state of confusion, she can invite him to begin problem identification through exploring it with her.

In Example 7.1 the nurse paused to ask Mrs. Thomas, "What is it that's concerning you?" (See Section 3.3 on the use of open questions.) By doing so she was able to ascertain that because Mrs. Thomas was overwhelmed by her anxiety, she was was unsure of her problem-solving path. The nurse's willingness to stop, look, and listen showed her interest in Mrs. Thomas' concerns and at the same time opened a door of communication whereby Mrs. Thomas might begin to explore the problem. Had Mrs. Thomas' response to the nurse's inquiry been "It's been six years since I had a baby and I would like to update my knowledge," the nurse would have been able to assess that Mrs. Thomas had reached the stage of understanding and was now ready to learn information upon which to base constructive action. In this case, helping Mrs. Thomas acquire the facts she sought would have been both appropriate and useful.

> In order for teaching to be effective, it must take account of the person's present level of problem solving and his readiness to learn.

The Ineffectiveness of Advice

Most people have had the experience of offering what they thought was helpful advice to someone with a problem, only to be disappointed and disillusioned when the advice was ignored. Even advice that is requested is seldom taken. Carkhuff's model helps to explain why this happens. Advice is a kind of prescription for action; when the person to whom it is directed is not yet at the stage of planning action to solve his problem, advice, like information, is of no use. Giving advice, however, is not as benign as giving information that is out of step with a person's stage of problem solving.

In order to understand why this is so, let us return to some of the ideas about stress presented in Section 2.5. In that section a crisis was defined as a situation in which a person's normal problem-solving capability is overwhelmed. Faced with an apparently insoluble set of problems, he is unable to mobilize either internal or external resources. His thought processes become jumbled, his perceptions are distorted, and he becomes unusually vulnerable to the influence of others.

The state of disorganization, uncertainty, and confusion described by Carkhuff as a typical response to a personal problem bears a strong resemblance to a crisis state. If the problem affects only one area of a person's life, it will not have the impact or extent of a full-blown crisis response, but the dynamics of coping with this period are very much the same. As in a crisis, a person in a state of confusion, seeing no clear way to solve the problem, is vulnerable to outside influence. To the extent that he feels powerless in the situation, he is tempted to give away, or even actively tries to get rid of, responsibility for the problem. In crisis this results in denial that the problem exists. In less severe forms of distress it may mean seeking or accepting advice and following a path that is not of one's own planning. If anything should go wrong, the person giving the advice can be held responsible. The well-intentioned advice will have become a trap for both the adviser and the person she was trying to help.

> Advice offered to a person in a state of confusion and uncertainty undermines his independence and self-responsibility and may delay, or even block, his ability to solve the problem of concern.

The following example demonstrates three of the possible responses to offers of advice.

Example 7.2   SOME CONSEQUENCES OF ADVICE

CASE 1. Patient: I'm so worried about my husband's health.

Nurse: Why don't you talk with your doctor about it.

Patient (later overheard talking with a friend): You know I'm really worried about Fred's health. I told my nurse about it, but she didn't want to get involved.

CASE 2. Patient: Do you think I ought to have my daughter stay with me for a while after I go home?

Nurse: Yes, I think that would be a good idea.

Patient (later overheard talking with daughter): The nurse said that you should come and look after me for at least a week after I go home.

CASE 3. Patient: Can you tell me why I feel so exhausted whenever I do anything, even walk to the bathroom. It's been nearly a week since my surgery and I really thought I'd be feeling better by now.

NURSE: Your doctor will be coming in to see you soon. Why don't you mention it to her.

PATIENT: (later overheard talking with doctor): The nurse suggested I tell you that I'm still feeling very tired. Maybe she thinks there's something wrong with me.

In each of these three situations the nurse's well-intentioned advice was misinterpreted. In the first case the patient heard the advice as a method of stopping discussion. Although this might not have been the nurse's intent, in fact, advice usually does lead to ending a conversation. In order to continue the patient would have to ignore the advice statement or begin a "Yes, but . . ." game, in which reasons for not being able to follow the advice are advanced. In cases 2 and 3 the advice offered was misinterpreted and the nurse was made responsible for the consequences. In both cases the patient seemed to be saying, "I'm just doing what I was told to do . . . ."

We usually give advice when we suspect that the person is unable to handle his problem situation. Sensing the person's confusion, we want to lend him our strength and wisdom. In our eagerness to see him reach constructive action, we seek to speed up the problem-solving process. Sometimes advice giving masquerades as spontaneous teaching; the person is instructed in a course of action that the caregiver, with the full weight of medical expertise, recommends to solve the problem. However, even well-founded recommendations seldom are useful if following them has no basis in patient understanding. Once the person has been labeled "noncompliant" by the caregiver and experiences the defensiveness of having "not done what he was told to do," the relationship of trust is usually so disturbed that effective teaching and learning are unlikely to occur.

When presented with a situation in which it is clear that the person has reached understanding and is searching for alternatives and resources to help him plan action, giving information is certainly justified, but even then advice is not really helpful. The only time the nurse knowingly and conscientiously takes over control and responsibility is during a medical emergency, when she gives others instructions based on her professional knowledge and authority. In such situations she also knowingly accepts legal responsibility for her actions.

In summary, we have seen that in order to serve as opportunities for spontaneous teaching, requests for advice and information must be carefully assessed. Carkhuff's work on personal problem solving has shown that when a person is in the initial stage of confusion and uncertainty, he needs help in exploring the problem and reaching awareness before he can effectively solve it and learn by it. Information offered as part of either prepared or spontaneous teaching is most useful when the learner has reached the planning stage of problem solving. Advice is not generally useful and can even be harmful when it takes self-responsibility away from the person affected by the problem. In spite of their anxiety to see problems resolved and confusion diminished, effective nurse teachers take the time to stop, look, and listen to the intent behind a request for help before attempting even spontaneous teaching.

> Even though a question may seem like a clear opportunity to teach by explanation, a more effective intervention is usually to help with exploration.

The nurse's use of CARE-ful listening and open questions, as discussed in Sections 3.2 and 3.3, will effectively guide the troubled person toward awareness.

7.2 RESPONDING TO REQUESTS FOR DIAGNOSIS

Nurses represent a special kind of problem-solving resource. They are seen as being more approachable, more willing to listen, and more accessible than doctors. For these and subtler reasons nurses are often consulted by people in their communities, by colleagues, and by relatives and friends about disturbing symptoms that might signify a health problem. "You're a nurse. What do you think . . ." is an approach that is familiar to all nurses. In responding, the nurse will consider her legal and ethical obligations and liabilities as well as the opportunity presented. It is this latter consideration that is discussed here.

Importance of Exploration

The vast majority of people who informally approach a nurse with a request for help in diagnosing a health problem are in the state of confusion and uncertainty discussed in the preceding section. Characteristically, their description of their experiences is incomplete, vague, somewhat disorganized, and focused on their discomfort rather than on the facts. Although these characteristics help the nurse determine that the person needs help, the description of symptoms is often medically unenlightening. The nurse's usual reaction to such an approach is either to feel annoyed or to feel flattered, and therefore willing to help the person solve the puzzle. Both of these reactions are likely to result in the nurse asking a series of closed questions (see Section 3.3). The answers to these questions give the nurse data that enable *her* to work on the problem, but they do not lead to any greater insight for the troubled person. By not listening fully to the person's perception of the problem before attempting to collect more medical data, the nurse may be led to make baseless assumptions about the problem. The social acceptability factor must also be kept in mind. The person with disturbing symptoms may initially dramatize the physical components of the complaint in order to attract the nurse's attention, even though he knows that this is not necessarily a balanced account of his experience.

It is much more helpful, when asked for diagnosis, to stop, look, and listen, as suggested previously.

> By using open responses that further explore, clarify, and summarize what the person is saying, the nurse has the best chance of helping him identify the true nature of

the problem. The nurse's goal is not to make an accurate medical diagnosis, but to help the person begin to work on his problem.

This kind of implicit acceptance of communication about distress gives the person "permission" to talk about it. Many such situations afford a valuable opportunity to teach: the nurse's acceptance and encouragement help the person learn that early diagnosis of health problems, even when symptoms are relatively minor, is important to responsible self-care.

Involvement of Both Mind and Body in Problems

When hearing the first attempts by a troubled person to describe what he is experiencing, health professionals are struck by the impossibility of clearly differentiating between mind and body. Most vague complaints can be labeled either mental or physical, depending on the listener's orientation. One of the reasons that nurses are consulted informally for diagnosis so frequently is an underlying anxiety about mental illness or fear that if symptoms are suspected as being of psychological origin, they will be considered "silly" or "neurotic" by the medical establishment. Although the symptoms of anxiety are well known, they are often dismissed as unimportant by even well-intentioned health professionals.

Because women are normally more alert to subtle changes in their body functions than are men—probably a result of sociological conditioning as much as biological differences—they become concerned about symptoms when they are still vague and nonspecific. A nurse who is also female is likely to be regarded as psychologically "safe" to talk with and yet able to separate dangerous from inconsequential symptoms. The earlier in its history a health problem is brought to the attention of a health professional, the more difficult it is to separate mind and body components, as the following example demonstrates.

Example 7.3   A PROBLEM OF BOTH MIND AND BODY

Sharon Usher recently presented herself to a large medical clinic with symptoms of early arthritis. She is in her mid-thirties and has an extensive family history of arthritic problems. The results of blood studies done to verify the diagnosis were inconclusive; however, the edema in Sharon's joints was clearly visible, especially in her knees. At one point in her work-up Sharon was sent for a psychiatric consultation. The examining psychiatrist discovered that Sharon had a troubling home situation involving an alcoholic husband. The psychiatrist interpreted Sharon's symptoms as representing her inability to escape from this victimizing home environment. A combination of anti-inflammatory medications and psychological counseling soon eliminated most of Sharon's symptoms, although it was never determined which therapy was more effective.

Regardless of whether the symptoms of distress experienced by a person are physical or psychological in origin, they represent a health problem that the nurse can use her skills to help solve. The first step is to help people learn to *identify problems early*, before they overwhelm the body's defenses. Being willing to listen through a description of symptoms is a major contribution that nurses can make to this educational goal.

Learning to Seek Medical Help

Once a person identifies that what he is experiencing is a departure from normal and a possible problem, he must first understand why it is important to *seek professional help* and then he must be able to approach and effectively use this help. Many people either do not know how to obtain medical care for themselves or their families, are frightened by it, or do not know the words to describe what they are feeling in such a way that they will be heard. These are all areas in which the nurse can contribute positively to learning through spontaneous teaching that is responsive to need. In the following example the mother's lack of effective medical communication skills endangered her young child.

Example 7.4   A PROBLEM OF MEDICAL COMMUNICATION

Dorothy Vickers, a young single mother living in a suburban apartment building with her four-year-old son, was out in the hallway when Don Norris, the night nursing supervisor at a local hospital, came home from work. After a short general conversation, Dorothy told Don that she wasn't sure what to do about her son. She explained that the child had been ill during the night and that she had called the doctor, but he had done nothing. In discussing the situation it became apparent that Dorothy had simply told the doctor that the child had not been feeling well since the evening meal. The doctor had responded by saying that it was probably not serious, but that she should come in if his condition worsened. What she had not told the doctor was that the child had had a temperature of 102°F orally and was complaining of abdominal pain. Resisting the temptation to tell Dorothy that she must take her son to the doctor immediately, Don spent a few minutes reviewing with her the information that the doctor would need once she got there and then helping her understand how important it was that her son get prompt medical attention. Together they planned and rehearsed what she would do and say to get that attention.

In this case example the mother had identified the problem, but when her initial attempt to get help failed, her strengths and resources were inadequate to allow her to cope with the problem in an alternative way. The nurse recognized that the mother needed help with understanding the need for medical care, understanding what the doctor would need to know in order to give that help, and developing some communication skills that would facilitate care. Although these seem to be major learning needs, a few minutes of carefully guided interaction helped the mother meet them in this instance. The nurse risked delaying care for those few minutes of investment in the mother's problem-solving capability, knowing that the effort was likely to save time in the long run.

In summary, when approached for a diagnosis of symptoms, the nurse can help with problem solving by taking the following steps:

1. Through exploration, careful listening, and open questions, help the person identify the nature and extent of the problem facing him.

2. Help the person understand why medical intervention in the early stages of illness is important to his future well-being.

3. Help the person assess his strengths and resources in the light of the demands being placed on him so that he can reach an understanding of the alternatives available.

4. Help the person make a plan for obtaining care, paying special attention to his skills in decision making and communication. Help him develop skills specific to his situation, if necessary.

5. Follow up on the episode to help the person make sense of the experience within his own frame of reference and reflect on how the experience contributed to learning.

The nurse's knowledge of medical care procedures and institutions make her a valuable resource to those in the community who are unable to bridge the gap between acknowledging a health problem and actually getting effective care.

7.3 HANDLING COMPLAINTS AND COMPLEX PROBLEMS

This section deals not only with helping the nurse take advantage of some special opportunities to teach, but also with helping her recognize some limitations that may be experienced. Two categories of requests for help are especially difficult to deal with objectively and creatively: complaints, and complex problems that seem to extend well beyond the present situation in duration and intensity. In both cases the nurse may come on the problem without warning and be expected to make a spontaneous contribution to the problem's solution. One of her most valuable contributions is to help with learning. We will begin by examining these situations separately, and then explore some of their similarities.

Understanding Complaints

We do not usually think of complaints as requests for help by someone who has a learning need. Yet a complaint is not voiced unless there is some expectation on the part of the complainer that something can be done to make his situation better. Nurses often are the recipients of complaints about medical care and medical personnel for some of the same reasons that information and advice are asked of them; nurses are available, approachable, and relatively psychologically "safe." Those who make the complaint may be assertively trying to maintain their rights and dignity or aggressively attempting to get the nurse to take over responsibility for the disturbing incident.

Like other kinds of communication, complaints are made up of both facts and feelings. Complaints are almost always presented as though the overriding feeling is anger and as though the "facts" of the situation are being discussed logically and objectively. The actual feelings being experienced, however, may range from helplessness to fear, from dismay to rage, and the facts are seldom objective. The first challenge for the nurse hearing a complaint is to detect something of the real situation underlying the public statement. She can do this most effectively through the stop-look-listen behavior described earlier. Stopping to pay attention to the communication is the first step, then looking for nonverbal behavior that may give some evidence of the underlying feelings being experienced, and finally listening carefully to the words to untangle the messages being communicated.

An important second step in handling a complaint is to acknowledge what the person is trying to say (Bramson, 1981, Chap. 3). This may be done by restating the main message. Rather than apologize or agree that it is a disturbing situation, the nurse might start her restatement by saying, "Then what you're saying is . . ." and then proceed to include both the facts and the feelings of the complaint. It is important to give specific verbal feedback that the listener is actually hearing the complaint.

No matter how legitimate, many complaints are met by impatience, patronizing dismissal, or physical avoidance. These negative behaviors increase the level of frustration and anger and reinforce the complainer's opinion that "no one cares." The angrier a person becomes, the less objective he is and the less he is able to problem solve effectively. Positive listening behavior on the part of the nurse reassures the person that his complaint is being heard, usually decreases the component of anger markedly, and is much more likely to result in problem solving.

If the nurse is going to contribute to the problem solution and use the opportunity she has to help the person learn, she must avoid becoming part of the problem. It is easy to become entangled in a problem by giving well-intentioned advice that makes the nurse responsible for the outcome, or by offering to intervene, or by apologizing and thereby accepting part of the blame. It is especially important to avoid involvement in the problem when the complaint is about the behavior of others. Presented with this kind of complaint, the nurse must first ask herself: "Whose problem is this?" When the complaint is on the behalf of other people, it is often useful to help the complainer clarify just how he is affected by the problem (see Elgin, 1983).

Suppose a patient's wife comes to a nurse with the complaint that "Ms. Jones is so impatient and abrupt with my husband." After listening carefully and restating the complaint, the nurse might ask the wife, "How is the nurse's behavior affecting you?" taking care that this is not said in an aggressive, confronting manner. The point is that the nurse can only hope to help with the problem of the person she is talking with, not that of a third or fourth party. Once the nurse helps the wife identify that she is irritated by the nurse's behavior and feels that it demeans her husband, then the wife's problem can be worked on. The wife may decide to talk with her husband about his feelings or possibly confront Ms. Jones about how the behavior is affecting her. Having been helped to shift her attention from solving someone else's problem to solving her own problem, some progress can be made.

Complaints are requests for help with problems that are generating anger, frustration, and increased stress. By actively listening to the complaint, the nurse helps to reduce the stress level. She then can help the person with problem solving, which includes the goals of awareness, understanding, constructive action, and learning.

Understanding Complex Problems

As discussed in Section 3.1, people seldom have simple, straightforward problems with which they need help. Rather, human problems tend to be complicated by strong emotions, a range of needs, and the involvement of other people. A medical problem superimposed on other life difficulties may push a person into a state of crisis. In his distress he may well reach out to a nurse, who he sees as a source of strength and caring. Like the case discussed in Example 7.1, the initial presentation of a problem to the nurse may be only the "tip of the iceberg." The troubled person may take care to phrase his difficulty in such a way as to be interesting and acceptable to the nurse in order to motivate her helping. The challenge for the nurse is to discover the true nature of the problem, or problems, and realistically assess her ability to help. As discussed several times now, a stop-look-listen behavior helps the nurse begin this procedure. Once the exploration process is established, the nurse can begin to clarify the meanings and messages behind the presented problem.

> In assessing her capabilities and limitations in helping with a problem, the nurse can be partially guided by two aspects of the problem situation: its duration and its intensity.

Duration has to do with the time interval involved. Relevant questions in determining duration are:

- How long has the *need* been unmet?
- How long have *stressors* persisted, and how long will they continue?
- How long have skills or *strengths* been lacking?
- Will social supports or *resources* become available in the near future?

If the nurse is already familiar with using the Health Balance model in patient assessment (Section 4.1), these questions will be easy to remember, even when she is surprised by a request for help.

The second aspect of a problem situation to be assessed is its intensity (Waring and McLennan, 1979). Remembering that a person experiencing a problem will probably not seek help with it unless he perceives it as extraordinarily intense, the nurse will be aided by estimating intensity from as objective a standpoint as possible. Relevant questions in determining intensity are:

- How severely out of *balance* are strengths and resources with needs and stressors?
- To what *extent* is the problem situation affecting other areas of life?
- How severely is *behavior* being affected by the problem?

The interaction between these two aspects of a problem situation are also important. The more intense and pervasive the disturbance to the health balance and the longer the time interval during which the imbalance has or will operate, the more likely it is that special help will be required. The nurse can do no harm by listening and exploring the problem situation with the person up to the point of determining whether her capabilities, time, and resources are adequate. If she should then find that the problem is so intense, of such long duration, or otherwise so complex that she thinks that special help is necessary, she can offer the person valuable assistance with motivation to seek such help. The following case is an example of a situation in which the nurse found that special help was needed.

Example 7.5   UPSETTING EVENT MASKS LONG-TERM PROBLEM

Cris Olson, head nurse on the surgical unit, first met Mr. and Mrs. West when she was doing her morning rounds. Ray West had been admitted to the unit the previous evening after his left arm had nearly been severed in an industrial accident. Aside from being in a great deal of pain, he was in stable condition. Connie West had apparently not left the hospital until late the previous evening and then returned early in the morning.

An hour or so after their initial meeting, Connie West appeared in the doorway of Cris's office, saying in an anxious manner that she just had to talk to someone and asking to come in. Cris put aside her paperwork, expecting to listen to and then reassure Connie about her husband's condition. Instead, Connie said: "I'm so worried about my daughter. I just don't know what to do!" There followed the story of how Mr. West and their 17-year-old daughter had had another in a long series of heated arguments three nights ago. It ended with the daughter gathering up an armload of belongings and leaving the house with her boyfriend, threatening never to return. She had not been in touch with her parents since. Connie West had contacted the police but had been told that, although they would look for the girl, they could not force her to return home.

It soon became obvious to Cris that the departure of the daughter so occupied Connie that she found it difficult to do more than tell and retell the events. Initially, Cris assumed that the girl's whereabouts was the major concern and inquired about what action had been taken other than contacting the police. Although Connie reported that she knew the boyfriend's parents and a number of her daughter's friends, whom she called "druggies," none of them had been contacted. She ended the session with Cris by saying that she might call some of them, but Cris doubted that she would.

The next morning Connie was again at her husband's bedside when Cris made rounds and again she came to Cris's office shortly thereafter. Once more she told and retold the story of the argument and the daughter's departure. With each retelling Mr. West's part in the drama was described as more violent and more unreasonable. At one point Connie suggested that her husband's accident was God's way of punishing him for his abuse of their daughter. It became increasingly clear to Cris that at least verbal battles had been part of Mr. and Mrs. West's relationship for a long time. Although she was certainly upset over her daughter's disappearance and her husband's accident, Connie seemed to see it as reinforcement of her view that her husband was an unreasonable man, given to fits of anger. She seemed so overwhelmed by events that, although she wanted to talk about them, she seemed unable to think through them or plan constructive action. Testing her hypothesis, Cris said to Connie: "You and your husband seem to have had some difficulty for a long time." Connie's response was to remain silent for a long moment, fidgeting nervously, and then to reply: "Yeh. Yeh, we have."

Cris could see that real help for the Wests would involve a time commitment and marriage counseling skills beyond her resources. The duration and present level of intensity of their problems suggested that their complex problems would take professional help. In the throes of the current crisis, however, she could see an opportunity to assist them in getting to another source of help. Her first step in this direction was to tell Connie that they had a staff psychologist who consulted with the nurses on a regular basis. She asked her permission to discuss their situation with him. Connie readily agreed to this. After the consultation Cris was able to report that the psychologist's opinion was that counseling could help them work through their problems. Connie not only agreed to meet with him to discuss resources and the likely goals of counseling, but also rewarded Cris with a rare smile and a warm "thank you."

Over the next several days Connie regularly stopped at Cris's office to talk, but she seemed a little less anxious. She reported that she liked the psychologist and that he was being helpful in suggesting how and where they could get extended help with their problems. She had been able to tell her husband that she thought they needed help, and even though he was not enthusiastic, he had agreed to "give it a try."

In this case example the nurse was presented with a complex set of problems. She was initially alerted to this complexity by Connie West's verbal behavior and by the confusingly mixed messages she seemed to be sending. As their interaction continued, the nurse was able to assess something of the duration and intensity of the problems confronting this couple and decide that they would need special help to find solutions. By recognizing the opportunity she had to help them learn how to get effective help, the nurse made a real contribution to this family's health.

Some Common Aspects of Complaints and Complex Problems

So far in this section we have suggested that careful listening, clarification, and assessment are appropriate first steps for the nurse presented with either complaints or complex problems. These requests for help share a number of commonalities aside from the nurse's initial behavior. One of these is that they both reflect *high stress levels or crisis*. The closer the troubled person is to crisis, the more he will want to "get rid" of the problem by having someone else take responsibility. One of the reasons nurses often have difficulty handling these kinds of requests for help is the underlying pressure for them to "take over." Appeals are made to their kindness, efficiency, and professional obligations. Even if he is not actively trying to get the nurse to solve the problem for him, a person in crisis is vulnerable to the influence of advice or suggestions. As discussed previously, advice can be harmful in such circumstances, since it leads a person away from, rather than toward, self-responsibility.

Occasionally the nurse encounters a person who seems to be trapped in a kind of crisis "cycle." His life is presented as being filled with dramatic crises from which he never quite recovers before being struck with another series. Indeed it does appear that some people develop special skills, although not very effective ones, for coping with crises. These skills usually include pleas for help to others willing to take over some of the responsibility for their woes. When confronted by a person who has suffered many crises over a long period, the nurse can suspect a seriously entrenched and complex problem. The most effective assistance she can offer is to help the person seek and accept the special help he needs to overcome this self-destructive cycle.

A variation of the person caught in a cycle of crises is the constant complainer. This person often feels helpless in his situation and uses complaints as a strategy for exercising some fleeting control over his life. Being ignored or placated reinforces his internal view that he is a helpless victim and makes him even angrier. Once again, really trying to hear what this person is saying, giving him feedback, and focusing on the needs that his complaints represent give the nurse the best chance of breaking through the complainer's hostile and defensive shield.

Sometimes *manipulation*, an attempt to control the behavior of the nurse in the person's behalf, is also a component of complaints or complex problems. When the nurse feels that she is being pressured into taking a specific action *for* the person, her best course is to confront the issue, saying, for example: "You seem to want me to talk to the doctor for you. I don't feel that I can do that, but I will help you decide how you can find out what you want to know." This kind of statement allows the person to know the limits of the help the nurse is willing to offer.

Finally, when presented with either a complaint or a complex problem, it is all right for the nurse to *delay* her attempt to hear the details of the problem situation. Careful listening is so important to the nurse's ability to help and teach that it may be necessary to put the problem on "hold" until adequate time is available for effective, uninterrupted listening. This can be done without alienating the troubled person by acknowledging the importance that he attaches to this difficulty and suggesting a specific time that the nurse will be available to listen fully.

In summary, complaints and complex problems have been discussed as representing special requests for the nurse's help. By giving the troubled person careful attention, the nurse can begin to assess the problem behind the angry feelings or the distortions of a crisis response. Her estimate of the duration and intensity of the underlying problem will guide her in setting realistic goals and offering appropriate help with problem solving and learning.

7.4 TEACHING WITHOUT PREPARATION

Questions, requests for advice or diagnosis, and even complaints are appeals for help. As such, they represent a need to learn. The learning need may range from minor pieces of information to complex skills, from conceptual understanding of a disease process to improved self-esteem. Sometimes the request for help comes from the confusion and uncertainty that precedes full awareness of a problem, and at other times it represents substantial progress toward problem solution.

All requests for help are opportunities to help with learning. They reflect a person's immediate interests, concerns, and needs and are therefore ideal starting points for effective teaching.

Whether or not the nurse chooses to use the opportunity to teach spontaneously, she should give attention to the subject of concern to the patient, since this will guide her teaching intervention whenever it occurs.

The skills for effective spontaneous teaching include the ability to assess the person and the problem situation quickly and accurately and the ability to connect her immediate response to the person's previous knowledge and to future problem solving. These skills demand that the nurse maintain perspective about how her answer to a question or response to a complaint fits in with the larger problem that these requests represent. In the following paragraphs we will discuss the skills of spontaneous teaching in more detail, using the Nursing Process steps of assessment, planning, and implementation as our framework.

Assessment

The best preparation for effective spontaneous teaching with a patient is to have completed a full patient assessment soon after admission to the facility. By becoming familiar with the details of his health balance, the nurse will be able to anticipate patient learning needs. When he begins to ask questions about his care or condition, this can be interpreted by the nurse as evidence of his motivation to begin the learning process. Her immediate response can then easily be directed toward meeting the already identified learning objectives and contributing to a larger learning program. Similarly, questions asked by the patient's family members are understandable in a larger context if the nurse is familiar with the patient's health balance.

Anticipation of needs based on a complete assessment does not mean that the nurse can safely make assumptions about the person's current interests or concerns. She must still stop, look, and listen carefully to determine the feelings and real messages behind his words.

Sometimes an opportunity to teach informally occurs without benefit of a previously completed assessment. In such instances the nurse's communication skills, sensitivity, and ability to assess problem situations quickly and accurately will be put to the test. The skills she has developed in making full patient assessments are useful in these instances, too, but cannot be used at the same depth. If a full assessment is like a color picture of the patient, showing many details of his world, the assessment that is possible in informal teaching situations is only a sketchy line drawing with few details. The nurse who has developed expertise at making patient assessments will be aware of how little information she has in informal teaching situations and will therefore not make any assumptions about the person's needs until she is able to clarify and confirm them.

Planning

At the same time the nurse is assessing a person's learning need in response to a request for help, she is planning how to approach the subject of concern.

Her ability to define objectives and organize material quickly is a challenge that makes spontaneous teaching especially enjoyable for many nurses.

> The key to effective informal teaching in which only minimal planning can be done is to help the person form connections with what he already knows and what he can use for problem solving in the future.

Previous patient assessment gives the nurse the background to be able to refer to prior experience and learning while anticipating how the person might make use of new learning in problem solving. She might use a patient's question to stimulate motivation for learning in a planned teaching session. Even when the nurse has no background information about the person requesting help, she can form a bridge between prior learning and experience and his current interest. After carefully listening to his request for help, she might inquire what it is that concerns him. When she finds out something about the nature of the problem, she might then ask what he already knows about the subject before proceeding. The time that it takes to be sure that one offers only appropriate help usually saves time in the long run and certainly improves the reward for both teacher and learner. As an example, consider the following simple exchange.

Example 7.6   ASKING DIRECTIONS TO THE LAB

PATIENT: Can you tell me how to get to the lab?

NURSE: (*Noting the person's anxious behavior*) Of course. Which lab are you looking for?

PATIENT: I don't know. They told me in the clinic to go have some blood taken and give this to them (*pointing to the pink requisition he was holding*).

NURSE: You want the clinic lab then. Have you been to the Medical Center before?

PATIENT: No. This is the first time.

NURSE: It's a little hard to find your way around at first. Do you know where the main clinic entrance is?

PATIENT: Yes. That's the way I came in. I know where that is.

NURSE: Good. Go to the clinic entrance. You'll see a sign that says "Clinic Lab" next to the elevators. Follow the arrow . . . (*telling him simply how to proceed*). You will get attention more promptly if you take that pink slip to the receptionist in the blue uniform right away.

Most people can recall an incident in which they asked for directions only to be given an impatient gesture, unintelligibly complex instructions, or directions to the wrong place. Although asking for directions does not seem like a typical opportunity for spontaneous teaching, the nurse in the example above used principles of good communication and teaching to help the patient learn how to get to the lab. She first clarified just what he was asking for. Next, she found out about his present level of knowledge and experience. Using this information, she directed him simply and offered the additional suggestion about getting attention. This suggestion was not offered as advice, but as a piece of information that was specific and included the reason for the suggested behavior. The nurse planned her response even as she was collecting enough assessment data to estimate his need.

Implementation

The choice of teaching strategy and materials is limited when one is unable to prepare ahead of time. Sometimes teachers limit themselves more than they need to; however, the most frequently used strategy for spontaneous teaching is explanation. When asked a question, it seems natural to respond with an explanation. To do so, however, treats the piece of information as though obtaining it were an end in itself, rather than part of a larger human concern, an attempt to solve a problem and a teaching opportunity. As in the case of Mrs. Thomas (Example 7.1), simply explaining when and where prenatal classes were held would have done little to solve her problem of anxiety and concern about her pregnancy.

> Explanation, the most commonly used strategy for responding to a request for information, can be much more effective if the nurse first assesses the need and plans the information to be offered.

Whenever a request for help has a greater component of feeling than of fact, or when the person is in a state of uncertainty and confusion and is himself unclear about the nature of his request, discussion is a more effective teaching strategy than explanation. By stopping, looking, and listening carefully to the person's request, the nurse has already initiated exploration of the problem. If the person is to be helped to reach the goal of awareness, he must be helped to talk about the problem. Through discussion, the nurse facilitates this process.

> Discussion is the initial strategy of choice whether the request for help is for advice, diagnosis, help with a complex problem, or a complaint. Through discussion, the nurse gathers data on which to base an assessment, plan a realistic approach, and get the person started on exploration.

Sometimes a request for help involves a manual skill or a procedure. The nurse may choose to simply explain the steps involved, but teaching will be more effective if she can show the person how to do it. Remember, however, that demonstrations are only as effective as the skill of the demonstrator and the availability of appropriate equipment (see Section 5.4). When teaching of this sort is spontaneous, these factors need to be carefully considered before choosing a demonstration strategy. If the procedure is simple and one with which the nurse is comfortably familiar, such as use of the call light, demonstration is the teaching strategy of choice. In order for it to be effective, time must be allowed for a return demonstration, practice, and coaching. If the procedure is complex and there is no available time for coaching, or the skills of the nurse are in doubt, or proper equipment is not readily available, use of this teaching strategy should be delayed until it can be included in a planned and thoroughly prepared teaching session.

Of the experiential teaching strategies, behavior rehearsal is by far the most useful in spontaneous teaching situations. If the informal teaching involves a person with whom the nurse has not had the chance to develop a relationship of trust, it is especially important that this strategy be introduced without any hint of condescension. Practicing in front of someone you know and trust is much less threatening than practicing in front of someone you do not know and have little reason to trust except in a general way. For example, after a discussion of the questions a patient might want to ask his doctor, the nurse might say: "Okay, let's go through the list of questions you want to ask once more," rather than "Now you tell me just what you're going to say to the doctor." In the first statement the nurse invites participation in the review, whereas in the second she demands performance. If introduced so as not to threaten the learner, behavior rehearsal can be extremely effective in helping a person take control of a situation, thereby increasing his self-esteem and sense of self-responsibility.

Even in the most impromptu of informal teaching situations, teaching materials can be included by the creative nurse teacher. Written materials such as pamphlets or instructions are often readily available, especially if the nurse has anticipated the patient's concern about a subject. As discussed in Section 6.1, written materials cannot effectively stand alone as a teaching method without verbal preparation, including explanation and discussion. The need for the nurse's attention to the individualization of written materials is no different in spontaneous teaching than it is in prepared teaching.

Probably the most useful teaching method in informal teaching is the diagram or drawing.

> Showing a person a picture or drawing a quick line sketch to accompany an explanation is effective because including visual as well as verbal channels of learning improves memory and comprehension.

The diagram or drawing need not be a work of art; the fact that it is immediate and a visual representation of the concept or idea being discussed is more important than its beauty.

Audiovisual and self-paced learning programs have limited usefulness as part of the teaching response to a request for help. If a question leads to further planned teaching, such a program can be a kind of learning bridge that prepares the learner for the more extensive teaching session. Without adequate preparation and follow-up, however, films, videos, and programmed learning are limited in effectiveness no matter when they are used. As discussed in Sections 6.3 and 6.4, such programs tend to be general. When responding to a spontaneous teaching opportunity, the nurse teacher would prefer to relate to the immediate interest and concern of the person by making her teaching specific and personally relevant to the learner.

In summary, assessment, planning, and implementation have been reviewed in this section as they apply to spontaneous teaching opportunities. The actions of the effective nurse teacher in approaching such an opportunity can be summarized in the following four steps:

1. Stop, look and listen.
2. Assess learning needs and realistic goals.
3. Anticipate needs and prepare when possible.

4. Connect new learning to past and future.

Many spontaneous teaching opportunities can be usefully responded to by acknowledging the person's concern and then delaying teaching until time is available and preparations have been made. Although questions and other requests for help indicate the person's motivation to learn, it is better to risk a slight decrease in enthusiasm for the subject by delaying teaching than it is to make an incomplete or insensitive attempt to help the person learn. In practical terms this means that if the nurse does not have time to listen carefully and teach effectively at the moment, she can tell the person that she hears his concern and when he can expect her to return.

Spontaneous or informal teaching makes up in immediacy what it lacks in preparation. It challenges the nurse's sensitivity to human needs as well as her teaching skills. It is one of the most important vehicles the nurse has available for helping others learn.

SUMMARY

In this chapter a number of different kinds of requests for help and the nurse's possible spontaneous teaching responses have been discussed. These have included requests for information, advice, or diagnosis; complaints; and requests for help with complex problem situations. Many such requests arise out of a person's state of uncertainty and confusion, which precedes actual problem solving. The nurse can help such a person by assisting him to explore the situation so that he can reach awareness of the true nature of the problem. As a way of assessing a person's learning need and as a method of facilitating beginning exploration, the nurse first needs to *stop* and pay attention to the person, *look* for nonverbal communication, and *listen* for the facts and feelings behind the request for help. Even as she is making an assessment of the learner's needs, she can begin to plan her teaching intervention.

In order for informal teaching to be effective in helping a person meet learning needs, connections need to be formed between what is already known, the new learning, and the ways in which this new learning can be used to solve the problem of concern. Helping to make these connections clearly and relevantly is a major challenge in spontaneous teaching. The skills that the nurse needs in order to use the many opportunities she has to teach informally are best developed through carrying out the steps of planned teaching. The skills of assessment are especially important because they help to develop the nurse's alertness to a person's perceptions of the problem behind a request for help.

The reader is encouraged to do some of the activities suggested in the Study Questions and Exercises section that follows. These will help the nurse more clearly identify opportunities to teach spontaneously and sharpen her skills in responding in ways that do indeed help people learn.

Study Questions and Exercises

For each of the situations described in exercises 1 through 3, note your immediate feeling reaction to the request for help and then decide what actions you would take, including your actual words to the person. Discuss your answers with your classmates or colleagues, role playing the situations if possible and allowing several people to respond. Discuss similarities and differences in approach.

1. Information and advice

- A patient who is recovering well after a hysterectomy says to you: "They were just in here to take more blood from me. Why are they doing that?"
- The same surgical patient later remarks: "You know, the most pain I have is way over here on my left side. What would they have done to me over there?"
- The patient's husband stops you at the desk and asks: "How limited is she going to be when she comes home?"
- A patient recently diagnosed as having emphysema asks you: "Do you think I should get another opinion about this?"
- A neighbor says to you: "My son Scott (a 12-year-old) is getting to be such a discipline problem. He won't listen to me or his father. What do you think we should do?"

2. Diagnosis.

- A nursing colleague says to you: "I'm so tired lately. I go to bed early and I still wake up tired. Do you think something's wrong with me?"
- A patient at a prenatal clinic, her 6-year-old daughter accompanying her, says to you: "Look at these red spots on Shelley's legs. She's had them for a week now. What do you think they are?"
- A friend in her early twenties says to you: "I don't know why I can't lose weight. I hardly eat anything. Not only do I not lose, but I feel bloated all the time. Do you think I have a hormone problem?"

3. Complaints.

- A patient remarks to you: "That night nurse is enough to make me want to sign myself out of here! I no sooner get to sleep than she wakes me up and wants to take my blood pressure. Then half an hour later she comes in and bangs equipment around. Between her coming in here all the time and my roommate making noise I'm not getting any rest at all."
- The daughter of an elderly patient tells you: "Momma's robe has disappeared again. I don't know what you people do with patients' personal belongings; do you take them home or something?"
- A doctor says to you: "I left orders yesterday that Mrs. Brown was to be gotten out of bed and helped to walk. She's lying there in bed now and says she hasn't been up at all. What's going on around here?"

4. Think of someone you know whom you regard as having (or had in the past) a complex problem situation. A social, marital, emotional, or medical problem, or combination of problems, may have been involved. Analyze the problem situation using the questions suggested in Section 7.3 to determine its duration and intensity. What kind(s) of help did this person need? What kind of help did he get? What do you think he learned from his experience? Discuss your analysis with colleagues or classmates.

5. Ask three persons for the same item of information or advice. How did they respond? Was their response helpful? Discuss your experiences with classmates or colleagues.

6. Keep a log for several days of requests for your help. Pick out several to analyze.

Who made the request? What type of request was it? What is your assessment of the person's learning need? How did you reach this conclusion? At what stage of personal problem solving was this person? How did you respond to the request? Discuss your experiences with colleagues or classmates.

7. Practice using the four steps in effective spontaneous teaching described on pages 188 and 189. Keep anecdotal notes periodically for several weeks about the teaching opportunities you identify. Review these notes. What progress have you made in your ability to identify opportunities, to stop, look, and listen first, to offer appropriate help? Discuss some of the situations with classmates or colleagues.

8. Review the initial patient assessment of a patient for whom you are caring, including his anticipated learning needs. Be on the alert for opportunities to teach spontaneously while caring for him. How are these experiences different from informal teaching you have not anticipated? Were you able to effectively connect the spontaneous teaching you did with previous knowledge and also planned patient teaching?

8

WHEN AND HOW TO USE LEARNING GROUPS

In this chapter we will depart from our focus on individual teaching in order to consider learning groups and their place in patient education.* Our major concern will be with small, interactive learning groups of three to twelve participants. We will initially review the dynamics of group learning and then proceed to the practicalities of how the nurse can plan, organize, and lead such a group. In the final section we will explore some different types of groups in the community and how the nurse might refer people to these for help with special kinds of learning needs.

The main points contained in this chapter are as follows:

- Small groups are effective settings for learning when attitude change, adjustments in life-style, and mutual support and encouragement are important aspects of learning goals. (Introduction)
- Group functions include concerns about accomplishment of tasks or goals and maintenance of positive interpersonal relationships between members. (Section 8.1)
- Groups progress through a predictable series of stages in reaching effective problem solving. (Section 8.1)
- The most successful groups are composed of members who have been selected for their similarity of learning objectives but diversity of experience. (Section 8.2)
- Organizational tasks to be completed before group meetings begin include arrangement of a room and needed equipment, determination of when and

---

*I am indebted to James P. McLennan, Counseling Psychologist, who has contributed his knowledge of group theory and expertise in group leadership to the writing of these pages.

how long the group is to meet, and notification of group members. (Section 8.2)
- The way in which a group is structured and conducted is determined by the category and complexity of its learning objectives. (Section 8.3)
- Whatever teaching strategy is used first in a group meeting will set the tone for group expectations and conduct thereafter. (Section 8.3)
- Community groups that may provide a valuable resource to patients and family members include community learning programs, self-help groups, and health service groups. (Section 8.4)
- Introducing a person to a representative of the community group to which he is to be referred means that he is helped to develop a personal relationship that will aid motivation to participate. (Section 8.4)

We all belong to a wide range of groups: work groups, family groups, interest groups, and social groups.

> A group is more than a collection of individuals; it is people in frequent face-to-face interaction who share a purpose or goal and whose behavior is guided by a set of roles and shared values.

Groups can be a powerful influence on the behavior of individual members. The degree of influence exerted by a group depends on how closely identified a person is with group values and beliefs and to what extent a person sees his personal needs met by the group.

For most people the group that has the most impact is the immediate family. This is the group with which a person is most likely to share values as well as a history of interaction and a bond of mutual caring. Groups that are organized to meet particular learning needs can also have considerable influence on an individual and lead to changes in behavior. Although most patient teaching occurs in one-to-one interaction, there are numerous instances when the powerful influence of the group is most effective in reaching learning goals. The nurse teacher with interest and skills in group leadership will find many opportunities to use groups to help her patients fulfill a range of needs.

In some ways today's medical care makes using groups to meet some learning needs even more attractive than it has been in the past. Patients in our medical facilities are more acutely ill when they arrive but stay for a shorter time than in past years. As one nurse recently put it: "We used to admit people when they were sick and send them home well. Now we admit people who are sicker and send them home still sick!" The implications of this trend are far-reaching. Seriously ill patients who have not fully recovered by the time they are discharged are likely to be undergoing an emotional as well as physical crisis. Because of pain, anxiety, and medications, their mental acuity may well be impaired during almost all of the time they are patients, making them less able to concentrate on details. Learning needs in these situations will be related to resolution of crises, basic information about the disease process, and beginning understanding and acceptance of events.

At the same time as these changes in medical care are affecting the patient, families have the burden of caring for the patient when he arrives home, still unable to adequately care for himself. Family members must therefore learn care procedures that would formerly have been done by hospital staff. In addition, family members must learn how to help the patient recover mentally and emotionally as well as physically. The combination of less available staff time, increased need to help family members learn how to care for patients at home, the increased psychosocial needs of patients, and a priority on reducing costs makes group approaches a viable alternative to individual teaching.

The first step toward making effective use of learning groups is to recognize the relative advantages and disadvantages of group and individual methods of helping with learning. Teaching that involves only one or two learners is the most common setting for teaching intervention by the nurse. The key to the success of individual teaching methods is the continuing feedback available from the learner.

> Helping with learning on a one-to-one basis has the advantage of continuing interaction and feedback, which makes the nurse constantly aware of the person's needs and progress and allows her to modify the structure, content, and presentation of material accordingly.

Because individual teaching activities are often embedded in other care activities, the length of time spent in explaining, coaching, reinforcing, and discussing a subject is variable, depending on need and progress. The evaluation of the success of various teaching strategies is immediate, so that the nurse is likely to feel rewarded for her efforts and motivated to continue trying to help with learning and problem solving. Individual teaching is most appropriate when learning needs involve complex skills and a unique combination of knowledge and attitudes, or when barriers to learning demand individual attention. Although the commitment of staff time, and therefore cost, is relatively high, so is the potential quality of learning that results.

The immediacy of feedback and personal attention to learning needs that characterizes one-to-one teaching is necessarily reduced in a learning group, even in one of only three to five persons. A group does, however, have some advantages that surpass individual approaches.

> Learning groups have the advantage of providing motivation, encouragement, support, and a wealth of models and resources to its members.

The advantages that groups have over individual teaching are related to the kind of support that people give one another when striving together to meet shared goals. The resulting interpersonal relationships give a person a strong sense of acceptance and belonging that can stimulate new motivation to overcome setbacks and solve problems. Group approaches are especially effective when the teaching-learning process is influenced by a sense of demoralization owing to a crisis situation, feelings of social alienation, or pressure to change major attitudes, values, and life-styles (Garvin, 1981). In addition to offering support and stimulating motivation for change, groups can provide valuable information for coping with a condition on a practical, day-to-day basis that one nurse teacher unaffected by the disorder herself cannot hope to equal.

The intent of this chapter is to help the nurse learn how to take the communication and relationship skills that are the basis of effective individual teaching and extend them to effective group leadership. We will first explore some of the basic principles of group dynamics and then show how these can be applied to planning, organizing, and leading learning groups. Finally, we will discuss some of the different kinds of community groups to which the nurse may refer patients and their families for continued learning.

8.1 HOW GROUPS PROMOTE LEARNING

Human beings are social animals; they live, work, and solve the problems of daily life in conjunction with others. Their preferences, choices, and actions bring change to others in their social worlds. If a person facing alterations in his physical, emotional, and spiritual functioning is to come to terms with reality in the broadest sense, he must do so within the context of his social environment. (See Section 2.4 for a discussion of the social and cultural aspects of learning.) The opportunity to meet the realities, identify the problems, and learn to change within a group setting helps him begin the process of well-balanced adaptation.

The nurse teacher may consider initiating such group learning opportunities whenever she identifies learning needs that are shared by several people. Participants in such a group may consist of several members of the same family, a group of patients, or a combination of patients and family members. The nurse may be the leader or facilitator of the group, or this role may be shared with other resource people. In this section the dynamic process that occurs in all groups and that can promote learning, problem solving, and behavior change is discussed in detail.

Characteristics of Groups

In order to understand how groups operate, it is important to recognize some of the characteristics that all kinds of groups have in common (see Douglas, 1979).

> Whatever its size, all groups have two basic and simultaneous concerns. One of these relates to the accomplishment of common goals or tasks, and the other has to do with the maintenance of the group as a functioning entity.

Some groups, such as staff meetings, action committees, or large classes, place a priority on task accomplishment; their purpose is to reach a goal or complete an assignment. Although the task involved is the most obvious concern, even these groups perform group maintenance functions in the form of being courteous to one another, obeying prescribed rules of protocol, and demonstrating their involvement in the subject through facial expression and other forms of nonverbal behavior. These actions ensure that the individuals in the group will continue to participate until the task is completed.

At the other end of the spectrum of group functioning, therapy groups or "encounter" groups seem almost totally devoted to group maintenance. The focus of their activities is on building personal, supportive, and caring relationships between members. Although sometimes overshadowed by the relationship aspects of group process, these groups also have a task or goal. The goal may be, for example, to help individuals become more in touch with their own strengths and needs by revealing themselves to others. Without the underlying current of some specific goals, these and all other kinds of groups would falter and die of lack of a sense of progress.

Learning groups such as those initiated by a nurse typically fall between these two extremes; task and maintenance functions have equal importance. The goal must be clearly identified, understood, and accepted as being personally relevant by each group member in order to motivate his willing participation. At the same time it is the interpersonal relationships that develop between members, forming a bond of mutual concern, that give learning groups their supportive strength (Waring and McLennan, 1979).

> Effective problem solving is usually the result of a combination of knowledge, attitudes, and skills. Learning groups facilitate these practical combinations and help members carry out constructive action by balancing group task and maintenance functions.

Stages of the Group Process

Given time, all groups progress through a number of predictable stages in their path toward accomplishing their intended goals. Although theorists differ in the terminology used for identifying these stages, the idea that a progression takes place in group development is commonly held. For example, Tuckman (1965) identified four stages, which he called "forming," "storming," "norming," and "performing." Social worker Helen Northen (1976) added a fifth stage which she called a "termination" stage. Whatever one chooses to call them, groups do progress through stages not unlike those identified by Carkhuff for personal problem solving (see Section 7.1). Groups as well as individuals approach a problem situation in a state of some uncertainty and confusion. It requires time and effort to be able to identify problems and priorities and to begin to formulate a plan of action. Only then can problem solving and learning take place. In the following paragraphs we will discuss each of the stages of the group problem-solving process even while recognizing that the stages described tend to overlap and blend with one another in actual group development.

Group Formation

Group formation, the first stage of a group's progression toward problem solving, strongly resembles Carkhuff's first goal of "awareness." In it a number of individuals who may well be confused and uncertain because of a troubling problem situation decide to come together and work on the problem for their mutual gain. In order for a group to develop out of a collection of individuals, each person must be convinced of the *potential benefit* that the group has for his own personal problem. The goals and purposes of the group must therefore be clear before individuals will choose to expend time and effort in participation.

Once group members are actually together in the same room, some ground rules are quickly established that dictate acceptable behavior within the group. The nurse can facilitate this early group development by helping participants talk about their expectations and their view of group goals. By providing some *structure* for the group's early activities and allowing them to focus on tasks and goals, the nurse gives a sense of direction and purpose to the group. Without some structure, most learning groups find it difficult to form a commitment to problem solving or to one another.

Initially, the individuals coming together in a small group usually share a sense of eager anticipation because of the group's promised rewards as well as some anxiety owing to the situation's unfamiliarity. A major challenge of group leadership is to help group members build on their positive anticipation while decreasing negative anxiety. Helping people become aware of what they can realistically gain through group participation is certainly one step in this direction. If people are going to stay with the group and allow a commitment to develop, two other conditions must be met. Individuals need to feel that they have something *in common* with other group members and they need to feel that they are recognized as *unique* individuals with their own needs, by the group leader and by one or two other group members.

> A combination of willingness to form bonds of mutual interest with others while maintaining one's own individuality characterizes group interaction throughout its development, but it is especially obvious and important during the earliest stages of group formation.

The length of time necessary for this first stage depends on the diversity of interests and concerns represented by group members and their combination of personalities. A carefully selected group of people who share a problem of importance to each of them will proceed through this stage quickly, taking only an hour or so to begin to develop a group identity. A very large, very diverse, or very task-oriented group will be slow to emerge from this stage.

Assessment and Testing

Once individual participants begin to feel as though they are members of the group and have a commitment to it, a stage of further assessment and some testing begins. Group goals are further explored and clarified during this time (see Garvin, 1981), but the major "work" of the group concerns the growing relationships between members. During this period group members seek to know and be known by other participants, to reach a clearer understanding of their own needs and those needs shared by the group. As interaction patterns begin to be established, it sometimes seems to group leaders that little progress is being made toward group goals. Groups need this period to establish interpersonal relationships between people, however, before they are able to move on with task functions. A group prevented from doing this finds it impossible to solve problems together.

During the assessment and testing stage, group members typically verbalize their concerns and beliefs. These exchanges allow members to assess the strengths, resources, needs, and weaknesses of other members and to form early identifications with some of them. People also attempt to measure themselves and their perception of their own needs against those of the majority of the group. By sharing their opinions and concerns they also "test" to what extent they will be accepted by others in active group membership.

People often "try out" group roles during this time. The roles they play within the group may not be ones that the nurse might anticipate from knowing the person on an individual basis. Sometimes people who are normally quiet take a leadership role in a group, and those who seem unaware of others' feelings may take it on themselves to consistently give encouragement and support to others.

In the process of assessment and testing, sometimes a conflict of attitudes or values arises. Although it may be upsetting to the leader to have conflict, it is a normal part of the group process. The nurse can help the group toward a resolution by acknowledging each individual as entitled to his views, trying to help the conflicting parties hear each other out, and not taking sides on issues.

> One important outcome of most successful small learning groups is the improved ability of members to accept points of view different from their own as having validity and merit.

The length of time needed by a group for the assessment and testing phase of group development will depend on the projected length of time the group will be meeting together and the complexity of group goals. The more deeply group members anticipate being involved with one another, the more time they will want to spend getting to know one another and feeling comfortable together.

Problem Solving

After what often seems like a long period devoted to group maintenance and the development of interpersonal relationships between members, a learning group is ready to consider alternative actions, plan, and solve problems related to their mutual goals. Groups that are helped to complete the assessment and testing stage tend to solve problems readily, whereas those groups whose leaders become impatient and push them on to problem solving take longer to accomplish it. Once established, groups seem to operate according to their own time schedule. An effective facilitator will not let the group get bogged down in side issues or conflicts, but at the same time will not insist on problem solving before participants are comfortable with one another.

It is in the problem-solving stage that a group's potential benefit to individual members becomes obvious.

> The creativity, concern, and intelligence that small learning groups often show in finding solutions to problems can surprise even seasoned group leaders.

The following case example demonstrates such creative problem solving.

Example 8.1   A GROUP TACKLES THE PROBLEM OF FEAR

A learning group had been initiated by Shirley Pierce, R.N., when she became aware that there were five patients on the unit who were receiving treatment for chronic heart disease. All had experienced an acute episode that led to hospitalization. Although they were in various stages of treatment and medication regulation, all were between 65 and 75 years of age and mentally alert. Each patient had been assessed by his or her nurse as having learning objectives associated with both treatment and developmental prevention.

Before the first meeting of the group, Ms. Pierce had talked with each patient to personally assess his or her needs and interest him or her in group attendance. The format of the group called for a half hour of explanation and discussion about a particular topic of mutual concern, followed by another half hour of social interaction among group members. As the group members became acquainted with one another, the social part of the meeting was used increasingly for group problem solving. On this particular day, their fourth session together, the topic had been "Stress and How It Affects Your Heart." During the session one of the group members had commented that her major stress was worry about having another heart attack, especially when she was alone. Others agreed that this was a source of anxiety for them as well.

The nurse had stayed with the group only for the first part of the meeting but returned at the time they normally would have adjourned. She found them in active discussion, and they asked to continue for a while. Twenty minutes later they called to her to come hear what they had decided. The discussion of their prevalent fear of another attack had led to a group decision to form a telephone network once they went home. They had exchanged telephone numbers and organized who would call whom. Each member would phone one other member on a daily basis between 8 and 9 A.M. to check that they were all right and had remembered to take their medication. They seemed delighted to have formed a continuing support group, and their growing concern and friendship with one another was evident.

In this example a group of people with similar needs was able to creatively solve a problem of mutual concern. Their solution was an outgrowth of the development of the group and was therefore enthusiastically endorsed by all.

Termination

If group members have formed close interpersonal relationships with one another and a commitment to group goals, they will experience a fourth stage, that of termination. Many people become anxious and sad when a group that has become a source of support and encouragement comes to an end. The group leader needs to be aware of these feelings and allow time for their expression. Groups sometimes decide to have a party or other social gathering to mark the completion of meetings. Such gatherings give members a chance to express the separation anxiety they are feeling and return to less intense interaction with one another in the social context. In effect, they reverse the group process by withdrawing from the group gradually.

Occasionally, groups that have met together intensively over a period of time suggest that they have a "reunion" at some future time. Unfortunately it is almost impossible to recapture the group feeling after other, unshared life experiences have intervened. At best, such a reunion will result in former group members feeling disappointed and, at worst, may lead them to devalue the accomplishments of the group and of themselves in the group (Waring and McLennan, 1979).

In summary, four stages of the group development process have been described. Whatever the purpose or composition of the group, these stages will occur in sequence.

> Members of learning groups in which task and interpersonal relationships are equally important will first acknowledge the group's purposes and goals as important for them individually (the group formation stage) and then spend time getting to know and relate comfortably to one another (the assessment and testing stage) before proceeding to problem solving.

These stages parallel Carkhuff's model of personal problem solving in which awareness and understanding precede constructive action (Carkhuff, 1980). Just as in individual teaching, problem solving and learning are facilitated in groups through the development of relationships based on trust and mutual understanding.

There are many approaches to understanding how groups function. For the nurse involved with task-oriented groups, such as staff groups and committees, books on personnel management offer guidance on increasing the effectiveness of such groups and on principles of leadership. In the field of psychology a number of theorists have used group settings to help people reach goals of personal growth and self-understanding. The interested reader is encouraged to investigate Carl Rogers' "encounter" group approach (1973), Eric Berne's "Transactional Analysis" approach (1974), Virginia Satir's work on communication within families (1972), and Fritz Perls' "Gestalt" approach (1973).

8.2 PLANNING AND ORGANIZING A LEARNING GROUP

In this section and the next we will be looking at some of the practicalities of initiating and conducting small learning groups. As with other kinds of nursing intervention, the effective use of groups begins with identifying the general goals and specific patient objectives to be met. In most instances the nurse will begin with an assessment of each individual who may become part of the learning group. Even when goals and objectives are determined for the group as a whole, without beginning with individuals, the knowledge and skills used by the nurse for the process are the same. The reader may wish to review the material contained in Chapter 4, especially Section 4.3, since we will be referring to these ideas as we explore group planning and organization.

In the following pages the identification of goals and objectives, the selection of group members, and the organization of group meetings will be discussed in detail. The nurse will find guidance on when to choose a group approach and how to initiate group learning.

Identifying Goals and Objectives

In Section 4.3 some general goals of care were outlined. Nursing assessment of a patient's need for treatment, maintenance, primary prevention, and developmental prevention helps the nurse identify specific patient objectives. These, in turn, guide the nurse in planning nursing interventions. One of the options open to the nurse is to offer the patient a group learning experience that will meet some of his specific objectives.

> When several people have similar learning objectives and when time and space suitable for having them meet together are realistically available, a group approach to learning can be educationally and economically sound.

In deciding which objectives might be effectively met through learning groups, the nurse will find that all four general goals are represented.

Treatment

Treatment is care that seeks to restore the health balance by eliminating or reducing the impact of negative factors in the person's life. Patients undergoing medical treatment in a hospital or outpatient facility commonly need to learn self-care procedures or have their family members learn care procedures so that treatment can be continued at home. Because many medical facilities are organized according to the nature of the health problem treated there (e.g., orthopedic, coronary, and pediatric units), a number of patients or members of their families with similar learning needs may be available at any one time. For example, a small learning group focused on treatment goals might meet to learn:

— why, how, and when to take prescribed medication;
— how to do diabetic urine or blood sugar testing;
— how to give medications by injection;
— how to change a dressing;
— how to care for an indwelling catheter;
— how to manage special diets.

Groups may also be organized to help patients and their family members learn about particular disease entities, for example, diabetes, heart disease, or emphysema.

Most of the groups organized by the nurse will focus on informational tasks. Given the opportunity to develop interpersonal relationships between members, they will also meet some of the individual's psychosocial needs. The sometimes dramatic realization that one is not alone with one's problem is a major benefit of learning groups. Participation in a group can be an important step toward accepting the realities of living with a chronic medical problem by reducing fear and promoting problem solving.

Maintenance

The general goal of maintenance means helping people keep and make use of the strengths and resources currently available to them. These kinds of goals and objectives are especially important if a person is to successfully make the transition from illness to wellness once he goes home. It often takes knowledge, commitment, and perseverance from caregivers at home to promote, or perhaps even insist on, the patient's maintenance of physical activity, mental agility, social relationships, and a sense of independence while he is still feeling less than well.

Some of the topics for group discussion that will help to meet maintenance objectives include:

— nutritional needs of the handicapped or elderly;
— support and social activity resources in the community;
— active and passive exercises for maintaining muscle tone;
— how to help with activities of daily living;
— how to recognize complications and get care;
— what to tell your friends about your illness.

In addition to the information that can be shared in a group setting, important positive attitudes can be supported. When a chronic disease or handicap will continue to be part of a person's life, it may be appropriate to refer him and his family to an available community support group to meet his need to maintain his strengths as well as to learn to prevent complications.

Primary Prevention

The goal of primary prevention seeks to avoid stressors that might cause a health imbalance. Because the exact nature of possible stressors may be hard to predict, the learning that will help patients and their caregivers carry out primary prevention is necessarily general. A group approach is an effective way to help several individuals learn basic knowledge and is conservative of the nurse's time. For example, patients who will return home with limited mobility need to be taught how to avoid falls. Without seeing the home, it is not possible for the nurse to predict which environmental factors might cause problems and which can be eliminated. She can, however, present general information to a group of patients or family members, encouraging them to evaluate their own situations. The group may well be even more effective in meeting primary prevention goals than individual teaching, since sharing views, opinions, and information with other group members will stimulate attention to and interest in the general goal. A group might come together to receive information and discuss such topics as:

— how to safely store medications and cleaning supplies;
— how and when to use asepsis;
— kitchen modifications for the arthritic;
— teaching children to avoid dangerous strangers;
— reducing allergens in the home.

The nurse may find that representatives of various community groups or agencies are valuable resources for specialized information on subjects such as those listed. Although it is important that the nurse identify the learning needs of her patients and their family members, she need not be totally responsible for the content of the resulting lesson. Although using outside resource people takes time and energy for coordination, the information that they can contribute can be extremely valuable to group members, including the nurse herself.

Developmental Prevention

The goal of developmental prevention involves helping a person become less vulnerable to possibly harmful stressors by strengthening his own defenses. It is an appropriate goal of care whenever negative factors in the person's environment cannot be eliminated or avoided. Because developmental prevention often means changes in one's habits and life-style, a high level of sustained motivation is needed in order to accomplish it. Learning groups are effective in helping people develop this kind of commitment to change by supporting their decisions, encouraging them when there are setbacks, and providing models for the new behaviors. Developmental prevention is the goal of most "health education" programs. Subjects that might be the focus of such a small learning group include:

— exercising for health and weight reduction;
— self-management of stress and anxiety;
— communication skills for parents;
— effective use of birth control;
— why low-salt, high-fiber diets are good for everyone;
— how to stop smoking.

As discussed in Section 2.5, people confronting a medical crisis have an increased motivation to make life-style changes that will help them avoid such problems in the future. Developmental prevention is therefore an important part of excellent patient care. Concerned family members may be included in a group approach and lend their support to the change process.

One valuable type of learning group for family members of patients who will require physical care at home focuses on some of the issues facing family caregivers. Groups might include discussion of alterations that need to be made in the home environment, the caregiver's own reduced independence, feelings of hostility and helplessness, or financial concerns. Through anticipating and sharing such issues in a group, the family member is helped to protect his own strengths and resources as well as those of the patient.

> The assessment of patient learning objectives within the general goals of treatment, maintenance, primary prevention, and developmental prevention help the nurse identify people who would benefit from a group approach to learning.

Groups offer a useful tool for nurse teachers in helping people acquire new knowledge, attitudes, and skills. They can be appropriately used in combination with one-to-one teaching, thereby giving patients the benefit of the support and added resources offered by a group while retaining the personal attention and help of an individual approach.

Selecting Group Members

The identification of similar learning needs is the first step toward initiating a group approach to learning. The next step ideally involves carefully selecting and preparing group members so that these needs will be met. Active selection of group members by the nurse is, however, not always possible. She may be able to designate certain patients to come to a stress management session but may not be able to predict who will actually come to a postpartum discussion group to which all patients on the unit are invited. Groups whose participants are not preselected will generally take longer to accomplish the group formation stage, since neither the nurse nor group participants are familiar with what they have in common. Because most of the groups initiated by nurses meet together for only a short time, a delay in group process can limit the group's success in solving problems.

> Because specific selection of group members and individual preparation before group attendance are such important factors in the facilitation of group process, the nurse is encouraged to take an active lead in group formation.

When the nurse teacher is able to select group members, *balance* is a key factor in the group's potential effectiveness. Although it is helpful to a group to have a range of points of view, experience, and knowledge represented among several members, it is not helpful to have one person in the group who is much more experienced or who has a vastly different point of view than the others. It is helpful if members are at similar levels of stress, have similar mental acuity, and share approximately similar socioeconomic backgrounds, since this will allow them to communicate more easily. It may be stimulating to a group, however, to have within it a range of ages, interests, and concerns. As the nurse gains experience with initiating groups, she will develop more confidence in the group process and its ability to handle diversity. On the other hand, she will be alert to the problem of including one person with overwhelming needs who is likely to monopolize group attention or someone who will feel frightened and intimidated by others.

Preparation of Group Members

If a small group is to work together quickly, all members must be active. Although this does not mean that they all need to be talkative extroverts, it does mean that they each need to know *in advance* what the group is intended to do and what kind of learning objectives can be met through this group experience and be willing to participate without coercion.

> With careful preparation by the nurse on an individual basis, group members can come together with clear goals and expectations in mind and not waste time trying to find a focus for their attention.

In an ideal situation the nurse will find it helpful to meet twice with each group member individually before convening the group itself. One of these meetings will be for the nurse to assess the person's reasonable learning objectives, major concerns, and present level of knowledge and experience related to his health imbalance. At the same time the nurse can evaluate personality factors that might influence participation in the group (see Section 3.4) and investigate practical factors, such as availability for group meetings. The second meeting can then be focused on motivating the person to participate and helping him learn what he can expect of the group experience. An important part of this nurse-patient interaction will be to establish a bond of trust that both the patient and the nurse can bring with them to the group. Establishing communication before the meeting of the group helps to facilitate the early stages of group process so that problem solving is reached more quickly.

When conditions are not ideal and the nurse is unable to select group participants or unable to meet with them individually before the first group meeting, she can at least give them written information. An introductory letter or information sheet should include a clear statement of the group's purpose and goals, an indication of how the group will be conducted, what resources are to be used, what degree of participation is expected, and data about when and where the group is scheduled to meet. As in the preparation of other written teaching materials, clarity of information should be emphasized and jargon avoided (see Section 6.1). If at all possible, the written information should be individualized. A letter signed by the nurse and directed toward a particular individual will stimulate attention and convey the intention of the nurse to be personally involved in the group process.

The importance of the preparation of group participants before their attendance is demonstrated in the following case example.

Example 8.2 POOR PREPARATION FOR AN ACTIVITY GROUP

Marsha Roberts, P.H.N., had served an older area of town for two years now. During that time, she had grown increasingly concerned about the large frail, aged population in the area. In discussions with the local senior citizens' group, it had been decided that an urgent community need was an activity group for some of the area's residents that would allow them social contacts and physical activity as well as give their caregivers some respite time. Marsha was to select group participants and act as co-leader and consultant to the once-a-week group. The senior citizens' organization would transport participants in their minibus and provide facilities and a trained activity director.

One of Marsha's choices for group membership was Mr. Young, who was 83 and was cared for by his 71-year-old wife. Both were in basically good health, but Mr. Young was often somewhat mentally disoriented. Both his doctor and the nurse felt that socialization would help his mental acuity and provide some "time out" for Mrs. Young to attend to her own needs and interests. Marsha met with both husband and wife to explain about the group and arrange for Mr. Young to attend.

After his first attendance Mr. Young reported the following experience to the nurse: "Right after lunch yesterday, just when I was going to take a nap, the police came and got me. They took me to a hall in town where there was a wedding. I know it was a wedding because we all had to sit down and have juice and fancy cakes, but I don't know whose wedding it was. Then a woman made us sing. She got very angry if we didn't. But we must have done it right because after a while, the police came and took us home again. I sure was glad to get home!"

Although Mr. Young's participation in the activity group was arranged with good intentions, it is clear that unless he was helped to understand why he was taken to the group and to see some advantage in it for himself, he would hardly be an enthusiastic participant in the future. In the case of such a patient, adequate preparation might include going with him to the group meeting the first time to explain what is happening and introduce him to others with whom he might interact.

Group Size

The size of the group selected to work together is critically important to the way in which objectives are met. In order for a group to give care and support to each member and to learn new knowledge, attitudes, and skills in a short time, the group must be limited in size.

> Extensive experience by many group leaders has shown that the upper limit for a "small" group is nine members. The minimum for group interaction to take place is three.

A larger group, such as the activity group described above, can be helped to function as a small group if it is broken down into sections of nine or less for discussion or specific activities.

When the nurse is unable to personally select group members, she can usually still specify how many "places" are available. If people are forewarned, the trauma of having to turn away people at the door is not so great. Nurses tend to be overly generous when placed in this situation, allowing all comers to participate. Unfortunately, a group that is too large will not accomplish its goals. There must be plenty of space and access to alternative group leaders if a large group is to be broken into smaller units.

The shorter a period of time the group has to meet together to accomplish its objectives, the more important it is to its functioning that the group membership be *unchanged*. It is particularly disruptive to time-limited learning or support groups for a nonparticipating observer to be present. Once a group is well into its development, it can tolerate the temporary absence of a member and his return, but the introduction of new members may cause the group process to regress to an earlier stage and interfere with the motivation of the old members.

Organizing Group Meetings

All groups require a certain amount of organizational time, effort, and coordination. These tasks generally break down into deciding where the group is to meet, when its meetings are to occur, how long each meeting is to be, and how many sessions will be planned. Once these kinds of decisions are made, the people involved must be contacted, directions given, and information about the group and its purpose reinforced. Use of a teaching outline such as that described in Section 4.4 will ensure that important details are not overlooked.

When considering *where* the group should meet, convenient access is an important factor. It may be that the nurse will want to use a room in the staff development unit or another area off her duty station so as to minimize distractions and interruptions.

A fact noted by many experienced group leaders is that the group process seems to be facilitated by a *small rather than large room*. A conference room is therefore more satisfactory as a meeting place for a small learning group than is one corner of a large classroom or auditorium. This phenomenon might be explained by the observation that people who are physically positioned within one another's "personal space" tend to relate to one another more quickly. Although there may be some initial discomfort in being close to others in a small room, this apprehension quickly disappears if the group leader helps the members interact in a nonthreatening way by focusing first on the task rather than on relationship aspects of the group.

Deciding at what *time of day* the group should meet will also be a matter of availability. It is often a real challenge to arrange that the nurse be free of other duties during the planned group meetings. This is best not left to chance. The nurse's supervisor and colleagues must be supportive of the nurse's participation in a group in order to avoid scheduling problems and responsibility conflicts. If family members are included in the group, evening hours may be preferable for meetings. To the extent possible, it is wise to avoid meeting times that immediately follow a meal so as to avoid the inattention that often accompanies digestion. Likewise, it is important to time the administration of pain medication so that the patient is neither in pain during the meeting nor overcome with sleepiness.

In the best of circumstances, one's attention span is limited to 45 minutes. When pain, anxiety, or other factors intervene, the ability of people to concentrate, learn, and remember is drastically reduced. For these reasons group activities should not be planned to continue for more than 30 minutes without a break or a change in activity. Even shorter intervals should be planned in the early stages of group process. As the group members become acquainted and more comfortable in the group, interest and attention span will increase.

One and a half hours is a generally useful length for learning group sessions. Enough can be accomplished in this time to justify getting the group together, while at the same time it is not so long as to risk fatigue or boredom. Other factors may, of course, influence the nurse's decision about length.

The more frequently a group is together, the more intense is their relationship with one another. If a central objective of a group is to provide emotional support for members, then frequent meetings will facilitate the closeness within which this objective can be met. Even when a group is focused on tasks, the relationships that develop between members will support the caring and sharing functions of groups. If a great deal of time elapses between meetings, members will feel that too many life events have occurred to adequately share them with others. In a clinical setting, where self-care or other care procedures or information about a disease are the chief reasons for a group's formation, daily meetings for three to five days will promote group development on both task and relationship functions. In some circumstances it may be feasible to have a group meet twice a day for two or three days, for example, to learn a skill, and then have a practice session together. In outpatient facilities weekly meetings are the most common. Because group members will have to bridge a week's worth of activities with one another before returning to group business each time, sometimes it is useful to start sessions with short social interaction periods.

In summary, a number of practical considerations for initiating group learning have been discussed in this section. The identification of learning objectives and the selection and preparation of group members have been emphasized as especially important. Some guidelines have been offered for determining the size of the group, the length of group meetings, and their frequency.

8.3 LEADING GROUP LEARNING

A learning group has been described in this chapter as one consisting of three to nine persons who share some common goals and learning objectives. Both the learning task and the development and maintenance of interpersonal relationships between group members are important to such a group. As the group develops an identity and a sense of commitment, it is increasingly able to give encouragement and support to individual members. At the same time it becomes able to use the diversity of knowledge and experience represented within it as resources for problem solving. The challenge for the leader of a small learning group is to facilitate the group process while helping it accomplish its learning objectives.

As stated repeatedly, the clear definition of goals and objectives is essential to successful learning. Just as with individual teaching, the nurse must identify the level of knowledge, attitudes, and skills to be learned in order to plan her teaching intervention (see Section 4.4).

Group learning is especially effective in helping members achieve complex levels of attitudes and skills. When learning in these categories is part of the group's objectives, the nurse-leader will want to pay special attention to facilitating group development and maintenance. Not surprisingly, the methods by which she can effectively do this parallel the methods and skills used to establish communication in individual interaction. The reader may wish to review the material in Chapter 3 on the attitudes and behaviors that encourage trust, how to use C-A-R-E in listening, and how to phrase open questions.

> The group leader is an important model of effective communication as she helps group members establish rapport and trust with one another.

At the same time it is important that a group be helped to move toward its task-related objectives. A sense of accomplishment is a powerful motivator for both groups and individuals. Table 8–1 summarizes some of the behaviors by the nurse-leader that contribute to the attainment of task and relationship objectives.

The exact combination of behaviors that the nurse might choose at any

TABLE 8–1. Behaviors That Promote Group Process

Task Functions	Relationship Functions
Initiating	Encouraging
Information seeking	Active listening
Clarifying	Showing respect, empathy, and warmth
Information giving	Expressing feelings
Summarizing	Seeking compromise
Consensus testing	

particular time will depend on the stage of a group's development, the roles played by various group members, and the learning objectives (see Glaser, Sarri and Vinter, 1974; Douglas, 1979). In the following paragraphs we will look at each stage of the group process and give the nurse some guidelines that she might follow in selecting teaching strategies and materials as well as interactional behaviors.

Group Formation

In the first stage of group process, group formation, a number of individuals come together to participate in a group experience and begin to form a group commitment and identity. An extended period of uncertainty and confusion can be avoided through careful preparation of group members. If people come to the first group meeting with a clear perception of the group's learning objectives, they will be much more likely to participate without hesitancy. If, in addition, a relationship of trust has been established with the nurse-leader, members will more quickly develop trust with one another.

Some priorities for the first meeting of a group are for people to become acquainted with one another and share their views of the group's potential importance to them. As they have a chance to hear and see one another, they begin to form perceptions of others' strengths and needs and estimate how they, as individuals, will fit into the group. The process is best accomplished by allowing discussion and encouraging active participation. It is usually helpful for the leader to focus attention on the group tasks during these early exchanges, even while being aware that the relationship aspects of group functioning are an underlying theme. Learning tasks and group objectives can usually be discussed without people feeling that they are being led to divulge more about themselves and their needs than they are comfortable sharing. It is important for group members to begin with a clear understanding of their purposes and goals and for early discussions and sharing to be psychologically "safe" and nonthreatening.

Drawing attention to the common goals, resources, and needs that group members share helps them begin to form a group commitment and identity.

A group that is meeting together for the first time will look to the nurse for strong leadership. The messages she gives during this initial period about how the group is to be conducted, what members are expected to do, and what her own role within the group is to be are important to the future accomplishment of objectives. If the nurse has initiated the group, members will probably expect her to be the sole source of information for it. If this is not to be the case and other people, including members themselves, are to function as resources for group problem solving, it is wise to clarify this point early. Otherwise, people can feel disappointed and uncertain when the nurse fails to maintain a high-profile leadership role. If the nurse is to be a facilitator rather than a lecturer, she needs to say this clearly and then demonstrate through her actions just what she means by the term facilitator.

The structure and level of formality that characterize the nurse-leader's early interaction with group members will set the pattern for the conduct of the group.

Most small learning groups benefit by being structured in the early stages but
conducted fairly informally. (See Chapter 5 Introduc ion for a discussion of styles
of teaching.) This combination gives participants the message that the acknowledged leader will give direction to the group, but that the active participation of
all members is expected and encouraged. The nurse might choose, for example,
to have each member introduce themselves to the group, including a general
statement of what they hope to gain through participation. Or she may choose to
conduct a discussion of group goals and objectives, rather than standing in front
of the group giving a formal explanation of group purpose.

During the group formation stage the attention span of group members is
reduced to 15 to 20 minutes. At the same time people are usually eager to receive
information that will prove useful to them individually. For these reasons the
structure of the first session or two can be designed to include a number of
activities and a reasonably high level of content. Short explanations, demonstrations, presentation of pictures or diagrams, and short audiovisual programs are
all useful methods for gaining the attention and involvement of participants and
stimulating initial learning. Frequent opportunities for discussion on topics related
to the content help group members begin to form bonds of communication with
one another. (See Section 5.3 on how to use a discussion strategy for teaching.)

The group formation stage has been achieved when group members feel
comfortable enough to interrupt the nurse's presentation of content with spontaneous questions or comments, when the noise level during discussions increases
because of eager participation, and when references are made by one group
member to another's contribution. These behaviors signify a growing involvement
with the group and a recognition of the other individuals within it.

Assessment and Testing

The second stage of group process is one in which members seek to know
and be known by others in the group. During this period the group typically
focuses on their relationship with one another rather than tasks. It is often
important that members be able to try out the expression of values and opinions
on their fellow members. Sometimes the nurse-leader may feel frustrated during
this stage because the initial eagerness to receive information suddenly slows. It
is, however, natural that a group of people who have learned enough to recognize
how much work the group will need to do in order to meet its objectives will want
to take a concentrated look at their fellow travelers.

This is usually a period of some tension in the group. The introductory
content helps individual group members become more acutely aware of their own
learning needs. As they discover the diversity of attitudes, values, knowledge, and
needs that exist within the group, they may perceive others as creating a barrier
to having their own needs fulfilled. These kinds of perceptions are the source of
the conflict that sometimes arises between individuals. If the group is to progress
to the point of seeing the diversity as a positive resource rather than as a negative

challenge to self-interest, they must explore the diversities and confront the conflicts.

There are two basic ways in which the nurse-leader can facilitate this progress. One of these is to actively practice effective listening techniques, clarifying and summarizing communication. In this way she serves as a model of cooperative, supportive group behavior. The aim of this behavior is to fully hear each individual in the group, acknowledging and accepting his or her point of view, although not necessarily agreeing with it. It is, in fact, important that the nurse refrain from taking sides on issues in which there are conflicting views.

A second way in which the nurse can facilitate group process during this stage is to continue to offer content related to the learning tasks within a known structure and provide opportunities for discussion and sharing at frequent intervals. The discussion of case studies, or group exercises that are oriented toward gathering information and applying ideas to practical situations rather than finding a single "right" answer allow people to share their diverse knowledge and opinions in a positive way. Highly contentious and emotional issues should be avoided until the group has reached problem solving.

> During the assessment and testing stage of group process, structure and content help to maintain the group's learning pace and momentum and the leader's modeling of effective listening behaviors helps members begin to accept the diversity within their midst.

It is tempting, especially for strongly "closure" nurse-leaders, to try to avoid conflict by pushing the group on to problem solving. Just as it is impossible to rush a person involved in a crisis into taking control of his life, it is impossible to rush a group into accepting one another and proceeding with effective problem solving. When a group is not allowed to resolve the relationship issues at this stage, members may withdraw from group interaction or lean increasingly on the leader to "give" them what they ought to know. If this should happen, learning will progress only at a low level of complexity and the growth of attitudes that could result in positive life-style changes will not occur.

Whatever the stage of group process, it is important for the leader to plan a positive activity for the end of a session, one in which participants feel a sense of accomplishment or enjoyment. Helping a group feel that they have made progress toward their objectives and ending on a positive note are especially important during the assessment and testing stage, when the group's pace and motivation may lag.

The end of this second stage of group process is marked by the ability of group members to practice effective listening and increasingly take over supportive relationship functions from the leader. In discussion the group will increasingly reach consensus on approaches or priorities and the nurse may sense that she is losing some control over the task functions and structure of the group.

> In a well-functioning small learning group the importance of the leadership role will diminish as the group progresses in development, with group members directing the flow and content of group learning.

An alternative leader may emerge from within the group who will become their spokesperson for either task or relationship functions.

As a group begins its problem-solving stage, a common perception by the nurse-leader is that it now takes at least twice as long to cover any item of content. This is due to the group's eagerness to talk about each point, apply it to their situations, and diverge into areas of special interest. The learning that will be taking place is at a much more complex level than it was previously, but during this time of transition and limited formal feedback, the nurse will be challenged to take on faith that the group knows best what it needs and wants. If learning objectives were clearly established at the beginning of a group's experience together, the nurse can applaud and encourage these developments.

As a general rule, the transition to problem solving occurs approximately one-third to one-half of the way through the expected life of the group. That is, a group meeting for four one-and-a-half-hour sessions could be expected to spend an hour in group development, followed by another one or two hours in the assessment and testing stage before being ready to solve problems efficiently. The time it takes for these early stages of group development is decreased when there are strong and obvious similarities between members and increased when there is marked diversity. The work that a group accomplishes toward its learning objectives during this first period lays the foundation for problem solving and should not be undervalued by the nurse teacher. Because of time constraints, some groups never progress to problem solving but still achieve important goals of knowledge and skills for their members.

Problem Solving

The problem-solving stage of group process is when in-depth work and learning are accomplished. Relying on the support and resources of other group members, each individual is able to come to terms with his own needs, solve problems in anticipation, and learn at complex levels. The role of the leader or facilitator becomes one of special resource to the group, presenting them with increasingly complex learning challenges to tackle and encouraging their creative efforts. If the practice of skills, the discussion of sensitive issues, or the planning of major changes are appropriate to the group's objectives, this is the period during which these can be approached. The facilitator who is able to let go of a controlling role and participate with the group as a problem-solving member will experience this stage as exciting and rewarding.

> During the problem-solving stage of the group process, the nurse-leader will continue to supply special resources to the group and act as "gate-keeper" by ensuring that all members participate, that the climate remains psychologically "safe" for all, and that the environmental limits of time and space are met. As the group takes self-responsibility for learning, the nurse can increasingly work with, rather than for, the group.

Many groups that are involved in problem solving find it difficult to stop. When the end of a session or the termination of the group is nearing, it is wise for the nurse to warn the group of the approaching time limit. They can, in this way, prepare for it rather than feeling emotionally "stranded" in the middle of a topic of concern. If the group has been working intensely, the nurse may wish to introduce a topic or activity that is less involving for the end of a session.

Termination

The more involved group members have been with the group process and the more complex the learning that has taken place, the more likely it is that they will need a period of gradual withdrawal from the group. Groups in which a strong emotional bond of caring has developed between members will experience the termination stage with real pain and feelings of anxiety. As with other kinds of crisis, it is important that the group be encouraged to talk about their feelings and how they anticipate the end of the group will affect them. This process is facilitated by helping group members evaluate group and individual progress in learning.

> If new behaviors have come about or are planned as a result of group learning, the termination stage is the time to evaluate and reinforce these with the strength of group approval and encouragement.

A variety of evaluation mechanisms might be used to help members make sense of their group experience, put it into the context of their larger experiences, and redirect their attention to their individual strengths, accomplishments, and remaining needs. Some of these evaluation instruments are discussed in detail in Chapter 9.

Table 8–2 summarizes some of the teaching strategies that are appropriate for each stage of group development. This list is not exhaustive, but it will give the nurse some starting points for planning her leadership approaches.

In summary, we have looked at the dual functions of task and relationship that occur in all groups and at the four stages of group process in terms of the leadership role. Some specific ways in which the nurse can facilitate the group process have been suggested so that group members can derive maximum support and learning from their group experience.

8.4 MAKING REFERRALS TO COMMUNITY GROUPS

The staff of a medical care facility interacts with a person for only a short interval in the span of a lifetime. Yet within this interval a sensitive professional is able to identify a wide range of human needs, many of which cannot be met in a clinical setting. When the fulfillment of these needs involves learning, support, socialization, or improved self-esteem, a referral to a group operating in the community is a realistic possibility. One need only look in the Yellow Pages of any metropolitan telephone book under "organizations" or "associations" to be impressed by the great number and variety of groups offering a wide range of services and opportunities. In this section we will look initially at some factors to be considered by the nurse in making such a referral and then explore a few of

TABLE 8–2. Summary of Group Leadership Strategies

For Group Development Stage
Introduction of members, emphasizing common goals and objectives.
Discussion of learning tasks and objectives.
Explanation of nurse's role as leader of group.
Explanation of "ground rules" or expectations of members' behavior.
Short explanations or information giving, followed by discussion of specific topics.
Skill demonstration and discussion.
Short audiovisual programs and discussion.
Presentation of diagrams, pictures, and examples.

For Assessment and Testing Stage
Case studies and discussion in which group can analyze problems.
Exercises in which ideas can be applied to real situations.
Role play of helping situations.
Explanation, followed by discussion focused on goal identification.
Practice of skills in which members help one another rather than observe, criticize, or compete.
Audiovisual programs that illustrate important principles or skills, followed by discussion of their
  application.

For Problem-Solving Stage
Consensus tasks, brain storming, and other creative thinking strategies.
Presentation of problems at increasing levels of complexity, helping group to spend time
  thoroughly investigating alternatives before making decisions.
Learning "games" or exercises, followed by discussion of principles and their application.
"What if . . ." problem scenarios and discussion.
Sharing of real-life problems experienced or anticipated by members and group input on
  solutions.

For Termination Stage
Review and reinforcement of main points and principles.
Evaluation of task achievements of group and progress toward group learning objectives.
Review of progress of individuals toward their own learning objectives.
Evaluation of impact on individuals of group relationship functions.
Information on resources for continued learning and support.
Encouragement of reduced intensity of relationships through "fun" activities or social interaction.

the major categories of groups in the community and the general purposes they serve.

Factors Influencing Referral

Telling people about groups in their communities and then suggesting that they attend suffers the same difficulty as any kind of well-intentioned advice (see Section 7.1).

> In order to be effective, referral to community groups for continued learning or support must be preceded by helping the person reach awareness of long-term goals and understanding of his needs.

Referral is one of the options open to the nurse in helping people make decisions and plan constructive action. Used within the context of the larger process of problem solving, it is an especially important option because people often have no knowledge of the kinds of resources in their communities that might be useful to them. Learning about them helps a person plan for his future in a positive way. When chronic disease or a long-term disability is involved, planning optimistically for the future is a vital step toward mental as well as physical well-being.

Because motivation to actually attend a community group can diminish when the medical crisis is past, a referral must be accompanied by careful preparation and planning. Just as with individual preparation for attendance at a nurse-initiated learning group, thorough information as to the group's goals and purpose and a personal relationship of trust with a group member are factors that increase motivation.

> The nurse will need basic information about the group's goals, structure, leadership, and entry procedures before attempting a referral.

It is helpful if a representative of the group can be introduced to the patient, or a family member, before he leaves the medical facility. In this way a source of immediate information is provided and a personal relationship is developed that will help to decrease the natural reluctance to approach an unfamiliar situation. If the nurse does not have detailed information about an apparently appropriate group or does not know how to reach a contact person, she can make a real contribution to future patient self-responsibility by helping him gather information and initiate contact. The person who has had experience with a small learning group within the medical care setting is an especially good candidate for referral to a community group for continued learning.

Other staff members within the medical facility may be good sources of information about community groups. These include psychologists, social workers, chaplains, and staff education personnel. Nurse practitioners and medical specialists may be able to direct the interested nurse to community resources for special needs.

Kinds of Community Groups

In the following paragraphs some major categories of community groups are briefly discussed in order to give the nurse an overview of the wealth of resources that exist for continuing learning and support.

Learning Programs

The organizations that offer opportunities to increase knowledge and skills include community colleges, adult education departments, and service groups, such as the Red Cross. Subjects range from the purely academic to physical education and fitness, hobby skills, language instruction, and job retraining. For a minimum fee people can participate in programs conducted especially for older adults, parents, caregivers, and the handicapped. Although oriented to helping participants acquire new knowledge and skills, such programs usually meet over a long enough time period and with a stable enough group that some of the other benefits of group membership can be realized such as support, socialization, and improved self-esteem.

Catalogs of course offerings are readily available by telephoning the organization involved. Patients and family members who have previous college or university experience may find such programs especially attractive, while those without a background of much formal education may find them frightening at first and need extra support and encouragement.

Human Relations and Therapy Groups

The term *therapy* usually indicates treatment for disturbed individuals. In recent years, however, a range of groups and programs devoted to helping well people function even more effectively in the areas of self-awareness, communication, and personal relationships have developed. Some of these use the basic structure and techniques of therapeutic groups, perhaps with an orientation toward one particular theoretical model. Most share an emphasis on honest communication with others in the group and feedback about a person's impact on others.

For the emotionally disturbed person, the nurse will want to consult with the individual's attending physician and perhaps a staff psychologist or psychiatrist before making any suggestions. They will be able to offer guidance on the kind of help that may benefit the person when he is discharged. Therapists and counselors in private practice are often good sources of general information.

For the well or temporarily distressed person who has identified some areas of intended personal growth, groups conducted by churches, private organizations, or even academic institutions may be appropriate. Because such groups are deeply involved with the attitudes and values of members, direct referral by the nurse is seldom appropriate. Rather, the nurse's role will be to give general information about a resource's availability and then to encourage and support the person while he thoroughly investigates its specific purposes and benefits.

Peer Self-Help Support and Rehabilitation Groups

There has been a long tradition of people with particular problems banding together to help one another. Often such groups reject the notion that direct help within the group from health professionals is appropriate or necessary. In most cases an underlying assumption of these groups is that the only person who can really help with this particular problem is someone who has had the problem himself. Some well-known groups are Alcoholics Anonymous, Recovery Incorporated, Narcotics Anonymous, and Parents Helping Parents. Although health professionals sometimes view such groups with some doubt and suspicion, there is good evidence that these groups help some people. They may not help all of the people who seek them out, but this can be said of virtually all helping services. At the same time self-help groups typically work in difficult problem areas, making their achievements impressive indeed.

The success of self-help groups varies from place to place. Before referring people to these groups, the nurse will want to investigate the apparent effectiveness of groups in her community by personal contact or consulting sources that can provide an immediate and objective appraisal of them. Once a person decides that he might be helped by such a group, the nurse can often arrange for a representative to meet with the person to give him additional information and encouragement.

Health Service Groups

For almost every major disease or disorder there is an association that seeks to give information and assistance to those who suffer from it. These range from large organizations with substantial research as well as service functions, such as the American Cancer Society, the American Heart Association, the Arthritis Foundation, and the Muscular Dystrophy Association, to small regional groups. As mentioned previously, these organizations are often good sources of public health education and patient-teaching materials. In addition, many sponsor community-based support groups for diagnosed patients or their family members. Because of their variety and accessibility to medical care facilities, such organizations form the largest category of resources for patient referrals. They offer valuable services to people after they leave inpatient care. Some institutions have arranged for representatives of such groups to regularly visit newly diagnosed patients or even to conduct learning groups in the facility. Every nurse owes it to her patients to find out what is offered by relevant health service groups in her community and strive to regularly update information.

In addition to the general categories of community groups outlined above, there are numerous others that may not be directly health related, but that offer valuable services or opportunities for particular individuals. Referrals to community groups that can offer education, support, and other kinds of assistance are an important contribution that the nurse can make to the well-being of her patients.

SUMMARY

In this chapter some of the principles and practicalities of initiating and conducting small learning groups have been described. Group learning offers participants support, encouragement, and resources that exceed those of individual learning situations. The nurse who recognizes the potential of small groups will find numerous opportunities to use them for patient education as an adjunct to individual approaches to learning. Many of the interpersonal communication skills that the nurse uses in one-to-one teaching are also appropriate to group leadership. Keeping in mind the sequence of stages of group development, the nurse can help a number of individuals with similar learning objectives become an effective group that stimulates complex learning and motivates change. Community groups also offer opportunities to patients or their family members for continued learning and services.

Study Questions and Exercises

In order to reach a greater understanding of groups and their development, the reader is encouraged to participate with a learning group in doing the following exercises.

1. Make a list of all of the groups to which you belong. If done as a group exercise,

this usually results in a lengthy list. Choose two or three groups to analyze. What are the objectives of these groups? What task functions are currently under way? How are maintenance functions carried out? What ground rules for behavior apply to group interaction? How is leadership determined and carried out? What has been accomplished by these groups?

2. Investigate the use of learning groups within a medical care facility. What are the objectives of these groups? How are members selected and by whom? Who initiates and leads these groups? What opportunities for group learning seem to exist that have not, so far, been taken? What restrictions apply to the initiation and leadership of group learning?

3. In a group of three to five persons, investigate material on group dynamics available in your library or in other textbooks. Prepare a report or article in which ideas about group process are contrasted and compared. Analyze the process of group development that has occurred in this project group.

4. Imagine that you work in an outpatient prenatal clinic. The following patients have come to your attention:

- Mrs. A, a young woman pregnant with her first child. She and her husband are happy about the baby but have some financial difficulties.

- Mrs. B, an older multipara whose youngest child is now eight years old. She is now awaiting results of chromosome studies.

- Ms. C, a young unmarried professional woman who is apprehensive about raising a child on her own but firm in her decision to do so.

- Mrs. D, aged 32, who is pregnant with her third child and would like to deliver this one vaginally, although she had a cesarean section with the last delivery three years ago.

- Mrs. E, aged 35, who is pregnant with her first child. She is only recently married and eager to start a family.

These five women are all nearing the third trimester of pregnancy and have all expressed some anxieties and fears related to the pregnancy. None has previously delivered in this facility.

Identify some possible learning objectives for each woman. Are there common needs that might be met through a learning group approach? What might be the learning objectives for such a group? What steps would you take in organizing and planning such a group? How would you go about selecting and preparing group members for their participation?

5. For the group described above, outline leadership strategies for the first two sessions. For each, note why you have selected the strategy, how it fits in with group objectives, and under what circumstances you would alter or delete using this strategy.

6. Survey several patients with similar diagnoses on a unit with which you are familiar. What are their identified learning needs within each of the four general goals of care? What do these patients have in common? In what ways are their experiences, knowledge levels, needs, or points of view dissimilar? Are there learning objectives that could be met through a learning group?

7. The best learning about group process and leadership occurs in actual groups. After identifying several people with similar learning needs, arrange for them to meet together for an informational session of one to one and a half hours. Carefully plan group objectives and leadership strategies. Conduct the group as planned. What task and relationship functions did you perform? What group development did you observe? Would the group have benefited by meeting for a shorter or longer time? Share your experiences and your feelings about them with a small group of colleagues or classmates.

9

HOW TO EVALUATE LEARNING

In this chapter we reach the final step in the Nursing Process: evaluating the impact and effectiveness of teaching and learning. Whether formal or informal, whether intended to assess the accomplishment of individual or group learning goals, evaluation is an important step in the teaching-learning process. Through it learners have the opportunity to look objectively at their achievements and feel rewarded by them and teachers learn how to improve the effectiveness of their teaching. This chapter begins with a section on feedback before proceeding to specific guidance for the nurse on using formal and planned evaluation methods. Also included is a section on avoiding common evaluation errors. The main points contained in this chapter are as follows:

- Evaluation is an essential part of the Nursing Process, allowing both nurse and patient to consider the progress made and formulate future goals. (Introduction)
- Evaluation is only as effective as the assessment that led to the setting of objectives. (Introduction)
- In individual teaching, feedback from the learner on progress made is a natural and frequent occurrence. (Section 9.1)
- Feedback allows teacher and learner to jointly adjust goals, set priorities, alter approaches, and reinforce progress on a continuing basis. (Section 9.1)
- Because the outcome of learning is the ability to change behavior, the observation of such changes is the most direct evidence of successful learning. (Section 9.2)
- Demonstrations, videotapes, and behavior rehearsal may be used to evaluate representative learned behaviors. (Section 9.2)
- Carefully constructed oral or written evaluation methods may be used to evaluate some aspects of learning. (Section 9.3)

219

- Patient-kept records and contracts are methods of involving and giving responsibility to the learner for his own progress. (Section 9.3)
- Evaluation methods that threaten or frighten the learner undermine the trust relationship between nurse and patient and may seriously jeopardize progress made toward important learning objectives. (Section 9.4)
- The attitudes and expectations of the nurse may influence the responses of the learner, and therefore the outcome of evaluation. (Section 9.4)

Evaluation is the last of the four steps described in Section 1.2 as part of the Nursing Process. Through evaluation the learner's progress toward goals that were identified during the assessment phase of the process is measured and interpreted. The basic questions to be answered during evaluation are:

— What has been accomplished?
— How are changes that have been made in the learner's knowledge, attitudes, and skills going to affect him in the future?
— How effective and efficient have teaching strategies been in helping this person learn?
— Were the objectives stated as a result of the nursing assessment realistic and appropriate?
— What more needs to be done in helping this person restore his health balance?

The answers to these questions must begin with the identification of goals and the statement of patient objectives. As suggested in Chapter 4, unless the destination is identified, one can hardly be expected to know when one gets there. For this reason evaluation can only be as complete as was the assessment of needs and the statement of objectives.

> Clearly stated, specific objectives provide the necessary basis for the effective evaluation of learning.

The complete evaluation of learning, however, does more than just measure the extent to which goals have been attained, as important as this is; it also identifies how this progress has occurred and points the way to future learning and change.

The determination of progress toward learning is done both by a discrete event during which progress is measured and through continuing interaction between teacher and learner. Within these pages *evaluation* will be used both as a general term and to specifically describe a planned and more or less formal method of measuring goal attainment. The term *feedback* will be used to refer to the informal interaction between teacher and learner that occurs throughout the teaching-learning process. Both are important aspects of teaching and learning.

The conditions and criteria as well as the specific behavior to be evaluated are part of well-constructed learning objectives. (See Section 4.3 for guidance on writing behavioral objectives and Section 4.4 for a discussion of levels of learning complexity.) There would be little point in identifying learning needs and goals if, at some point, these were not to be looked at carefully to decide whether progress had been made.

The more specifically learning objectives are identified as a reflection of learning needs and the more carefully the desired learning complexity is defined, the more helpful to both nurse and learner will be the evaluation in noting progress and directing further learning.

In addition to the event in which progress is measured through demonstration of a behavior, feedback between teacher and learner is a continuing part of personalized, interactive teaching. If evaluation is like determining whether one has reached the desired destination, then feedback is like installing signs along the way to let the travelers know they are on the right road and continuing to make progress.

We will begin our discussion of evaluation by outlining some of the advantages and practical aspects of giving and correctly interpreting informal feedback during teaching. This is followed by two sections devoted to different kinds of formal evaluation methods. The final section of this chapter contains specific guidance for avoiding some of the common pitfalls of evaluation.

9.1 MAKING USE OF FEEDBACK DURING TEACHING

Because of its place in systems theory, the term feedback has become part of the English language. Within this context it refers to that portion of a system's output or result that returns to the system and acts to modify further output. In an electrical system, for example, a portion of the signal generated is "fed back" into the system, so that the signal can then be amplified, diminished, or otherwise modified. A diagrammatic representation of feedback within the system of Nursing Process is shown in Figure 9–1.

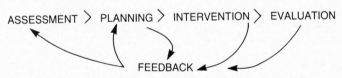

Figure 9–1. Feedback and the Nursing Process "system."

Feedback may occur at any time during the Nursing Process and acts to modify an earlier step in the process. For example, feedback in the form of new information given to the nurse during the planning stage might alter her assessment of the patient's needs. Similarly, feedback such as the patient's responses observed by the nurse during her nursing care or teaching might affect her plan for future intervention.

Feedback is an informal and interactive mechanism whereby both nurse and patient continually monitor the Nursing Process and its impact on the patient.

Even when only two persons are involved in interaction, there are a number of sources of feedback. These sources can be grouped into three general categories: internal, another person, and the environment (see Table 9–1).

TABLE 9–1. Sources of Feedback

Internal	• The experience of feelings such as interest, fatigue, or anxiety • Self-observation of own behavior
Another person	• Nonverbal behaviors, such as impatience, approval, or attention • Verbal responses, such as praise, criticism, questions, or coaching
The environment	• Observation of changes in objects • Awareness of changes in the expected sequence of events

In individual teaching these three general sources of feedback are operating for both teacher and learner; in a learning group they are operating for each person present. Through attention to feedback, the following modifications might be made to the teaching-learning process:

- *Objectives* may be altered, corrected, clarified, or given a different priority.
- The nurse's *plan* for intervention may be altered so that it is more effective.
- Verbal and nonverbal *interaction* may be modified.
- Problems of *motivation* may be identified.

Like other aspects of dynamic interaction, feedback occurs whether or not it is recognized and correctly interpreted or initiated purposely. It can be used intentionally by the nurse teacher to analyze what has happened so far, to influence what is happening now, and to motivate what will happen next. In order to do this she will need to pay special attention to the learner's responses and take care in monitoring her own verbal and nonverbal responses during their interaction. For the sake of discussion the nurse's role in using feedback has been divided into three categories: interpreting feedback, using feedback to correct and coach, and using positive feedback to motivate and reinforce.

Interpreting Feedback

As part of communication, feedback is not objective and quantifiable. Rather, it reflects moods, attitudes, values, and unplanned reactions to events. Because it is often so spontaneous, being able to recognize and correctly interpret feedback are valuable skills that can guide the nurse in assessing needs, modifying intervention, and monitoring progress.

The learner gives feedback in several ways—some are verbal and others are nonverbal. A starting point is for the nurse to give her full attention to all aspects of communication with the learner. The reader may wish to review Section 3.2 on the use of nonverbal communication skills, particularly the use of C-A-R-E in effective listening. By using such skills the nurse will be able to sense the feelings being experienced by the learner in relation to the learning task. The congruence, or lack of it, between verbal and nonverbal communication can be especially important feedback. For example, suppose a nurse has just taken a sheet of

written instructions to two patients. Both were expecting her to do this and had been prepared by her to receive them.

RESPONSE OF PATIENT 1: (*Leans forward in bed to accept the sheet from the nurse.*) Oh, thanks. I'll go over this now. Will you be around a bit later in case I have questions?

RESPONSE OF PATIENT 2: (*Frowns as the nurse approaches.*) Oh, thanks. I'll go over that later. (*Carelessly tosses sheet on a pile of papers at his bedside.*)

Both patients said "thanks" and both promised to give attention to the sheet of instructions, but the feedback received by the nurse was quite different.

The nurse may want to clarify her interpretations of feedback by checking them out with the learner. In this way she gives him feedback about the effect his behavior has had on the nurse. To patient 1 she might say, "You seem really eager to get on with doing things for yourself. That's really nice to see. Can I do anything else to help you?" This kind of positive feedback gives the patient the nurse's approval and offers further support.

In clarifying her interpretation of patient 2's feelings, the nurse might say, "You seem a bit less than enthusiastic about dealing with those instructions right now. Does something about them trouble you?" In this instance confronting apparently negative feedback from the patient helps the nurse find out whether a different kind of intervention is appropriate. It also lets her know where the patient stands in relation to the learning objective represented by the sheet of instructions.

> The correct interpretation of feedback by the nurse depends on her willingness to give full attention to the person's communications and then to immediately clarify perceptions verbally.

These actions will ensure that the nurse has the opportunity to correct her interpretations or to alter her approach to more fully meet the needs of the learner.

One further note: Nurses who are "personalizers" in Jung's terms (see Section 3.4) can tend to interpret negative feedback as being directed at them, personally. Seemingly negative feedback needs to be clarified immediately so that the real problem can be identified and the nurse's helping does not become clouded by inappropriate defensiveness.

Giving Feedback That Corrects and Coaches

There is a strong argument for consciously using feedback during teaching rather than waiting for a formal evaluation to measure progress. This argument has to do with the potential of feedback for correcting errors before they become serious and for coaching a learner in the development of complex skills. To use feedback in this way tests the sensitivity and communications skills of the nurse. To avoid corrective feedback while learning is in progress, however, is to make the evaluation phase more difficult for all concerned. It takes skill to help a patient recognize that his attempts to draw insulin into a syringe are not good enough to ensure the sterility of the needle. Waiting to inform the patient of a problem of

this magnitude until the end of the teaching session is much less effective, educationally.

Coaching that includes both encouragement and correction involves the following steps:

1. Be sure that the person *understands and agrees* with both the general goal of learning and the specific learning objectives. If his feedback indicates that he does not thoroughly understand the objectives, they may need to be restated or subdivided for clarity.

2. Talk through the specific *procedures* to be used in the present learning session, including the criteria to be used in judging acceptable progress.

3. Start with giving *positive feedback* that focuses on specific behaviors.

4. Next, identify *problem behaviors*, encouraging the learner to evaluate them himself and think through how they might be changed. Avoid directing general criticism at the person; instead help him correct an item of behavior by pointing out the criteria for success. Deal with only one item at a time and do not generalize.

5. *Praise* his efforts to change even if the behavior is still not completely successful.

6. *Summarize* specific progress toward the objective with positive feedback before ending the session.

Note that these steps emphasize the positive but still allow the nurse to actively correct unacceptable behaviors without threatening the learner.

> Giving the learner immediate feedback on progress made and problems remaining gives him important information with which to guide his behavior and helps him to more fully participate in the learning process.

Giving Feedback That Motivates and Reinforces

In comparison with giving feedback that seeks to correct an error, positive feedback and praise are easily given and willingly accepted. For the nurse teacher who is striving to make her teaching as effective as possible, it is important to realize how powerful positive feedback is.

As discussed in Chapter 2, the factors that affect learning include the role of previous experience and learning, perception of present need, the social and cultural context of learning, and stress. Nurse-patient interaction was shown as a central factor in the learning process; feedback is a key component of that interaction. Positive feedback contributes to the learning process by telling the learner that he is successful at his current stage of learning and can move on to the next stage. It lets him know that he is working on an important problem. It provides approval within a social context. It may reduce his anxiety and stress level and help him "move" toward desired behavior and continue it until he is able to "re-freeze" into a new habit pattern (see Section 2.4). Like applying a splint to a weak limb, positive feedback reinforces and helps to strengthen desired behavior and progress in learning.

Positive feedback is central to "behavior modification," a strategy used in special circumstances to influence the teaching-learning process. Based on the

work of B. F. Skinner (1938), behavior modification theory holds that, although any problem involves thoughts and feelings as well as actions, it is the action component that can be modified and relearned in more positive directions. When actions or behavior is changed, attitudes and feelings also change. Although some people regard behavior modification as a manipulative and exploitative technique, it is endorsed by others as a highly effective therapeutic method. It has received wide attention as a useful tool for managers in solving a variety of personnel problems (Honey, 1980).

To the extent that behavior modification has the effect of motivating a person to change problem behaviors to more desirable behaviors through use of positive feedback and reinforcement, it is also a useful tool for the nurse teacher. The ethical problem raised by behavior modification is one of deciding whether the ends justify the means. The conscious and regulated use of positive feedback makes a powerful technique out of a naturally occurring but usually not pre-planned process. Most parents have discovered that positive reinforcement is much more effective for stimulating desirable behavior than is punishment. Most parents also feel justified in deciding what is "good" and "desirable" for their children and therefore manage to circumvent the ethical problem. The role of nurses in these kinds of decisions for patients is not so clear.

> Successful behavior modification consists of carefully analyzing the problem behavior before attempting to modify it through positive reinforcement.

The purposeful use of at least the analysis part of this technique can be helpful to the nurse who is confronted with a situation in which the patient needs and wants to replace or remove destructive habits such as smoking, compulsive eating, or argumentative or hostile verbal response patterns. The key steps in this analysis are listed in Table 9–2. They may be jointly followed by patient and nurse in an effort to reach a mutually acceptable plan of action to solve a problem. Active participation by the learner removes the coercive or manipulative element from this approach.

The four steps represent only the analysis, or assessment phase, of behavior modification. Planning and implementation need to follow if change is to occur. Even going as far as the analysis of problem behavior, however, has merit. Doing so allows intensely specific attention to and communication about a problem. Done in conjunction with the patient, this attention and communication is itself positive feedback that gives the message that the person is important and his problem soluble. The focus on "triggers" and "payoffs" greatly increases a person's insight into his priorities, needs, and motivations as well as his own behavior. If the process of behavior analysis can be carried far enough for the person to take responsibility for a change and plan a system of new rewards and satisfactions for the new behavior, he will be well on the way toward actually implementing it.

So far we have discussed the use of positive feedback in unplanned and spontaneous communication and as part of a procedure aimed at behavior change. In addition, positive feedback can be initiated by the nurse teacher as a kind of interim evaluation of progress made. At the end of a lesson or discussion, the nurse might say to the learner, "Let's see what we've done so far." She may then

TABLE 9–2. Steps in Analyzing a Problem Behavior

Step 1. Identify the Problem Behavior.
Thorough and specific identification of the troubling behavior is essential to successfully changing it. Write down the details of the behavior, specifying the exact actions that are taken. Do not attempt to include feelings, thoughts, or reasons associated with the behavior.

Step 2. Identify What Triggers the Problem Behavior.
Habitual behaviors are often triggered by certain events, the presence of certain people acting in specific ways, or other kinds of stressors. These stressors may not seem to have any direct relationship to the problem behavior, but are consistently present before it occurs. Record the triggering event or events in as much detail as possible. If time and the cooperation of the person are available, stop the modification procedure at this point while the person observes his own behavior to check out whether the event recorded does, in fact, seem to be the correct trigger for the problem behavior.

Step 3. Identify What Reinforces the Problem Behavior.
When a behavior is habitually repeated, it is because there is some kind of "payoff" that reinforces it. This payoff may be a feeling, a response by another person, or an altered perception of oneself. Write down, in as much detail as possible, what makes the problem behavior satisfying. Beware of judgmental attitudes at this point. It is easy for an observer to consider the payoffs silly, trivial, or inappropriate. If the nurse gives the person verbal or nonverbal feedback that embarrasses him, the effectiveness of the modification procedure will be greatly reduced.

Step 4. Identify What Should Replace the Problem Behavior.
It is not usually possible to just eradicate a problem behavior. Rather, it is more effective to actively replace it with an acceptable alternative. Write down what behavior is desirable as a replacement for the problem behavior. Pay special attention to how this new behavior will be triggered and what the payoff will be to reinforce it. The new behavior must be as immediately satisfying as the old one, although not necessarily in the same way. It is advantageous if the new behavior results in some longer-term rewards as well, which can be additionally reinforced by positive feedback.

summarize the learning that has been completed and restate the learning objective. By doing this she reinforces the fact that progress has been made, encourages the learner to evaluate and feel satisfied about that progress, and helps him mobilize his resources to continue. This kind of positive recognition of learning may be used effectively both in individual teaching and in learning groups.

> Positive feedback acts to reinforce behavior and stimulate motivation whether used spontaneously or as a planned part of the communication between nurse and patient.

In summary, feedback has been discussed as an important aspect of the continuing evaluation of learning progress. Correctly interpreted, feedback from the patient lets the nurse know whether her intervention is contributing to learning and helps her better understand the learner's feelings, attitudes, and values. Initiated by the nurse, feedback is useful in guiding, correcting, and reinforcing learner behaviors. Used frequently during interactive teaching, feedback helps the learner to participate more fully in the learning process and helps the nurse to adjust her teaching approaches more sensitively to his needs.

9.2 EVALUATING LEARNING BY OBSERVING BEHAVIOR

Learning has been defined throughout this text not only as the acquisition of new knowledge, attitudes, and skills, but also as the ability to take action as a

result of them. If successful learning results in changed behavior, the most direct method of evaluation is in the observation of these changes. Unfortunately, because of the limited time available to the nurse to help with the learning process, the changed behavior that reflects a successfully met objective may not occur within the nurse's view. Despite this difficulty, the observation of behavior, even representative or intended behavior, is the most direct and valid evaluation method. In the paragraphs that follow several approaches to the observation of behavior will be discussed, including "return" demonstrations, videotapes, and behavior rehearsal.

Direct Observation of Learned Behavior

The best of all possible circumstances for evaluating learning is to be able to observe the learner putting new knowledge, attitudes, and skills to work in real-life situations. Unfortunately, the nurse teacher seldom has an opportunity to make such observations firsthand. Most of the learning with which the nurse helps will be put to use outside the immediate clinical situation or is preventative in nature, and therefore results in no obvious behavior changes. For example, the nurse who has successfully helped a patient understand presurgical procedures may observe that he shows no obvious anxiety, but this observation is hardly diagnostic of effective teaching or successful learning. The absence of behavior or other available data is not conclusive evidence.

> The situations in which there is an opportunity to directly observe learned behavior are characteristically those in which the patient has learned and subsequently takes self-responsibility for actions.

Examples of these kinds of situations include the patient who has been taught to, and subsequently does, collect his urine for measurement; the patient who takes responsibility for his own medication schedule by initiating contact with the nurse at the prescribed times; and the rehabilitation patient who is observed feeding himself or safely transferring from bed to chair. Self-responsibility is a key factor in each of these behaviors. The nurse's observations help her evaluate not only whether the patient has learned how to do the procedure adequately, but also whether he is motivated enough to initiate it himself.

Although there are limitations to the amount of self-responsibility that can be assumed by patients or their family members within clinical environments, the alert nurse teacher working in this setting will take every possible opportunity to allow learning to develop to this point. This usually means that specific target behaviors be identified during the assessment phase of the Nursing Process, provisions made for their practice under supervision, and the learner helped to take increasing responsibility for the behavior and its consequences. The problem of legal liability if the patient does something for himself needs to be considered but should not be used to exclude creative attempts to promote learning.

The thorough evaluation of learned behavior often needs to go beyond simple observation. Once again, the evaluation process depends on specific learning

objectives having been recorded during the assessment and planning stage. In some instances checklists or rating scales are useful in clearly evaluating behaviors.

Using Demonstrations and Videotapes in Evaluation

Demonstrations that are set up with the specific intent of evaluating motor behaviors tell the nurse little about the learner's motivation to carry out the behavior on his own as demonstrated. They are effective, however, in evaluating whether or not the person does indeed know *how* to perform the behavior or procedure. Lacking this capability, it is certain that he will not carry it out on his own. Videotaping a demonstration adds another dimension to evaluation, since the learner can thereby participate in evaluation by reviewing the tape. In the following case study, videotapes of demonstrated skills were used to determine the learner's level of competence in performing a complex procedure.

Example 9.1   EVALUATING RESUSCITATION COMPETENCE

Susan Staples had been the R.N. in charge of the medical department of Zymox Industries for three years. This large, heavy-machinery manufacturer had a corporate policy that all supervisors must have demonstrated competence in first aid and, especially, cardiopulmonary resuscitation procedures. To date, this had meant that supervisors were scheduled to attend a review course every year. In the time Sue had worked at Zymox, she had observed that the supervisors seemed bored by the repeated classes and that on the occasions when they were called on to perform in an emergency, their skill level was questionable. She therefore gained approval for the following change in procedure.

As each supervisor neared the anniversary of the last class attended, he would be called, without warning, to a staff education classroom. In that room an "emergency" would be set up using the Resusci-Ann model and a videotape recorder. The supervisor was given details of the mock emergency just before he entered the room and was told he was to give aid. His performance was video tape recorded. After the demonstration he sat down with a nurse to review the tape. Together they evaluated his performance according to a standardized checklist and decided whether he needed to attend supplemental classes. Several kinds of situations were used in rotation, so that an individual could not prepare his response ahead of the demonstration.

The experience of Sue and the medical department in conducting these demonstrations was positive. The supervisors, although anxious about being called, could see that the real point of their training was that they be able to perform in a real emergency. The number of people having to be taken away from duties to attend classes decreased so that the workload of the nurses was about the same. Both nurses and supervisors liked the personal attention and opportunity for joint evaluation that the demonstrations provided.

In this example an evaluation method was devised that allowed the learners to demonstrate their skills in a situation that was as close to reality as possible. Their ability to make decisions based on circumstances, and their motor skills were tested.

Whenever demonstrations are used to evaluate behavior, it is important that

TABLE 9–3. A CPR Checklist Used in Evaluations

(Check each behavior performed correctly and in sequence. Mark each behavior performed correctly but *not* in sequence with an "*." Describe variations from procedure and performance weakness at the bottom of the evaluation sheet.)

_____ Visually observes entire accident scene.
_____ Removes dangerous items from vicinity or
Safely transports victim away from immediate danger.
_____ Gives appropriate directions to others and/or
Uses the assistance of others appropriately.
_____ Clears victim's airway and
_____ Positions head to facilitate respiration.
_____ Quickly examines victim for injuries and
_____ Loosens tight clothing.
_____ Checks for pulse and respirations.

a clear set of criteria be used by the observer. There are two basic forms for this criteria: the checklist and the rating scale. A portion of the checklist used during the Zymox demonstrations is shown in Table 9–3. This kind of checklist identifies the sequence of behaviors that are considered important to the satisfactory performance of CPR in this particular industrial setting. It does not, however, allow the observer to objectively measure those behaviors; the definitions of words like "safely," "appropriately," and "quickly" are left to subjective judgment. Because the demonstration is videotaped, it was decided, in this instance, that the demonstrator and nurse could jointly resolve differences of opinion with the backup of a detailed procedure manual used during training. In other instances the checklist might need to be detailed enough to allow the nurse to make a much more specific critique of the behavior observed. For example, the item that reads: "Gives appropriate directions to others" could be altered to read: "Singles out one bystander and attracts his attention. Tells him that he is to call the paramedics. Gives clear directions to the nearest telephone and tells him to call extension 111."

Another useful method for evaluating specific behaviors is the rating scale. Although they are somewhat time-consuming to construct and validate, they help the nurse evaluate a number of levels of attainment for a single learning objective. In this way both learner and observer are clear about what has been accomplished and what needs further attention in order to meet the desired objective. Typically, rating scales identify three to five levels of performance for the same objective. Each of these levels may be assigned a numerical rating.

The key to using rating scales for evaluating behavior is to define each of the levels of performance in clear, unambiguous language. The validity of the scale can be determined by having several people observe the same behavior; they should each identify it as the same level on the scale.

If these conditions are met, the nurse will find that rating scales allow her to evaluate behavior much more objectively than other methods.

Rating scales are usually used for items of overt and easily observed behavior. Some work has been done, however, on rating the much more difficult areas of interpersonal relationships and emotional functioning (White and Mitchell, 1975;

TABLE 9–4. A Rating Scale for Two Learning Objectives

Subject of Learning:		Self-confidence	Initiating CPR
Outcome	Rating	Levels of Functioning	
Most desirable	+2	Gives evidence of comprehending preliminary information by asking pertinent questions. Approaches accident scene confidently. Uses all available information in assessing situation. Calmly gives clear and specific instructions to bystanders to ensure safety and get help.	Quickly assesses general situation, taking safety precautions as needed. Then focuses full attention on victim. Clears airway and examines victim quickly to determine extent of injury. Positions victim carefully, checks vital signs, and correctly initiates CPR within 45 seconds of arrival at scene.
Desirable	+1	Listens carefully to preliminary information. Approaches accident without evidence of anxiety. Uses most of information to assess situation. Gives clear instructions to bystanders to ensure safety and get help.	Quickly assesses general safety and assesses victim for major injuries. Performs clearing of airway, positioning, and checking of vital signs in correct sequence and begins CPR within 60 seconds of arrival.
Acceptable	0	Listens to preliminary information. Exhibits some anxiety but does not hesitate to approach accident scene. Uses most important bits of information to assess situation. Immediately gives clear instruction to call for help.	Assesses general situation, including safety. Assesses condition of victim. Clears airway, checks for pulse and respiration. Begins CPR correctly within 90 seconds of arrival.
Undesirable	−1	Demonstrates anxiety by nervous gestures. Asks for pertinent information to be repeated. Hesitates before approaching accident. Gives only general instruction to call for help.	Takes longer than 90 seconds to assess situation and victim's condition. Distracted by bystanders. Performs procedures correctly with no more than two errors in sequence.
Least desirable	−2	Reports that anxiety interfered with performance. Shows reluctance to approach accident. Does not use available information in assessing situation. Delays instructing someone to call for help.	Fails to adequately position victim, clear airway, or take vital signs before beginning CPR.

Waring and McLennan, 1979). For these uses the scale is made up of a statement representing the *present* level of functioning with a rating value of 0. Two levels are then identified that reflect goal attainment, and these are rated either "Desirable: + 1" or "Most desirable: + 2." A further two levels are identified that reflect diminished functioning, and these are rated either "Undesirable: − 1" or "Least desirable: − 2." At specified times behavior is rated and progress noted.

In Table 9–4 this procedure for constructing a rating scale has been adapted to a learning objective that has an attitudinal component and to one that does not. In both cases the level of functioning rated 0 is judged to be a *minimally acceptable* level.

Rating scales are most effectively used when there is time for repeated attempts at performing a behavior or set of behaviors and when the learner is able to compare his current performance with previous ones. Psychiatric, rehabilitation, and outpatient settings provide this kind of longer-term relationship between nurse and learner and allow for intermittent evaluation of specific objectives. Rating scales used in these circumstances help motivate learners to continue striving to achieve a high level of performance.

Using Behavior Rehearsal in Evaluation

In Section 5.5 behavior rehearsal was described as one of the "experiential" strategies for teaching. In behavior rehearsal the learner "plays" himself in response to a set of simulated circumstances. Whereas demonstrations are appropriate for evaluating motor skills, behavior rehearsal may be used to evaluate decision-making skills or attitudes.

> For the purpose of evaluation, behavior rehearsal is useful in determining whether the learner is able to make appropriate decisions based on a set of conditions as well as to carry out procedures correctly or perform motor skills.

In evaluating decision-making capability the nurse might present several situations to the learner that require different approaches. For example, behavior rehearsal might be used in the evaluation of mothers' behavior in response to a number of different kinds of threats to their children's safety. Each situation would require that specific kinds of decisions be made and quickly acted on.

Behavior rehearsal allows nurse and learner to compress time for the sake of convenience. One would hope that the responses judged to be correct during behavior rehearsal would, in fact, be those carried out during a "real" situation. Rehearsal is limited, however, to an evaluation of whether the learner knows *how he should perform* in the set of circumstances, not whether he actually will. Once again, checklists and rating scales are helpful in making observations more objective and for increasing the involvement of the learner in the evaluation process.

In summary, several approaches to observing behavior in the evaluation of learning have been outlined. The observation of behavior, whether in response to real or simulated situations, is enhanced by the use of videotaping. Observation can also be improved by including the details of target behaviors and their performance criteria in the nursing record so that other caregivers can share in the evaluation. When computerized records are used, it is relatively easy to include a question for each caregiver relating to target behaviors so that each is alert to the learning taking place and can easily record their observations with regularity.

9.3 USING VERBAL METHODS OF EVALUATION

Words are frequently the vehicle by which progress toward learning is evaluated. In the following paragraphs the use of oral questions, written tests and questionnaires, and patient-kept records and contracts is discussed.

Using Oral Questions and Answers to Evaluate Learning

In Sections 3.3, 4.2, and 5.3 we have discussed the use of questions as they relate to the development of a trusting relationship between nurse and patient, the gathering of assessment data, and the use of a discussion strategy for teaching. Questions may also be used effectively to help evaluate learning progress. These kinds of questions go beyond the informal queries posed by the nurse in order to obtain feedback from the learner. Rather, evaluation questions are carefully constructed so that the learner has the opportunity to verbalize the complexity as well as the content of his learning (see Table 4–5, Levels of Learning).

If, for example, the nurse is attempting to evaluate the patient's ability to "remember" information, she might ask him: "What is the name and dosage of the medication you will be taking at home?" If she is evaluating his ability to "apply" his knowledge, she might ask: "In what circumstances would you call your doctor?" And if she is interested in the patient's ability to "analyze" his knowledge, she might ask: "How do insulin and the carbohydrates in food interact in your body?"

Similarly, the following questions might be used to evaluate different levels of attitude formation: "What kind of attitudes do you expect to encounter about cancer?" (Recognition) "What might you say to a person who believes they can catch cancer from you?" (Response) "What is your present attitude toward your disease? How did you develop that attitude?" (Verbalization)

In order to effectively evaluate learning progress, oral questions must be as carefully planned and phrased as written ones so that they test the level of learning attained. In using oral methods of evaluation the learner must be prepared for the fact that these particular questions are being asked specifically to determine progress, not to open the subject for discussion. Because we use questions in so many contexts, the quality of the evaluation will depend on the learner's cooperation with this special kind of "testing" procedure.

Although the answers to oral questions are not permanent, they do have the advantage of containing nonverbal as well as verbal elements. To the sensitive nurse teacher, these elements may be as important in determining what has been learned, especially in the area of attitudes, as the spoken or written message. On the other hand, nurse teachers may be so anxious to have learners succeed that their phrasing of oral questions suggests the answer they want, or their nonverbal communication gives important clues to the learner.

Using Written Tests and Questionnaires

The pen-and-paper test is the most common form for evaluating what knowledge has been learned. Because responses to questions are permanently recorded, they can be carefully analyzed and reread, thus making evaluation more objective than it can be with oral responses. The most important aspect of test construction is the careful wording of questions to reflect the level of learning that is being evaluated. In addition to all levels of knowledge, the less complex levels of attitudes and the "perception" level of skill learning can be tested through use of questions (see Table 4–5).

Written tests may be constructed to require different kinds of responses from the learner: designation of true or false statements, multiple choice, filling in words or phrases, and writing sentences, paragraphs, or essays about a given topic. The length of the answer required is generally an indication of the complexity of learning required to answer it correctly.

Questionnaires are usually used to evaluate attitudes, preferences, and opinions. The questions on them are often open-ended and have no "correct" answer. Questionnaires seldom give reliably objective data on the learning that has been achieved, although they may give important subjective information.

One of the most important uses of tests and questionnaires is to provide data for research and program evaluation activities. When answers to written questions are to be contributed by a number of learners for statistical analysis, their construction is especially important. The interested reader is referred to texts on research methodology for guidance in this area. Polit and Hungler (1983) include particularly readable chapters on observational methods as well as use of interviews and questionnaires in the recent edition of their nursing research text.

There are two major disadvantages in using written tests and questionnaires in the evaluation of learning. One of these is the liability they share with all written materials: their usefulness is directly related to the visual acuity and the reading and writing abilities of the learner. (See Section 6.2 for a more detailed discussion of the use of written materials in teaching.) Written tests also suffer because they are so commonly used in classroom situations; adult learners often feel threatened by the nurse teacher's implicit demand that they perform correctly to "prove" they have learned. Avoiding the first problem requires careful assessment by the nurse before presenting written materials of any kind. The second problem of threat can be lessened by using effective feedback throughout learning so that the learner knows in advance what will be tested, by allowing the learner to correct his answers himself before going over the test with the nurse, or by using a pretest and posttest format so that the learner is already familiar with the form of the test. In addition, testing should be conducted in the privacy of the teaching-learning environment without subjecting the learner to publicly defending his answers or receiving public criticism.

> In constructing and administering tests, the nurse must keep in mind that if the learner fails to answer questions correctly, the nurse must be prepared to give time and caring involvement to dealing with the crisis of self-confidence that will result.

Whenever a person is unable to answer test questions correctly, the test instrument itself should be examined for clarity and the verbal capabilities of the learner reassessed. Alternative methods of evaluating learning may help. When the problem is not the test, but rather that the person has been unable to meet important learning objectives, further instruction may be feasible. A change of teaching strategy or teacher are well worth considering at this point.

Using Patient-Kept Records and Contracts to Evaluate Learning

When patients or their family members are actively involved in the writing of learning objectives, the evaluation of whether or not they have been met is also an appropriately shared task.

Sometimes such learning objectives are put in "contract" form; the learner writes down exactly what he will attempt to accomplish, when he expects to meet his goal, how his accomplishment will be measured, and what he is to gain by doing this. Formal patient contracts can be an effective motivational tool in helping to change long-held behavior patterns or to relearn behaviors during rehabilitation. Herje (1980) points out that a good patient contract must be realistic, measurable, focused on a positive behavior (rather than the absence of a behavior), time limited, and rewardable. At the end of the specified time, progress should be measured by the stated method. The analysis of behavior outlined in Table 9–2 is useful as a preparation to the writing of a patient contract.

Whether or not a formal contract is written, patients can often actively participate in the evaluation of their learning as well as in the setting of objectives. One method of patient self-evaluation is the keeping of records that reflect target behaviors. The patient may, for example, keep a diary of what he eats as an indication of his progress toward learning to lessen his intake of cholesterol or carbohydrates. He might record his pulse rate after each exercise session or write down his physical response to certain kinds of environmental stressors. This kind of approach increases the learner's responsibility for his own progress.

When patient-kept records are part of the evaluation of learning, two factors should be borne in mind by the nurse. One is that in order for such approaches to be successful, she must first help the person learn how to keep the record. This learning is in addition to the knowledge, attitude, or skill "content" of target behaviors. A record form may need to be designed for the convenience of the learner and attention given to the record-keeping skills required. Another factor that is important to successful patient self-evaluation is that progress should be reviewed frequently at prescribed intervals. Nothing is quite so annoying or disappointing as painstakingly keeping a record and then finding that no one is interested in helping you use it for evaluation. Review intervals should, at first, be short so that errors in the mechanics of recording behaviors can be corrected and positive feedback given about accomplishments.

In summary, the use of oral and written approaches to evaluating learning has been described in this section. Although these methods are less direct than the observation of learned behaviors, they have an important place in determining the degree to which new knowledge, in particular, has been acquired. They are necessarily limited by the learner's verbal comprehension and expression, but by using carefully phrased questions, the nurse can learn a great deal about learner progress as well as the effectiveness of her teaching strategies.

9.4 AVOIDING EVALUATION ERRORS

As the final step in a carefully planned process of helping a person learn, evaluation should be a high point in which successful teaching and successful learning are celebrated. Problems with the evaluation phase of learning are especially disheartening to the nurse teacher who has put considerable time and effort into helping with learning; there is no closure and only restricted opportunity to learn from the experience. Like most potential problems about which one has some warning, there is more wisdom in avoiding evaluation problems than there is in belatedly trying to correct them and the errors they represent. In the following paragraphs three of the most common problems in evaluation are discussed: unclear objectives, teacher expectations, and learner stress.

The Problem of Unclear Objectives

Throughout these pages the necessity of clearly defining goals and objectives as a prerequisite for effective teaching has been stressed. By the time one reaches the point of trying to evaluate what learning has taken place, the reorganization of objectives is pointless. This problem cannot be easily treated; it must be prevented. Some of the specific ways in which the problem can be avoided are as follows:

1. Be sure that teaching is preceded by a thorough assessment of learner needs.

2. To the degree possible, involve the learner in the definition of these needs and the identification of learning objectives.

3. Write down learning objectives. Having objectives in black and white helps the nurse teacher more clearly judge whether they adequately include a time frame for learning, an anticipated behavior that is to result from learning, and criteria by which to evaluate success.

4. In acute care situations limit objectives to those that can be reached in short periods of time, recognizing the facts that teaching time is limited, the condition and needs of patients change quickly, and total length of stay is generally short.

5. Encourage and pay attention to feedback from the learner as teaching progresses. Do not hesitate to alter or "fine tune" objectives so that they more clearly reflect current learner needs, but make these changes in writing so that other caregivers are aware of the needs and the efforts being made to meet them.

6. Start evaluation of learning as a specific activity early, well before the patient's discharge. Successful evaluation not only clarifies what progress has been made, but also provides information about other needs and future goals. The opportunity to help the learner make further learning plans is too important to his future well-being to be missed because of a last-minute flurry of other activities.

The Problem of Teacher Expectations

Because the teaching in which the nurse is involved is highly interactive, the expectations and perceptions of the nurse teacher influence the teaching-learning process as much as do those of the learner. Sometimes those expectations and perceptions get in the way of learning progress or lead the nurse to misinterpret or even unintentionally alter events. The phenomenon by which a person's expectations act to change outcomes was first called the "self-fulfilling prophecy" by Merton (1957). It is also sometimes called the "Pygmalion Effect," after the ancient legend of a statue that came to life when its creator fell in love with it.

The phenomenon begins with a false perception of a situation. This results in behaviors based on that perception, which in turn make the "prophecy" come true in what Merton calls a "reign of error."

There are several well-known examples of this phenomemon, including the bank failures during the Great Depression. The perception by members of the public that certain, actually solvent banks might fail led to a "run" of withdrawals, which created in reality what was expected.

The self-fulfilling prophecy affects everyone from time to time. Whenever either good or bad stereotypes or strong beliefs influence interaction between people, expectations do alter reality. Behavioral scientists have been concerned about this problem as it affects social change and counseling relationships. (See, for example, Muldary, 1983, Ch. 10 on "Protecting Impressions.") The following example summarizes some research conducted on self-fulfilling prophecy in an educational setting.

Example 9.2   SELF-FULFILLING PROPHECY IN A CLASSROOM

In 1968, Rosenthal and Jacobson reported a study conducted in an elementary school classroom. Intelligence tests were first given to all of the children. The teacher was then told that certain of her students were "intellectual bloomers" and that in the next few months they could be expected to make rapid progress. In fact, these children had been chosen at random. Over a six-month period the "bloomers" actually gained several points over their peers on I.Q. tests; the expectation had become reality. The teacher was unaware that she had treated any of the children differently. To her, the process seemed magical.

The researchers identified several kinds of behavior that could have resulted in the findings: nonverbal behavior, such as smiling, touching, and nodding approval, verbal feedback on the students' successes, and the teacher's expectation that they could do well on a particular task.

For the nurse teacher, this effect must be considered when evaluating learning progress. One cannot avoid entering a teaching situation with certain expectations about one's own abilities and the likelihood of the learner's success or failure. Sometimes negative expectations are based on nothing more than stereotypes, prejudices, and unfounded beliefs. Yet they risk becoming true if supported by the behavior of the nurse. Positive expectations based on optimistic views of learner capability also have a way of becoming true. The nurse teacher is encouraged to examine her own attitudes and become aware of how she can use the self-fulfilling prophecy in a positive way by approaching learners optimistically even while maintaining realistic objectives.

The Problem of Learner Stress

Several times in this text stress has been discussed as altering the teaching-learning process. In some cases the stress of recognizing a need can stimulate interest in learning. In other cases stress can be a barrier to effective learning. Because high levels are known to decrease objectivity, stress is not a useful companion to evaluation. There are two basic ways to avoid this problem. One is to choose the time for evaluating learning progress carefully, taking into account the learner's stress level owing to factors such as impending discharge, changes in environment or treatment, and the presence of other people. A second is to adequately prepare both the evaluation procedure and the expectation of the learner so that stress is not induced by the process itself. We have already mentioned the problem of giving tests to adult learners. Barbara Narrow (1979) goes so far as to make the following statement:

> It is inexcusable, in my opinion, to evaluate any person in such a manner that he feels dumb, stupid, inept, put down, or inferior. I feel that the psychological damage done to a patient by lessening his self-confidence and self-esteem is equal to, or greater than, any physical damage that can be inflicted by negligence or mistreatment. (p. 185)

This opinion is one with which I wholeheartedly concur.

The problems of evaluation discussed here are ones that any well-intentioned nurse teacher can experience if active precautions have not been taken to avoid them. Other problems occur when the focus of evaluation inadvertently shifts from evaluating progress made by the learner to the activities of the teacher. It is relatively easy to fall into the trap of confusing an evaluation of what the learner has learned with what the teacher has taught. If the learner has acquired new knowledge, attitudes, and skills as a result of teaching, we then know something about the effectiveness of that teaching. If we simply know that the teacher tried to teach, we have evaluated nothing of teaching effectiveness or learner progress. For this reason the number of people attending a teaching session or the apparent interest of the learner may tell us something about motivation to learn, but they are not valid criteria by which to judge teaching or learning effectiveness.

In summary, we have looked at three common errors in evaluation that can be made by the nurse teacher. For the problems of unclear objectives and learner stress, preventive action and thorough planning are much more effective than attempting to "treat" the situation once it has arisen. Avoiding the negative effects of the self-fulfilling prophecy demands that the nurse teacher be aware of the impact her behavior has on others and be willing to alter stereotypes that may get in the way of learning.

SUMMARY

In this chapter a number of aspects of evaluation have been considered. The part evaluation plays in the teaching-learning process is to verify progress in learning and point the way to further learning objectives. Feedback, as an important part of evaluation, has been described as the continuing and dynamic assessment of whether the selection of objectives, plans, strategies, and materials is effectively contributing to progress. In addition, a formal evaluation that is separated from other aspects of the learning process allows both teacher and learner to review progress, reach closure on that particular part of their interaction, and put progress into the larger context of needs, hopes, and plans.

Study Questions and Exercises

1. Review the learning objectives for several patients with whom you are familiar. Do these objectives clearly state what behavior is expected as a result of learning, a date by which the behavior should occur, and a method of evaluation? In consultation with classmates or colleagues, rephrase these objectives so that they are more specific, more realistic, and easier to evaluate.

2. Analyze a short conversation with someone you know. What kinds of feedback were given and received? What were the sources of this feedback? Was feedback initiated by you interpreted correctly? In a subsequent conversation with this person or in a role play done in the classroom, verbally check out your interpretation of feedback you are receiving from the other person.

3. Analyze a problem behavior that affects you according to the steps in Table 9–2. In consultation with classmates or colleagues, decide how you might alter the "triggers" or "payoffs" such that the behavior is changed. If resources permit, discuss your analysis with the person whose behavior has been analyzed. Use careful listening and open questions to obtain his perceptions of the problem. Together plan how to proceed to change the behavior.

4. Observe several children at play, or, together with colleagues or classmates, view a videotape of several children. Identify behaviors that are the result of a learning process. How do you think this learning occurred? Who was the "teacher"? In what ways do you think the behavior might change if the child was aware that his "learning" was being evaluated? What implications do these observations have for patient teaching and learning evaluation?

5. Choose a skill that you have had some experience in helping patients or family members learn. Construct a checklist and a rating scale for evaluating the learning of this skill. If resources permit, use these instruments when you next teach the skill.

6. Choose an article in a health-related magazine. Read the article and then write what you think were the author's objectives. Construct a written test to reflect these objectives. Ask a colleague or classmate to read the article and then administer your test. What was the reader's opinion of the test? How might the questions have been changed if the test had been given orally? Did the reader's abilities in comprehension and expression influence the test results?

7. Think of someone you like very much. List their good qualities that you especially appreciate. Now think of someone you dislike. List their negative qualities that you especially dislike. Share your lists with a small group of colleagues or classmates. How might your opinion of these two persons be perpetuated by your own behavior?

8. Ask several nurse teachers of your acquaintance what their experience has been with the evaluation of patient learning. What are their preferred approaches and methods for evaluation? What can you learn from their experiences?

10

HOW TO DEVELOP A PATIENT EDUCATION PROGRAM

Most of the teaching carried out by nurses within the context of patient care is planned and implemented in response to individual patient needs. However, when many individuals have the same kinds of learning needs, there exists the opportunity to develop a patient education program of broader scope and wider dimension. In this chapter we will explore the processes and procedures of developing such a program. In particular we will look at what to consider when assessing, planning, organizing, and implementing patient education. Special attention will be given to program management. The final section of the chapter provides a checklist for the nurse who is involved in program development. The main points contained in this chapter are as follows:

- The process of developing a patient education program consists of four phases: assessment, planning, organizing, and implementing/managing. (Introduction)
- Both patient needs and an analysis of available resources are part of the initial phase of assessing the feasibility of a patient education program. (Section 10.1)
- The careful organization of the planning phase is one of the most important aspects of ensuring a successful program. (Section 10.1)
- Program planning is a decision-making process that benefits from the contribution of a variety of points of view and concerns. (Section 10.2)
- Planning includes making decisions regarding program philosophy and objectives, evaluation methods, and management responsibilities. (Section 10.2)

- The preparation of teaching staff and the marketing of the program are two of the major activities to be started during program organization. (Section 10.3)
- During the organizational phase of program development, session content, teaching materials and methods, and operating procedures are decided. (Section 10.3)
- Program management, the coordination of resources, and feedback to the sponsoring organization often demand as much or more time than actual program delivery. (Section 10.4)
- An important aspect of successful program implementation is clear lines of authority for managing problems as they arise. (Section 10.4)

Nurses are in an ideal position to assist in the development of patient education programs. Their awareness of frequently occurring gaps in patient knowledge, attitudes, or skills alert them to areas in which a program approach may be effective. In addition, their developed teaching skills make them valuable resources for all phases of program development.

Two common reasons for developing patient education programs are to *standardize* some aspects of one-to-one teaching offered to individuals with learning needs in common, such as diabetics or new mothers, and to provide *repeatable* learning experiences for groups of individuals with similar health needs. Programs may be developed to meet a full range of goals from treatment and health maintenance to primary and developmental prevention. (See Section 4.3 for examples of each of these.)

The challenge in developing patient education programs is to make special learning resources available to a group of patients while maintaining the flexibility to meet individual needs.

Consequently, patient education programs that result in effective learning require careful planning, organizing, and management. This chapter focuses on these behind-the-scenes activities. They have been divided into four phases, the major aspects of which are shown in Table 10–1.

TABLE 10–1. Phases of Educational Program Development

Assessment Phase	Planning Phase	Organizational Phase	Implementation/ Management Phase
Identify and assess health needs of individuals	Agree Upon: Philosophy of program	Carry out: Marketing	Coordinate people, time schedules, equipment, and materials
Identify and assess resources available:	Curriculum/objectives	Materials development	
Sponsorship	Benefit to/impact on sponsor	Staff development	Conduct program
Funding	Methods of evaluation/research	Plan details of: Operating procedures	Carry out planned quality control and accountability procedures
Time			
People	Participants (learners, teachers, consultants)	Follow-up procedures	
Equipment	Responsibilities for program organization and management		Manage problems as they arise
Materials			
Plan planning phase	Plan organizational phase		

In the sections that follow we will look at the components of each of these four phases. These pages are intended as an introduction to a complex subject; the interested reader will find a wealth of additional learning resources in texts from the fields of organizational and educational psychology, health education, personnel management, and nursing leadership.

10.1 THE ASSESSMENT PHASE OF PROGRAM DEVELOPMENT

This first phase of the program development process is one in which awareness of a frequently occurring or general health education need is brought into focus and exploration begins on what might be done about it. This dawning awareness often occurs in informal discussion between health care co-workers about problems they have encountered or observations they have made. The conversation might then take the form of: "Wouldn't it be nice if...?" For example, wouldn't it be nice if:

— all our newly diagnosed diabetics could avoid such a period of dismay and depression over the diagnosis;

— teenagers who drank alcohol at a party could get a safe ride home without embarrassment or punishment;

— frail elderly people who are likely to fall or who live alone had an easy way to call for attention when they need help;

— post-cardiac patients were helped to see themselves as "well" again?

These kinds of creative ideas and general concerns, based on nurses' observations and awareness of needs, have, in fact, led to innovative health education programs (Waring and McLennan, 1979). In some instances they were inspired by the questions and interest of a health educator, and in others nurses themselves took the initiative in beginning the assessment of a potential program.

Having come up with what seems like a good idea, the next major hurdle is deciding where to begin in making it a reality. A popular planning model, called the PRECEDE model, encourages starting exactly the way the nurses did in the examples above: with concern about quality of life. PRECEDE, suggested by Green and others in 1980, is an acronym for *P*redisposing, *R*einforcing, and *E*nabling *C*auses in *E*ducational *D*iagnosis and *E*valuation. According to Green, the name of the model was chosen partly to emphasize the need for health educators to analyze what behaviors and causes "precede" improvement in the quality of life. As indicated in Figure 10–1, the planning of a health education program begins with determining what factors are affecting an individual's or group's quality of life and working backward from there, carefully diagnosing contributing factors at each level. The result is a health education program that takes the complexity of health behaviors into account as part of a logically sequenced planning process. In Section 10.5 the questions posed relating to the assessment phase of program development follow this model.

An important aspect of the PRECEDE model is consideration of "enabling factors" leading, in part, to an "administrative diagnosis." If nurses are to actively

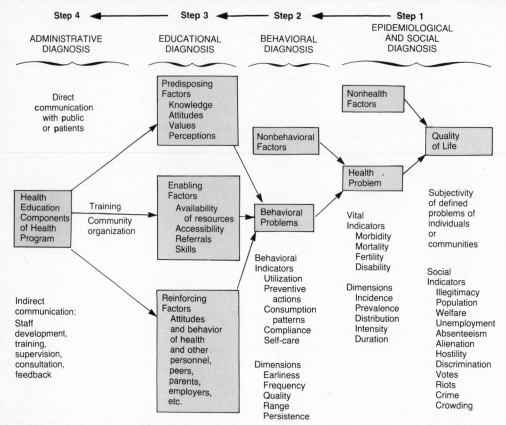

Figure 10–1. The "PRECEDE" model for health education planning. (Reprinted from Squyres W, et al: Patient Education and Health Promotion in Medical Care. Palo Alto, CA, Mayfield Publishing Company, 1985, p. 219, as adapted from Green L, et al: Health Education Planning: A Diagnostic Approach. Palo Alto, CA, Mayfield Publishing Company, 1980.)

participate in the development of educational programs, they must take early account of the organizational realities affecting them and the patients to be educated. They must look carefully and dispassionately at what resources exist that will help convert their good idea into a functioning program and what administrative barriers might stand in the way of program development. A thorough assessment of resources will include investigation of the following:

- Organizational policies and objectives related to patient education
- Protocol for obtaining approval for educational activities
- Funding sources to cover time and material expenditures
- Amount of time realistically available to the nurse for planning and development activities
- People with special skills, such as health educators or medical experts, who can contribute to the project

- The existence of other similar educational programs
- The availability of teaching equipment and already prepared materials in the subject area of concern

As suggested in Section 1.3, economic issues force medical and health care facilities to be careful about their sponsorship of activities that do not directly improve patient care. Although the nurse may be able to see clearly why an educational program should be instituted, she cannot expect that decision-makers not immediately involved in the delivery of patient care will share her enthusiasm.

Gaining administrative support for educational programs demands that nurses first help decision-makers learn why and how the program will benefit the organization.

This principle of first helping organizations learn why a program will benefit them applies to gaining support from volunteer, community, or governmental agencies as well as from medical care facilities. Without sponsorship, few educational programs survive beyond the assessment phase of development (Squyres and associates, 1985). It is therefore critically important that the nurse approach this issue early in the process. Organizations are at least as likely to respond to a request for help to solve a problem and participate in program development as they are to respond to a request for sponsorship of a fully planned program in which they have had no guiding role. Just like individuals, institutions have difficulty responding positively to a fait accompli; they would rather feel as though they have some control over the change. (See, for example, Klein's chapter on organizational resistance to change [pp. 117-124] in Bennis, Benne, Chin, and Corey, 1976.)

Once information has been gathered and assessed about patient needs and available resources, the nurse is ready to organize the planning process. A major mistake is made by concerned caregivers who fail to adequately plan a patient education program and instead rush into implementing what they think ought to work.

The more people that will be affected by a program as participants, leaders, or sponsors, the more complex will be the program that results and the more time and care will need to be devoted to the planning process.

Breckon, Harvey, and Lancaster (1985, pp. 88-93) suggest several principles of planning, which include "Plan with People," "Plan with Data," and "Plan for Priorities." The first principle they list, however, is "Plan the Process." The PERT method (*Program Evaluation and Review Technique*) is proposed as a useful approach for doing this. Not unlike the PRECEDE model, it starts with a statement of intended goal and then works backward, listing all the steps that must be taken or tasks accomplished in order to reach that goal. The list is then diagrammed on a flow chart to show the sequence of activities and the amount of time allotted to a task or group of tasks. The following example shows how this scheme works in practice.

Example 10.1 AN EDUCATIONAL PROGRAM FOR FAMILY MEMBERS

The idea for an educational program for family members of terminally ill patients developed out of a staff meeting on the oncology unit. The charge nurses, clinical psychologist, social worker, and clergy present all agreed that they spent a great deal of time talking with family members about things that might be handled in a group setting. They decided that a three or four session program repeated every month or six weeks would satisfy some of the needs of family members they were unable to adequately meet on a one-to-one basis. The initial list of objectives for program participants included:

— understanding what community resources were available to help them cope with the situation,

— understanding what to expect concerning hospital procedures and personnel,

— becoming acquainted with resource people and services in the hospital,

— understanding basic legal rights and obligations when a family member dies, and

— gaining mutual emotional support from group members.

These objectives would subsequently be refined, and in several instances changed, before the program was implemented, but this initial statement gave them a starting point. A list was made of activities that would be necessary to complete their assessment and begin the planning phase of program development. The prioritized list read in part as follows:

1. Review other support programs in the area.
2. Review experience of professional staff in similar programs.
3. Talk with staff of other units about their perception of need and ideas about proposal.
4. Meet with the director of nurses and the assistant administrator to gain approval to explore idea.
5. Investigate possible funding sources.
6. Set up multidisciplinary guidance committee, which would then decide on:
7. Feasibility of program,
8. Program philosophy, objectives, and format,
9. Framework of administrative responsibilities, and
10. Apply for sponsorship/funding.

The initial time schedule looked like this:

May	June	July/Aug.	Sept.-Oct.	Nov. 1st
1		7	Organizational phase and final	Target starting date
2	5	8	implementation planning	
3	6	9		
4		10		

In this example, program development had the advantage of initial input from a multidisciplinary group and the possibility of introducing the idea to decision-makers as one that would save staff time. Instead of rushing ahead, they recognized that in order for the program to succeed, they needed to do a thorough job of assessing, planning, and organizing their approach.

In summary, the initial assessment phase of educational program development involves a careful analysis of patient learning needs and available resources. If the resulting "diagnosis" indicates that a program approach is realistic, detailed plans should then be made for the "planning" phase of development. Just as the nurse teaches more successfully when she takes the time to investigate learner needs and preferences, so, too, program developers are well advised to take the time to do their "homework."

> The assessment phase lays the foundation of communication, cooperation, and information on which the remainder of program development depends.

The challenge for the nurse who can easily see the benefits of a proposed program is to maintain her enthusiasm during what almost always seems like slow progress toward the goal. Impatience is controlled and the final quality of the program improved by organizing the process into a series of steps, each of which makes its contribution to overall development but can be appreciated as a goal itself.

10.2 THE PLANNING PHASE OF PROGRAM DEVELOPMENT

During the planning phase work begins in earnest on the proposed program. At this time the "nuts-and-bolts" decisions are made that will shape the program. If the goal of the assessment phase was to lay a foundation, then the planning phase builds the basic framework and structure of the project. In this section we will explore some general considerations when working with a planning committee and then focus on the specific kinds of decisions that lead to a strong program framework.

Working with a Planning Committee

The design, or planning, phase of most educational programs is carried out in a working group or committee. This occurs for the very good reason that the success of most educational efforts demands a "horizontal" flow of communication between a number of individuals, functional units, or professional disciplines. Committees are a well-established mechanism used in health care organizations to provide horizontal (as opposed to hierarchical) communication for solving problems of coordination and integration (Rakich, Longest, and O'Donovan, 1977).

For the individual nurse, working with a committee is often both a positive and a negative experience. On the one hand, committees, by representing a range of views, concerns, and interests, provide the opportunity to resolve potential conflicts and make acceptable decisions that effectively reduce problems for the program later. On the other hand, committee work can be time-consuming and the group's tendency toward compromise, frustrating. There is an old saying that a camel is a horse invented by a committee. Most individuals working in a committee at some stage wonder whether a camel is being invented! Five "rules" for enhancing the effectiveness of committees concerned with planning an educational program are as follows:

1. *Limit the size* of the committee. An ideal number is five, with a reasonable

range of three to seven. This number gives the group access to varied resources without adversely affecting open communication. (See Section 8.2 for discussion of group dynamics related to size.)

2. *Do not discriminate* against divergent views within the committee. As long as the committee members are willing to commit themselves to problem solving and have no longstanding personal feuds with other members, it is healthier to work out potential conflicts in the planning stage rather than wait for implementation.

3. *Establish realistic time limits* for decision making and stick with them. As suggested in Section 10.1, a comprehensive list of activities that must be done and a time schedule for completing them greatly facilitates the committee process.

4. *Establish methods of reporting* or recording the committee's work. Making reports publicly available gives credibility to the committee as a representative group and shows that progress is being made.

5. *Start with easily made decisions* or those of a general nature, such as elements of the basic philosophy of the program. Starting with items that allow committee members to get to know one another and reach consensus easily will promote group development. Time will be required before the committee will be able to handle contentious issues well.

These suggestions are appropriate to a committee that has the authority to make decisions about the proposed program. Occasionally the nurse is involved in an "advisory" committee, the members of which are expert resource people for a program or project led usually by a health educator. The five rules also apply to this kind of committee. In addition, it is especially important that the specific goals and objectives of the committee be clear, both to the group itself and to the organization.

At their best, advisory committees can be an excellent means of gathering together the wisdom and experience of a group of people who would not have time to work on the program intensively. They give credibility to a program because they often hold key positions in the organization. In addition, their visible support of the program increases general acceptance of it.

At their worst, advisory committees can be merely part of a public relations game, with no real interest in the program by group members and no real intent to use their advice by program leaders. A health educator I know has, on several occasions, organized an advisory committee for programs consisting of 15 to 18 persons. Because this size group has trouble reaching consensus on any issue, they give no effective advice and the educator can proceed with running the programs the way she wants to run them. Although she does retain power, her manipulative behavior also generates considerable frustration.

Planning committees or advisory committees that function during the planning phase can contribute valuable information, coordination, communication, and credibility to a program's development.

> The keys to a committee's effectiveness are clearly stated goals, a commitment to the educational program's intent by individual members, and the group's ability to solve problems.

A number of critical decisions must be made, either by a planning committee or by program leaders, before an educational program can move into its organizational and implementation phases. The most important of these decisions are reviewed below.

Decisions to Be Made During the Planning Phase

The first and foremost questions to be answered by those developing a patient education program are, What exactly are we trying to accomplish? and How are we to do that? When examined in detail, these apparently simple and straightforward questions can quickly become complex. There is a prime opportunity to investigate these complexities and make major decisions about an educational program while it is in the planning stage, well before program implementation. If decisions concerning direction, evaluation, and management should be deferred, program leaders who are immersed in start-up details will find themselves trying to manage crises precipitated by this lack without the time or the objectivity to logically think through the consequences of decisions.

Categories of important decisions to be made during the planning phase of program development are:

- what form the program will take to reflect its philosophy, goals, and objectives;
- what methods will be used to determine the results or outcomes of the program;
- what benefits the program will have for its sponsors;
- who the participants are to be (learners, teachers, and advisors); and
- how responsibilities, authority, and resources are to be distributed.

In the following paragraphs we will look briefly at each of these categories.

Educational programs that are developed under the auspices of an educational institution usually begin with a "curriculum plan." The principle of starting with a clear overall statement of what the program intends to do applies to much smaller patient education programs as well. A curriculum plan states the general goal of the program and shows how various elements of content further that goal. For example, a school of nursing might have a curriculum plan that includes a statement of what kind of nurse is to be prepared in the school and then describes how various courses and their content contribute to that goal.

> Making decisions about a program's philosophy, general goals, and purposes early in the planning process allows the program to be developed with a coherent form and structure.

An analogy to this principle is that it is helpful to a person constructing a jigsaw puzzle to know what the overall picture looks like. If the picture is not available, the person spends extra time attempting to fit pieces together in error and contrary to the intended design.

The *form* that a patient education program takes is determined by its basic philosophy or intended outcome. The example below shows portions of the philosophy statement from several programs.

Example 10.2   PROGRAM PHILOSOPHIES

Program 1: (from a post-coronary support program) It is important that the program foster self-help and independence.

Program 2: (from a weight loss program) This program is based on the belief that increased activity as well as altered eating patterns will lead to improved health and self-esteem.

Program 3: (from a parenting program) Improved ability to express feelings and handle conflict will positively affect relationships within the marriage as well as the parent-child relationship.

Each of these statements of philosophy or belief about what the program intends to do suggests some specific learning objectives. For example, in program 3, the participant will need to learn skills in communicating feelings and handling conflict as well as develop a positive attitude toward using these skills in at least two kinds of relationships. These objectives, in turn, suggest what kinds of instructional content and activities might be included. Taken together, the philosophy, objectives, and content determine the form of the program.

A natural extension of the question "What is it that we are really trying to do?" is "How will we know when we get there?" As noted in Section 4.3 and in Chapter 10, clearly stated teaching goals and objectives are essential to useful *evaluation* of learning. Likewise, in a patient education program, the stated goals and objectives form the basis of an approach to evaluation. There are three related reasons for making decisions about specific program evaluation methods during the planning phase of program development.

Perhaps the most obvious of these is that in "selling" the idea of an educational program to a sponsor and to program participants, one wants to be able to identify what will happen as a result. To be able to say what the program intends to do is important; to be able to say how that result is to be measured greatly strengthens a program's appeal.

A second reason for deciding questions of evaluation early is also related to sponsorship. As discussed in Section 10.1, most educational programs begin with an idea about what will improve the quality of life for participants. Organizations, especially those that are contributing financial or staff support for a program, are interested in seeing results in quantifiable terms. Translating quality into quantity, and vice versa, takes determined effort by planners who are thoroughly acquainted with the goals of the program and who have a variety of options available for implementation. Once a program has begun, it is difficult to add unexpected and unplanned recording devices or financial justification procedures that are not disruptive or meaningless.

A third reason for planning evaluation well in advance has to do with the opportunity for research presented by large-scale or continuing programs in patient education. Well-planned and well-executed research not only adds information to our knowledge about the teaching-learning process, but also has implications for future nursing practice and, as Polit and Hungler (1983) phrase it, the nurse's "scientific accountability."

An area of decision making related to the evaluation of program results is the determination of what *benefits* the program holds for its sponsors. At the most basic level, sponsors want to be sure that the program is planned in such a way that its results will be clear. A further consideration is how those results translate into improved business, better public relations, professional credibility, or other benefit for the sponsor. Identifying such potential benefits early in program development allows planners to learn details of organizational protocol and procedures and choose strategies for presentation of the program.

Once the general form, evaluation methods, and benefits of the proposed program have been determined, planners can turn their attention to the program's *audience* and *resource personnel*. Such questions as "Who will come?" "How will they get there?" "Who will teach?" and "Who can help us?" will need to be answered. Careful consideration must be given to how participants are to be attracted or referred to the program, what is likely to motivate their involvement, and what caregivers need to be convinced of the program's worth in order to reinforce a would-be participant's interest. The companion set of considerations are "Who is most qualified to teach or manage the program?" and "What other kinds of help will be needed?" Many times the planning group also becomes the personnel selection group at this stage.

> As details of the patient education program become clearer, it is increasingly important to include the major teaching, leadership, and resource people in the process.

A final major area of decision making during the planning phase of program development has to do with how *responsibilities, authority*, and *resources* will be distributed. As the planning group completes its task, decision making passes to those who will be leading the organizational and implementation phases. The lines of authority to be followed, procedures of accountability, the use of funds, and the channels for getting help if needed all should be determined. To do this clearly and in writing avoids confusion and power struggles later and helps maintain the momentum needed to get a program working.

In summary, the planning phase of program development is one in which major decisions are made regarding the program's form, evaluation methods, benefits, participants, personnel, and future management. Because of the complexity of these decisions and the need for "horizontal" communication between departments, disciplines, or functional groups, a committee approach to planning is advantageous. Some ideas about how to improve the effectiveness of a planning committee have been discussed and a possible decision-making agenda suggested. Thorough planning is essential to program effectiveness.

10.3 THE ORGANIZATIONAL PHASE OF PROGRAM DEVELOPMENT

As was discussed in Section 10.2 the what, why, and who of the proposed patient education program are decided during the planning phase. By the time

TABLE 10–2. Elements of Marketing and Their Application to Education

Product/Service	An educational program is a service that offers consumers the opportunity to gain knowledge, attitudes, or skills that lead to their recovery or maintenance of health or the prevention of future health problems.
Pricing/Cost	Patient education has both direct and indirect costs to the participant. Direct costs include registration fees and purchase of supplies. When the education program is part of prescribed treatment, third parties may be billed for reimbursement, either as a separate item or included in "auxiliary" services. Indirect costs to the patient include time, any inconvenience caused by participation, and travel costs. The stress induced by learning and change can also be considered (see Section 2.5).
Distribution	The availability of the program to potential consumers is a major marketing concern. This factor includes investigation of other similar or competing programs in the geographical area, timing the program to match current interest and convenience of participants, and reviewing the characteristics of the facility in which the program is offered, such as access, comfort, and amenities.
Communication	The most important element of marketing has to do with communicating information about the planned program to identified target groups so that they will be motivated to participate in spite of costs. They must be given specific information about how to join the program and must believe that the program will meet their own health needs. (See discussion of Health Belief model in Section 2.3.)

the organizational phase begins, developers are ready to consider the specifics of where, when, and how. The major tasks of this phase include marketing the program to its anticipated audience, preparing teaching staff, assembling or developing teaching materials, and determining the details of operating and follow-up procedures. In the paragraphs that follow we will look at each of these tasks briefly.

Marketing the Program

The term marketing is so frequently associated with the commercial world that its application to patient education programs is often overlooked. Marketing has to do with products, pricing, distribution, and communication (Quelch, 1980). It begins with research into what people perceive as a need and what previous experiences have influenced their present attitudes, knowledge, and skills, a process that is similar to the nurse's assessment of an individual's readiness to learn (see Sections 2.2 and 2.3). A marketing approach then seeks to match a product (or service) to identified consumer groups, "teaching" them, through communication, how to obtain and use that product. Each of the major elements of marketing are listed in Table 10–2, together with notes as to their application to patient education.

The gathering of information that will form the basis of a marketing strategy begins in the assessment phase of program development, when the health needs of a group of individuals are determined. By the time the organizational phase has been reached, information that has been accumulating is brought together and decisions are made about how best to inform and motivate those for whom the program has been designed.

> The challenge of successful marketing is to present the opportunity for program participation in the most attractive, interesting, and stimulating way possible, appealing to the target group's perceived health needs.

This presentation must be made whether the program is directed at currently hospitalized patients, or well individuals in the community; whether people are expected to attend, or must arrange to come of their own volition. In all cases the role of marketing is to prepare participants to learn what will be offered during the program.

The choices regarding the use of various media approaches to get the message out are similar to those made by the nurse teacher in deciding on teaching materials. Health education texts are a good resource for information about media use, especially for public education programs. (See, for example, Chapter 18, "Using the Media to Achieve Maximum Impact," in Breckon, Harvey, and Lancaster, 1985.) During the organizational phase of program development, these choices will need to be made, materials prepared, and a time schedule for their distribution planned.

Preparing Teaching Staff

Most patient education programs involve several teachers, assistants, or resource people. The organizational phase of program development is a good time for them to get together to begin working cooperatively. Preparatory sessions are held in order to:

- develop an interpersonal relationship between staff members, so that a high level of cooperation is achieved;
- distribute information about the planned program with opportunity given to clarify details;
- update knowledge or skills that are the subject matter of the program; and
- plan specific teaching approaches and methods.

The staff development or nursing education unit in medical facilities can be a valuable resource for preparing program staff.

Many patient education programs use members of several different disciplines as teachers in order to present a comprehensive approach to the subject.

> The use of multidisciplinary teaching staff greatly enriches an educational program but demands that careful attention be paid to cooperation, coordination, and continuing communication between staff members.

One of the most effective ways of achieving these goals is to provide the opportunity for teaching staff to participate in a group process of their own. If they can get to the point of accepting differences of background and attitudes while genuinely respecting one another as individuals, the presentation of the program will go smoothly. (See Section 8.1 on stages of group process.)

Even when a program's design involves standardized presentation of material to patients over a period of time by different teachers, it is important to prepare staff for the program's introduction during the organizational phase.

Assembling and Preparing Teaching Materials

Finding out what possibly useful materials already exist, reviewing them, and developing new materials take much more time than is usually planned for these tasks. This process should be started even before exact teaching methods and approaches are decided. In fact, knowing what is available may positively influence these decisions. The resources listed in Appendix B are good starting points, as are telephone calls to organizations devoted to subjects associated with the content of the planned program. (See Chapter 6 for guidance on developing educational materials.)

Deciding on Operating and Follow-Up Procedures

The organizational phase of program development is the appropriate time for decisions to be made about how people, materials, and records are to be handled. Many of these details are reflected in the questions posed in the checklist in Section 10.5. Imagining an individual participant as he moves into, through, and away from the program is one useful device for ensuring that all "bases are covered." It is especially important to consider the mechanics for completing evaluation tests and questionnaires, how observations are to be made and recorded, and how research measurements are to be conducted. Polit and Hungler's book *Nursing Research* (1983) gives helpful guidance for the latter.

Whenever the planned program will be ongoing or have multiple sessions, procedures should be written down for the sake of consistency as well as program evaluation. If a written guide is to be the major source of information for teaching staff, this task should be approached with all the care of preparing teaching materials; it will in fact be used to teach the teachers. (See Section 6.2 for notes on writing instructions.)

As long as enough time is available before the program begins, anticipated procedural problems can be creatively overcome. The following are examples of such problem solving.

Example 10.3   SOLVING PROCEDURAL PROBLEMS

Problem 1. How to divide a large group into small discussion groups with a minimum of confusion.

Solution. Name tags were color coded and appropriately colored signs were posted around the room. The instructor could then direct participants to go to the sign that matched their name tag to form small groups.

Problem 2. How to maintain the quality of teaching in a standardized program of postoperative pre-discharge instruction conducted by the patient's primary nurse.

Solution. Checklists were prepared for assessment of patient learning needs and for lesson content. The patient evaluation questionnaire included questions about whether specific information had been given. In addition, a short videotape was prepared showing a demonstration lesson. This was used as an orientation for new staff members and as a refresher for others. Nurses had easy access to this tape, which included answers to commonly asked questions.

Problem 3. A group program for newly diagnosed diabetic patients and their families was to be partially evaluated through use of a research instrument. The researcher wanted the questionnaire to be individually administered in an interview format. The program's teaching staff, however, was apprehensive about using the questionnaire and felt that its administration would take up too much valuable teaching time.

Solution. All patients were visited at home, shortly after discharge, by a representative of the local diabetic association. When the problem was made known to the group, they volunteered to give the questionnaire at the time of the representative's visit, since this also gave the representative valuable information about the person's future learning needs. The researcher went to the association's regular meeting to teach them how to use the questionnaire.

The clear definition of operating and follow-up procedures is an important organizational challenge. Every effort should be made to make them as complete as possible. At the same time the initial procedural outline should not be regarded as "cast in concrete."

> Having clear guidelines on procedures helps to smooth the implementation of a new program, but even the most carefully constructed procedures will need to be modified as the program matures.

In summary, the organizational phase of program development consists of deciding and acting on the when, where, and how of the planned program. In this section we have discussed marketing, preparing staff, assembling or developing teaching materials, and outlining operating and follow-up procedures. As much time as possible should be allowed for organization, since its careful completion will greatly reduce confusion and conflict once the program begins.

10.4 THE IMPLEMENTATION PHASE OF PROGRAM DEVELOPMENT

After what seems like a long preparatory period, the program is finally ready to start. Rather than coming to an end, behind-the-scenes activities now increase dramatically in number and pace.

> The program manager or coordinator can expect to spend at least twice the amount of actual patient contact time in management activities. The time necessary for coordination is increased by program size and complexity.

If thorough assessment, planning, and organization have been completed, a person will have been appointed to the position of program manager or coordinator, with undisputed authority to make day-to-day decisions concerning implementation. Although specific tasks may be delegated, having one person with management authority and responsibility is crucial to a program's success (Rakich, Longest, and O'Donovan, 1977, Ch. 7). Once implementation begins, this person's major job is to ensure communication to and from participants, to and from teaching staff, and to and from the sponsoring organization. Her activities divide into four basic areas: coordinating, conducting the program, ensuring quality control and accountability, and managing problems.

Coordinating

Clark and Shea (1979) describe coordination as gathering together and then synchronizing different work efforts so that they function harmoniously in meeting goals. Whether conducting an orchestra or leading a patient education program, coordination is not a simple task. In addition to harmonizing the efforts of the people involved in a program, the coordinator must balance time schedules, equipment, and materials. She may also need to coordinate the marketing and public relations aspects of program implementation.

Most patient education programs are difficult to coordinate because they cannot be "managed" in a traditional hierarchical fashion. They often depend on the use of talent from a number of groups, departments, or personnel classifications. Synchronizing these talents depends more on good will, good timing, and good communication skills than it does on the formal structure of the sponsoring organization. Most decisions made are negotiated ones, balancing the priorities of other people and units with the needs of the program.

> Three factors make successful coordination possible: the thorough assessment, planning, and organization of the program; clear lines of authority and responsibility so that decision making and action are not delayed; and the effective communication skills of the coordinator.

Throughout this chapter the importance of the assessment, planning, and organizational steps has been emphasized. Without these steps and the decisions that are made within them, the coordinator faces an impossible task. In order to survive the conflicting needs, desires, and priorities of the people and organizational units involved, the program must first have clearly established goals and capable management.

In addition, there must be clear lines of decision-making authority and responsibility. At best, the program director or coordinator is able to make all but the most major decisions in a climate of trust and support from organizational administration. This kind of situation allows the coordinator the best chance of negotiating decisions quickly with other decision-makers involved in the program. At the very least the lines of authority should be carefully planned and structured so that the coordinator can contact the responsible person without delay when need for a decision occurs. If decision making is a slow process, implementation of the program will lose momentum, support, and the confidence of the very people on whom its success depends.

There are a variety of styles of coordination, just as there are styles of other kinds of leadership. Some people prefer to establish a relationship of mutual liking and trust before they begin to resolve questions of activities, roles, or viewpoints. Others put a priority on establishing their credibility as an intelligent decision-maker during the organizational phase of program development, before approaching negotiations with other decision-makers.

Whatever the personal style of the coordinator, he does not usually have direct administrative control over the people or material resources that the program will use. His decisions will therefore necessarily be negotiated ones and his general approach, to lead and convince, rather than to direct and control. The program coordinator needs to have well-developed communication skills and a thorough understanding of and commitment to the proposed program. Without these characteristics, he will be unable to grasp an opportunity to advance the program through an offer of help from resources. He will also lack a firm knowledge of what elements of the program are essential and not negotiable.

An important aspect of the coordinator's job concerns timing. Not only do decisions need to be made and resources brought together, but these things need to happen at the right time. Successfully doing this requires careful planning, the preparation of other people involved, investigation of alternatives in case of emergency, and some degree of intuition on the part of the coordinator. It means sending reminder notes, storing supplies in places where they can be found, and sharing information with others who can "back-up" the coordinator. Good coordination pays dividends when it is time to conduct the program.

Conducting the Program

Until participants are thoroughly familiar with operating procedures, the program manager needs to be immediately involved with the actual running of the program. In a program with group sessions, there is furniture to arrange, power outlets to be found, patients to be greeted and registered, and many other seemingly minor details that take time, knowledge of program goals, and sometimes on-the-spot decisions. In a standardized one-to-one teaching program, staff will need reminders of what resources are available to them and where supplies are stored, as well as support and encouragement when they try the program for the first few times.

Involvement in the early implementation of the program also allows the program director to assess the completeness of the planning and organizing phases of program development and make necessary modification in operating procedures.

Maintaining Quality Control and Accountability Procedures

Once a patient education program has actually begun to offer services, the program director's principal task becomes one of liaison between the sponsoring organization and program participants. This liaison role takes the form of maintaining the quality of the program through staff supervision, receiving feedback from patients regarding the program's effectiveness in meeting its goals, and reporting on the program's needs, accomplishments, and financial status to sponsors.

If several teachers or staff members are involved in conducting the program, one important responsibility of the director or manager is to supervise them and help them maintain the quality of program that was envisioned by the planners. There are few patient education programs, especially those using multidisciplinary approaches, in which the manager has the power to hire and fire staff. Therefore, her relationship to teachers in the program is more one of coordination and consultation than one of formal supervision. The informality of this relationship does not preclude the development of standards of performance and periodic evaluation. An effective and widely accepted approach is a cooperative one. In it personnel participate in setting their own goals in line with program standards and periodically evaluate their own performance (Barrett, Gessner, and Phelps, 1975).

> In patient education the role of the program manager is to help the teacher learn to do the best possible job, just as she is helping patients learn. A cooperative approach to supervision is both useful as a role model and effective as a management approach.

Another important aspect of the program manager's job is to receive feedback from patient participants about whether the program is meeting their needs as intended, to what extent it is accomplishing its goals, and what the overall impact and outcome of the program are (Squyres and associates, 1985, Ch. 7). This kind of feedback may take several forms, ranging from subjective questionnaires to findings from formal research or testing procedures. Although much more difficult to quantify, informal conversation with patients is an excellent source of immediate feedback. Their satisfaction with the program and the suggestions they offer for improvement should be taken seriously.

Finally, the program manager acts as a conduit of communication and accountability between the program and the sponsoring organization. Although most programs that are thoroughly planned have periodic reporting procedures for which the manager is responsible, sponsors welcome additional information about how the program is going and what impact it is having on the organization's public relations. This kind of communication with sponsors helps to maintain interest in the program and makes continued support much more likely.

Managing Problems

Although thorough program development lessens the occurrence of major problems during the start-up phase of patient education, there are always a few "bugs" to be worked out. One of the most important reasons for appointing a program manager and giving her decision-making authority is to quickly and decisively resolve the problems that arise. A relatively minor problem, such as an equipment failure, can cause needless confusion, loss of teaching time, and an erosion of the teacher's credibility with patients. Problems that need the help of the manager fall into three general areas: policy, personnel, and procedures.

Despite the care taken by the planning committee, policy problems can be discovered as a program begins. In one such situation the hospital's central supply department was to make available equipment to be used in the program. As the program was about to begin, it was discovered that policy forbade the equipment's being removed from the hospital building. The education program was being conducted in an adjoining building.

The key to solving such problems is to present the issue to decision-makers and help them understand how the problem affects the program. If they or their staff have not been made defensive by frustrated program staff, a resolution can usually be negotiated. Occasionally the program manager will need to arrange a meeting of higher level decision-makers to settle the issue.

The most common personnel problems involve conflicts in schedules. As discussed earlier, staff members should be given the opportunity to build rapport with one another so that responsibility for resolving such issues can be given to the group. The program manager will find it useful to have developed his own conflict resolution skills so that personality clashes, poor performance, or complaints can be handled confidently and without delay. Continuing education courses offer one of the best opportunities to gain and practice conflict resolution skills. Personnel management texts, such as that edited by Beach (1975), also are a good resource for the program manager.

The anticipation of procedural problems was discussed in Section 10.3, along with the caution that as the program begins, modifications in procedures will almost certainly have to be made. Gathering the staff group together to resolve procedure problems is a useful approach for two reasons. The first is that those most directly involved are the most likely to see a solution to a problem. The second is that having been involved in the decision making, staff members are more likely to carry out the change.

In summary, effective leadership is of prime importance during the implementation phase of program development. In this section we have explored the role of the program director or manager in terms of coordinating, conducting the program, maintaining quality control and accountability procedures, and managing problems as they arise. The importance of the manager's immediate involvement in program details and her ability to communicate effectively have been emphasized.

10.5 A CHECKLIST FOR PROGRAM DEVELOPMENT

Involvement in the development of patient education programs gives the nurse the opportunity to make an important contribution to patients' future health and well-being. At the same time she can develop her own organizational, communication, teaching, and leadership skills through such involvement. The following checklist is offered as a guide to the nurse as she progresses through the four phases of program development. It is formulated as a series of questions in order to stimulate discussion. Not all questions will be appropriate to all programs. Conversely, with a specific project in mind, many more questions will occur to the reader. It is helpful to make as comprehensive and specific a list of questions for oneself as early in a program's development as possible, to use as a guide. As the project progresses, more can be added so as to decrease the possibility of overlooking important developmental areas.

Phase 1: Assessment

Needs

- What kinds of learning would improve the *quality of patients' lives*? What problems would be solved or goals met through this learning?
- What has contributed to this lack of knowledge, attitudes, or skills? What is the incidence of the need? How prevalent is it? How is the need distributed in the general or patient population?
- Is the *need* currently perceived by patients in the affected group? In what ways? Is need urgent and short term, or important but longer term? What contributed to the perception of need?
- Does the need involve a present *behavior*? Will this behavior change or stop as a result of learning? What factors reinforce the behavior? How powerful are these factors?
- What *attitudes* are currently held by those with the learning need? What factors reinforce those attitudes? How powerful are these factors?

Resources

- What *other learning opportunities* on similar subjects already exist in the community? Do these fulfill the need you have identified? If so, in what ways? If not, why not?
- Are there realistic ways to expand or alter already-existing programs to meet the need? What would have to be done?
- If a new program is developed, what can be learned from existing programs?
- Are there *people* in your organization or community who have skills, knowledge, experience, or time to contribute to program development? Who are they? How could they be contacted? Are there regulations or protocol to be followed in contacting them? How would you interest them in your project?
- What resources exist for financial *support* of a new program? What are the procedures for application? What criteria are used to approve a project? Are there other projects or groups funded by this/these organization(s)? What has been their experience in gaining approval and working with the organization?
- To what degree would your employing organization support such a program? Would operating funds, staff time, materials, or expert consultation be available?
- What patient education programs currently exist with the support of your organization? How did they gain that support?

- What is the *protocol* for gaining approval for educational activities? Who needs to approve, and how might you interest them in your project?
- Are there other organizations in your community that could contribute support to your program? Have they been involved in similar programs in the past? To what extent and with what result?
- How much *time* do you and other nursing staff realistically have available for program development activities?
- What patient teaching *materials* are available or could be obtained within the subject area of concern? Are there resources available for the development of new materials?
- What teaching *equipment* would be available to the program? Who is skilled in the use of this equipment? How might additional equipment be obtained? Approximately what cost is involved?

Plans for the Development Process

- What would be the major goals of a program developed to meet the identified patient needs?
- What steps, tasks, or activities would be necessary in order to thoroughly plan a program that accomplishes those goals? What is their order of priority? What is a realistic time frame for doing these things?

Phase 2: Planning

Organizing the Planning Group

- What *people*, within the sponsoring organization, seem the most appropriate to be part of the planning group? Who is the most involved in or concerned about the patient need that has been identified? Who can contribute planning or other skills to the group? Who holds a key position that would give the program access to special resources? Who is available to spend time in planning activities?
- What people have been recommended to be part of a planning or advisory group by others? What were their reasons for these recommendations? To what degree is it important that these recommendations be followed?
- What people outside the sponsoring organization would appropriately be members of a planning or advisory group? What special skills or knowledge would they bring to the project? What protocol would be involved in an invitation to join the group?
- How will the planning group be *structured*? Has a leader for this group already been identified, or will the group appoint one? How can power struggles within the group be avoided?
- On what *time schedule* will the group operate? How often will they meet? For how long? How will an agenda be constructed? Where will they meet? Will transportation to and from meetings be a problem?

- What *records* will be kept of the group's activities? Who will be responsible for transcribing and distributing them? To whom will they be distributed and in what detail? How can corrections be made? How will questions from those outside the committee be handled?

Planning Decisions

- In concise terms, what are the *general goals and purposes* of the proposed program? What beliefs and philosophies underlie this statement of purpose? In what ways can these beliefs be supported by research or experience? To what degree can planners reach consensus on these beliefs?

- What *form* should the program take to accomplish its goals? What general subjects or content areas could be included? What kind of communication processes will be involved (individual, group, media, etc.)?

- How will the program's outcome be evaluated? How will this evaluation be received by the sponsoring organization? Will the method of evaluation assist in gaining support for the project? Will evaluation include financial justification? Will it give quantitative as well as qualitative results of the program?

- Will research be conducted on program results or process? Who will take responsibility for this research? What audience will be interested in the results? What will need to be done to plan, organize, and execute the research project?

- How will the sponsoring organization benefit from the proposed program? Can the program reasonably be expected to produce revenue, increase business, or improve public relations for the organization? How will sponsorship of the program be viewed by similar organizations, by the community, by professional groups?

- Who will be the program's *participants*? How will potential learners be identified? How will they know about the program? What is likely to motivate them to participate?

- Who will teach? What is the level of preparation of available teachers? Will other assistance be needed to conduct the program? How will this be arranged?

- Who will take *responsibility* for organizing and implementing the program? What special knowledge, attitudes, and skills are required or desired of program leaders? How are they to be selected and appointed? What will be their relationship to the sponsoring organization? How will accountability be demonstrated?

- How will the program manager's position fit within the organization's lines of authority? How will this influence her decision making? Who will supervise the program manager? What will be the manager's relationship to other program staff members? What influence will members of the planning group continue to have on the program?

Phase 3: Organization

Marketing

- How will the program's *service(s)* be presented to potential consumers? What identified needs, perceptions, previous experience will be appealed to? What details of the program's process and expected results will be used in marketing it?
- Will there be *direct costs* to the consumer in the form of registration fees or purchase of materials or supplies? What concessions will be made (if any) to low-income participants? What criteria will be used to determine eligibility?
- Will reimbursement of costs be possible through insurance companies or other third parties? What criteria are used to determine whether costs are reimbursable? What procedure will be followed in applying for reimbursement? Who will take responsibility for this?
- What *indirect costs* might consumers experience? How can inconvenience, travel costs, and time spent be minimized? Will learning content or the program's process be stressful for participants? How can this be controlled or minimized?
- How will information about and accessibility to the program be *distributed* in the community/organization? What options will be given to participants about timing and venue of the program? What facilities will be used in program presentation? What amenities contribute to the comfort of participants? What negative factors can be removed or minimized?
- What groups have been targeted to receive *communication* about the program? Is there more than one category of motivation to participate? How will publicity target these specific motivations? What percentage of those who receive information about the program can be expected to participate?
- What methods and materials will be used to convey program information? What has to be done to prepare these materials? How will they be distributed? Who will be responsible for distribution? How will those who are interested contact the program? How will they register? How will the questions of potential consumers be answered?

Staff Preparation

- What personal characteristics, attitudes, knowledge, and skills can staff be expected to already have? How were/will they be selected? How much time is available for their preparation? Who will supervise their performance? What will their relationship be to one another and to the program manager?
- What in particular must program staff know, believe, or be able to do in order to be effective? Which of these are priorities? How are they to be helped to meet these objectives? What materials and methods will be used to prepare staff? Will clinical experience be provided as part of their preparation? Who will supervise their performance?

- Who will be responsible for staff preparation? How will their capabilities be measured? By whom? What will happen to those who do not meet minimum standards? Will the performance of teaching staff be monitored? By whom and in what way?
- Is continuing education for staff members planned? What are its objectives and priorities? Who will take responsibility for this?

Preparation of Materials

- What known patient-education materials are *available* on the subjects of concern? What sources of information might be consulted about additional materials? What materials are being used by similar programs elsewhere?
- *How many* copies of various teaching materials will be needed? How are these ordered and with what expected delay? What copyright restrictions apply to available materials?
- What materials that are not available or are *unique* to this program are needed or desired? What objectives would the use of such materials help to meet? What would have to be done to develop new materials? What equipment, supplies, and creative abilities would be required? Who would be responsible for their development? What costs are involved? How much time is required?
- Will new materials be tested before use in the program? How will this be done? Who will review materials for accuracy? To what extent will these materials be publicly distributed? Should they be protected by copyright?

Organizing Operating Procedures

- How and by whom will operating and follow-up procedures be decided? Will these be written? By whom will they be reviewed? Who has overall responsibility for procedures? How general/specific and flexible/standardized are these procedures?
- Will program participants have direct individual contact (by telephone or in person) with program staff *before* the program begins? What information will they be asked to give? What information or instructions will they be given?
- How will a would-be participant *register* for the program? Will he be given or sent preprogram materials? Will he be given or sent a reminder about attendance?
- What needs to be done to *set up* the program venue? What is the preferred furniture arrangement? Where are directional signs to be placed? Are restrooms conveniently located and clearly marked? What arrangements must be made for refreshments? Will smoking be permitted? How will required teaching equipment be transported to the teaching venue? How and by whom will its working order be checked? How are teaching materials to be organized and made available? How much time will be required for set-up?

- How will a participant be greeted at the beginning of the program's *first session*? What will he be expected to do? How will this be made clear to him? Are participants to be introduced to one another and to staff members? What messages will intentionally be given about the expected relationship of participants to one another and to staff? What messages will be given about the relative formality or informality with which the program is to be conducted?

- Does the choice of the first teaching methods used reflect the intended formality/informality of the program? Will interaction with the teacher or between participants be invited/facilitated? How will the goals and objectives of the program be made clear to participants? How are the form, process, and evaluation of the program to be made clear to participants? How are the responsibilities of participants for practicing skills, completing homework or assignments, and so on to be outlined?

- *As the program progresses*, what flexibility is planned in terms of interests and concerns of participants, teacher preferences of methods and materials, and time limits for discussion or activities? How is the participants' progress toward program goals to be assessed? What feedback is to be given to them about this assessment? If the group process is important to program goals, how is progress to be assessed and what feedback is to be given?

- *As the program concludes*, how will attainment of program goals be evaluated? What tests, questionnaires, or discussion will be part of this evaluation? How much time should be allowed for these? Is withdrawal from the group process expected to take extra time? How will participants be helped to focus on their future health responsibilities?

- Is there a provision for the *follow-up* of program participants? When is this to be done and by whom? What are the objectives of follow-up and how is their attainment to be measured? Are "advanced" educational programs being planned?

Phase 4: Implementation/Management

Coordination

- What are the lines of authority and *responsibility* for decision making? What are the characteristics of the current relationship between program staff members and between staff and program administration? How could/should these relationships be modified to promote cooperation? How will communication to and from staff members be facilitated?

- What level of *cooperation* will be necessary between staff members? How will this be maintained? What level of input will staff members have in decision making, planning of teaching methods and material, and modifying procedures? What kinds of responsibilities can be delegated to staff members by the program manager?

- What *equipment and teaching materials* need to be obtained? How much time is required for their arrival? What storage space is available for the program's use? How will additional supplies be ordered as needed and by whom? What alternatives will be provided in case of equipment breakdown or shortage of materials?

• Who will have responsibility for *marketing* the program, contacting media, and sending out materials? How and by whom will the impact of marketing be evaluated and approaches modified?

Conducting the Program

• What role will the program *manager* play in the initial stages of the program? What kinds of decisions can be made immediately? In what ways will the manager help staff members follow planned procedures?

• How and by whom will *procedures* be reviewed? How and by whom will modifications be made? What provision is there for immediate feedback from participants or staff members about their satisfaction with the program and the achievement of goals?

Maintaining Quality Control and Accountability

• What criteria will be used to evaluate *teacher performance*? When and by whom will this evaluation be made? How will excellent performance be rewarded? How will poor performance be handled? With whom will performance evaluations be shared?

• What *channels of authority* exist for making suggestions for policy change or having complaints heard? What kinds of incidents will be reported to authorities? How will decisions made by administrators be communicated to the program manager and staff?

• What *records* will be kept regarding participants, staff time, management time, use of materials, and expenditure of funds? By whom will records be kept, and what channels will be used for their submission?

• How will the effectiveness of the program be judged by decision-makers/ sponsors? What criteria will be used for determining the program's benefits to the sponsoring organization? How are data to be collected and submitted for these evaluations?

Problem Management

• To what degree is the program director able to negotiate with other units or departments regarding program needs? What are the channels for modifying program policies, and how is the need for this presented?

• What authority do the program director and staff members have to make on-the-spot decisions to resolve problems as they arise? How are these decisions reported and to whom? How is information about the occurrence of minor problems collected? What input do staff members have in resolving these or temporarily modifying operating procedures?

• What mechanism is there for improving the quality of the program? How often is the program reviewed with the intent of improving it, and who is involved in this process?

In summary, a checklist of questions appropriate to each of the four phases of program development have been presented. For any specific program additional questions may be added and others deleted in order to reflect a complete overview of what must be done and decided in order to make the program operational.

SUMMARY

In this chapter guidelines for the development of patient education programs have been explored. The tasks and decisions that go into program development were divided into four phases and discussed separately. In the final section a series of questions were posed as a guide to program developers. A point that has been emphasized throughout the chapter is that successful patient education programs depend on thorough assessment, planning, and organization before implementation.

For the nurse who has not previously had experience in program development, the time and effort required may not seem to balance with benefits. Yet we would urge nurses to participate in program development for three reasons. One reason is that no other resource provides patients with the quality of teaching and support during learning as do well-planned programs. Essentially, they make available to many patients the opportunity for learning provided individual patients by a committed nurse teacher. Second, by participating in the development of patient education programs, the nurse is able to experience the satisfaction of contributing directly to the patient's wellness. Finally, program development provides the nurse with the opportunity to learn, too, and to sharpen her skills in communication, decision making, interpersonal relationships, organization, and leadership.

Study Questions and Exercises

1. Investigate what patient education programs are sponsored by your employer or a health care facility with which you are familiar. Discover, if possible, what led to the development of these programs. Does this organization have stated policies about the sponsorship and approval of proposals for health education? Discuss your findings with classmates or colleagues.

2. Talk with a nurse who has been involved in the development of a patient-education program. (Those in nursing administration, the education department, or staff development will be able to help you find a source of information.) Talk with this person about the development process. In what ways was it similar to or different from that outlined in this chapter? Discuss your findings with classmates or colleagues.

3. In discussion with colleagues or classmates, identify a number of patient learning needs that you have observed to occur frequently. How would a program developed to meet these needs improve the quality of life of the patient participants? Choosing one of

the less complex ideas, list the steps that would need to be taken or tasks accomplished in order to thoroughly assess and begin to plan such a program. (See discussion of PERT model and example in Section 10.1.) How feasible do you think this program is?

4. Write what you think would be an appropriate statement of philosophy for your own school of nursing, another professional program, or a well-established patient education program with which you are familiar. You are encouraged to collaborate with others on this task. Your aim is to answer the question "What does this program intend to do?" Be sure to define any adjectives you might use as carefully as possible.

Search out the curriculum, statement of philosophy, or statement of intent for the same program. Compare it with your own. When in the development process were these written and by whom? What relationship do they have to program content and evaluation? Have they ever been updated or modified? Discuss your findings with classmates or colleagues.

5. Attend at least one session of a health education program in your community. What are its goals and purpose? Talk with a program leader about the evaluation methods used. What has evaluation shown about the program's success so far? Talk with several participants in the program. What do they feel are the most positive and least positive aspects of the program? What is their general level of satisfaction with it? Do they intend to continue with the program or follow the ideas or principles it encourages? Discuss your findings with classmates or colleagues.

Appendix A

APPROACHES TO COMMON PATIENT-TEACHING SITUATIONS

This appendix presents material that has been organized around four commonly occurring teaching situations. This material may be used as a reference for the nurse planning individual or small-group teaching or as a starting point for the development of patient education programs. The four sections are:

App 1. Admission Teaching
App 2. Preoperative or Pretreatment Teaching
App 3. Teaching Patient Care Procedures
App 4. Discharge Teaching

Each of the four sections includes a list of background information that is especially useful to the nurse in planning teaching, some possible learning goals and objectives, useful teaching strategies and materials, and notes on evaluation methods.

All patients have learning needs. Teaching is one of several kinds of nursing intervention planned within the framework of the Nursing Process in response to these needs. Certain events occur during a patient's care that give rise to particular kinds of knowledge deficits. These events are usually transitional; that is, they represent a new set of goals and behaviors for the patient and his family members. The nurse who seeks to teach effectively will anticipate these events and strive to intervene with her teaching before their occurrence, or at the earliest opportunity. We begin with the event of admission to a medical care facility and explore the teaching that is appropriate to the person as he adapts to the role of patient.

App 1. ADMISSION TEACHING

The most frequent reason for seeking medical care is the existence of a health problem that the person feels he cannot manage without additional resources. Entrance to care may generate feelings of fear, apprehension, confusion, and a reduced sense of independence. These negative feelings emanate from the person's past experience with being cared for, his present anxiety about what is happening to him, and his estimate of the future consequences of this medical episode. For the same reasons he may also experience a range of positive feelings, such as relief, hope, and an increased sense of confidence in his decision to seek help. Whether the entry point for care is a hospital admission office, an emergency room, the scene of an accident, a doctor's office, or a clinic, positive and negative feelings are usually mixed and result in an inability to concentrate or clearly perceive the details of events. (See description of Carkhuff model in Section 7.1.)

The general goal of caregivers is to help the person through this transitional period by ensuring his physical safety and then helping to reduce his stress level sufficiently that he is able to effectively use the resources offered to him.

> Helping the newly admitted patient learn what is being done on his behalf, what is expected of him, what he can expect of caregivers, and how to manage his immediate environment adds to his sense of control and individuality while reducing his stress level.

Similar teaching intervention directed at the other significant people who accompany the patient increases the effectiveness of his personal and social support network. Some of the major factors to be considered by the nurse as she plans and implements teaching intervention during the patient's entrance to care are outlined in the following paragraphs.

Background Information

Whatever the nurse knows about the patient's previous experiences with medical care, his perceptions about his present situation, his expectations about his future well-being, and his current health balance is useful as she gives physical care and begins her teaching intervention. It is always helpful to stop, look, and listen to the patient and the people with him before attempting an explanation or direction. The answers to the following questions may be especially helpful to the nurse when planning admission teaching.

- What is the patient's native language?
- To what degree is the person currently limited in his ability to hear, see, or think clearly?
- Are other people accompanying the patient? What are their names and how significant is their relationship to the patient? To what degree will they continue to be involved in his care?
- What has been the patient's previous experience with medical care? Has he formerly been a patient at this facility, or one like it? How recently has he seen a doctor for examination or treatment? Does he have a chronic illness that necessitates regular treatment?
- What is the perception of the patient and those accompanying him of events that led to his seeking medical intervention?
- What is the stress level of the patient and those with him? (See Section 2.5.)

The answers to these kinds of questions give the nurse information about the patient's ability to use help with learning, his present level of knowledge about admission procedures, his mental state, and the structure of his support group.

TABLE A–1. Sample Plan for Admission Teaching

Learning Objectives—For the learner to:	Teaching Content
General Goal: Treatment	
Identify members of the medical team by name.	Identity and role of medical team members.
Describe the role of each in relation to his care.	
Describe what he needs to do to cooperate with procedures and treatments.	Expectations of medical team regarding cooperative behavior.
Actively choose to cooperate with treatment.	
General Goal: Maintenance	
Describe the importance or reason for various aspects of his care.	What is being done on his behalf.
Ask questions about care.	Involvement of patient and family in care to maintain sense of control and self-esteem.
Respond to verbal coaching by family member(s) regarding cooperative behavior.	
General Goal: Primary Prevention	
Demonstrate safe use of equipment.	Safe use of equipment, such as lights, bed adjustments, and bathroom.
Describe and practice limitations of physical movement.	Nature of and reasons for physical limitations.
General Goal: Developmental Prevention	
Describe events and procedures to take place as part of treatment.	Nature of and reasons for anticipated events and procedures.
Describe or demonstrate how and when to call for assistance.	Use of signal light.
	Availability and appropriate use of assistance.
Demonstrate through nonverbal behavior or describe lessened levels of stress.	Stress reduction as a result of knowing what to expect.

Learning Goals and Objectives for Admission Teaching

A number of constraints affect admission teaching and necessarily limit goals and objectives. Major among these is that nursing care needs often are more urgent than learning needs, making the time available for teaching minimal. A part of the limited-time problem is that, by its nature, admission teaching occurs before the nurse has the opportunity to fully assess the patient and his needs, and she must therefore teach more or less spontaneously and without preplanning (see Section 7.4). The nurse who is able to take even a few moments to determine the patient's communication abilities, mental state, and background knowledge will find that her attempts to help him learn will be more focused and require less time. Fortunately, early learning needs are generally restricted to the least complex levels of learning: remembering or understanding knowledge, recognizing attitudes, and perceiving skills. Table A–1 shows some of the learning objectives and relevant teaching content that may form part of admission teaching.

Relevant objectives vary from patient to patient and from situation to situation. The public health nurse visiting a family for the first time may emphasize her role as teacher and consultant and reassure the person about the confidentiality of their exchanges, while the emergency room nurse would need to focus on helping the patient understand what is being done for him now and how he can cooperate with the efforts of the medical team.

Teaching Strategies and Materials for Admission Teaching

Given the pressure of time, the most commonly used strategy for admission teaching is *explanation*. Yet, without an established interpersonal relationship with the patient and knowing little about his needs and perceptions, this is the strategy that is most likely to fail. If this strategy is chosen because of the pressure of time, it can be made most effective by keeping explanations short and language simple and without jargon. Feedback should be encouraged because it helps the nurse determine whether she is meeting patient needs.

A *discussion* strategy is especially useful for admission teaching, since it allows the patient to share information with the nurse as well as the opportunity for him to learn what he currently needs to know. Likewise, *demonstration* is appropriate when there is a need to learn manual skills.

Many hospitals and large clinics have prepared *pamphlets or short videotapes* which serve as introduction to the facility. Although these are valuable for outlining the scope of available resources or rules for behavior, such as visiting hours, their contribution to patient knowledge is necessarily general. They may be supplemented by individual attention that might include more interactive teaching strategies, such as discussion and demonstration.

Because people are often in or near a state of crisis at the time admission teaching begins, *written materials* that are personalized for the learner and designed to help him recall important pieces of information, such as the name of the doctor who cared for him in the emergency department, are valuable adjuncts to teaching. Seeing his diagnosis written on a slip of paper sometimes makes it seem less frightening and foreign to the patient. A card given to relatives of a person in surgery noting what room he will be in later in the day is reassuring as well as informational.

Admission teaching gives the nurse the opportunity to begin a *relationship of trust* with the patient and his family that will continue to influence his interaction with her and other caregivers (see Section 3.1). In addition to the information contained in the teaching, these early exchanges:

— indicate to the patient and his family to what degree he is regarded as a unique and responsible individual by caregivers,

— give the patient clues as to whether and to what degree he will be involved in decisions about his care,

— set a precedent for future teaching content and strategies, and

— inform the patient about how welcome other significant people are in the clinical setting and whether they will be encouraged to give him support.

Most of these messages are conveyed in subtle ways; they are communicated in the display of the nurse's attitudes and willingness to listen and inform. The more interactive the teaching strategy used, the more effectively can the nurse's warmth, respect, and empathy help the patient regard his encounter with medical care positively and nondefensively.

Notes on Evaluating Admission Teaching

In the absence of thorough assessment information or time to formulate individualized learning objectives, the use of feedback during teaching intervention is essential. Only by carefully *stopping* other activities, *looking* for nonverbal signals, and *listening* can the nurse determine whether she is even close to meeting a patient's needs. Using the analogy of a journey, even though the nurse might be clear about the intended destination, she must be certain that the patient is accompanying her on the same road and that her pace matches his.

It is at the end of rushed explanations that one so often hears: "Do you understand?" or "Do you have any questions?" The speaker undoubtedly thinks she is inviting useful feedback. In fact, it is the uncommon learner who is assertive enough to be able to use such "opportunities" (see Section 3.3). The person is much more likely to ask questions if the nurse gives permission, gives thinking time, and then gives the opportunity to have questions answered. She might say something like: "I've tried to fill you in on what to expect, but I know you will have some questions. Why don't I come back in about ten minutes and we'll talk about anything that was unclear or that you'd like more information about." The responses of the patient or his family when she does return give the nurse valuable information about their most urgent concerns and the success of her explanation strategy in meeting their needs.

Because admission teaching has more to do with knowledge and attitudes than with skills, the *observation of behavior* as an evaluation method is seldom clearly definitive. If teaching has been successful, then the patient and family members will be less anxious than they might have been and more cooperative with medical care procedures. The best that the nurse can do is to observe the learner and subjectively judge signs of stress and anxiety and signs of cooperation. In fact, when one is involved at this level with a patient and his situation, it is indeed possible to judge fairly reliably whether he is unduly frightened or attempting to cooperate. Unfortunately, these observations, although helpful, are not quantifiable; they constitute a form of *feedback* rather than formal evaluation.

Oral evaluation of specific learning objectives is the most common and readily available form of evaluation. In it, the learner is asked to "repeat back" what he has learned. Just as with oral evaluation in other circumstances, care must be taken in phrasing questions so that they obtain the necessary data without implying the desired answers (see Section 9.3). Under the condition of anxiety that so often marks admission teaching, it is especially important that the nurse, even though interested in evaluating the learner's level of progress, not threaten him, add to his anxiety, or talk to him condescendingly. The patient may have temporarily lost some of his independence, but the nurse cannot afford to have him imagine that she thinks he has lost his mind as well.

One method of oral evaluation that often works well is to ask the learner to explain the subject of concern to a family member who did not hear the original explanation or discussion. Either by listening in on this "replay" or by coming back to answer questions later, the nurse is able to judge the learner's comprehension of material presented.

Written questionnaires have often been used in medical facilities to evaluate the quality of admission teaching as well as the patient's response to other aspects of the facility. Such questionnaires are usually administered after the immediate crisis has passed, when the patient is well on the road to recovery. It is instructive for nurses who are doing admission teaching to later ask patients such questions as "What do you remember most clearly about your admission?" "What do you now wish you had known about then that you did not learn until later?" or "What kinds of information were you given at admission that helped you or your family later?" Although the answers to these kinds of questions are subjective, they will help guide the sensitive nurse in planning further admission teaching.

In summary, this section has presented guidance for teaching during the admission of a patient to a medical care facility. Similar ideas could be applied to admission to a health resource as well. Although not comprehensive, the material here has dealt with background information, the organization of a teaching plan, strategies and materials for teaching, and evaluation methods. The nurse who is anticipating doing admission teaching as a regular part of her patient responsibilities is encouraged to gather information from previously admitted patients, their family members, and colleagues about what they see as important aspects of this particular learning process. Such data will assist her in planning a realistic approach to admission teaching that is sensitive to both patient and organizational needs.

App 2. PREOPERATIVE OR PRETREATMENT TEACHING

Preoperative or pretreatment teaching may precede events as major as transplant surgery or as minor as a dressing change. The nurse can, of course, anticipate that the patient and his family members are anxious and concerned about the outcome of major procedures. It is not as obvious that many people feel a great deal of apprehension about procedures that caregivers view as minor. The starting of an intravenous line, the installation of a urinary catheter, or the passage of a nasogastric tube are examples of procedures that are especially anxiety-producing because they "invade" the body. Generally speaking, the more stressful and complex the procedure, the more preparation the patient will need.

> The goal of preoperative or pretreatment teaching is to help the patient learn what to expect and understand why the procedure is being done.

On the basis of such information he can then participate actively in whatever decision making is possible and cooperate as the procedure is carried out. Knowing what to expect reduces his fear of the unknown and makes him feel less helpless in the face of events that are not within his control. Making the effort to help the patient *understand the "why"* behind procedures reassures him that his individuality is being respected, allows him to ask more perceptive questions as events progress, and permits him more flexibility in accepting what happens even if it is not exactly as described. As discussed in Section 2.5, research evidence shows that when stress is reduced through teaching before surgery or treatment, less anesthetic and less analgesia are required, hospital stays are shorter, and healing is improved.

Although major barriers to learning can certainly reduce the effectiveness of teaching in the period before surgery or the beginning of treatment, it is by far preferable to help the patient learn *in anticipation* rather than during or after the procedure. For example, deep breathing and coughing routines that the patient will be expected to carry out after surgery must be taught in advance. Once the patient is drowsy from medication and in acute pain he is not only unable to fully understand the reasons behind the routine, but also naturally reluctant to cause more pain. Ideally, the nurse will have helped him understand the importance of these routines when motivation was not such a problem, allowing her to simply reinforce the learning later.

When major procedures or surgery is anticipated, it is especially important for the nurse to include the *other people* who are providing significant support to the patient in the preparatory teaching. Knowing what will happen and why will allow them to reinforce teaching with the patient and provide continuing intelligent support of him when he most needs it.

Occasionally the nurse encounters a patient who really does not want to be taught about surgery or treatment procedures. This person is usually acutely aware of his stress level and makes the judgment that he will be "better off" (i.e., less stressed) without information. Although it is the nurse's responsibility to offer preparatory teaching, it is also her obligation to respect a decision to refuse it. When this occurs the patient is usually just speaking for himself. Family members may want and need preparation in order to provide support to the patient. They should be offered teaching in a setting apart from the patient. They, then, will be able to participate in giving information to the patient as he is ready for it. In the following paragraphs some of the major factors to be considered by the nurse in planning and implementing preoperative or pretreatment teaching are outlined.

Background Information

The kinds of information needed by the nurse before beginning preoperative or pretreatment teaching falls into two general categories. One of these is her knowledge of the patient's health balance and learning needs. The other is her knowledge of the procedure to be performed. Because a major reason for preparatory teaching is to inspire confidence in caregivers, the teacher must be able to give detailed, specific, and correct information as well as be able to answer the learner's questions with assurance.

When a patient is admitted to a facility just before surgery or a treatment procedure and the nurse's time for assessment and teaching is limited, her approach may be much like that described for admission teaching. The basic background information listed in Section App. 1 will be essential to the success of her teaching effort.

The nurse's teaching approach to the patient who was previously admitted and for whom a thorough nursing assessment is available can be much more specific and focused on his particular learning needs. The planning of teaching intervention is benefited by knowing answers to the following questions.

- To what degree is the person currently limited in his ability to hear, see, or think clearly?
- Are there other people who have been involved in his care and who are providing support to the patient? Should they participate in the patient's preparatory learning session(s), or should they receive information in a setting apart from the patient?
- To what degree has the patient's doctor already given him preoperative or pretreatment information? What is the patient's perception of what he has been told?
- What has been the patient's previous experience with procedures such as the one he is about to undergo? What are his positive and negative perceptions of that experience and how does he now regard the outcome of it?
- What has the patient's apparent attitude toward care been since his admission? What seems to be his stress level? Has he indicated concern or anxiety about the anticipated surgery or procedure to caregivers?
- What level of trust have you been able to establish with the patient and his significant others?

Answers to these kinds of questions help the nurse determine how best to approach the teaching situation, taking into account the patient's perceptions and concerns as well as his current level of knowledge. The completeness with which the nurse is able to gather this information will, in large measure, depend on the interpersonal relationship she has been able to establish with him.

Learning Goals and Objectives

One of the major concerns of nurse teachers as they plan preoperative and pretreatment teaching is to determine how much information to include and how specific to make it. This kind of teaching presents the nurse with one of the most common of patient education challenges: how to balance what the nurse thinks the patient *ought* to know with what the patient *wants* to know. As discussed in Section 2.1, successful teaching must at least begin with the patient's current interests and concerns. The extent to which teaching can proceed beyond these immediate subjects will depend on the nurse's ability to motivate his interest and communicate skillfully. The availability of time and limitations of the nurse's own knowledge will also affect the content of teaching.

In general terms, the nurse teacher's goal will be to help the patient learn why the procedure is being done, what he can expect to happen during it, and how he will be affected by it. When a potentially life-threatening procedure is involved, the nurse will want to take special care to prepare the patient for what will happen after the procedure is completed. Not only is this information

TABLE A–2. Sample Plan for Preoperative or Pretreatment Teaching

Learning Objectives—For the patient to:	Teaching Content
General Goal: Treatment	
Name the procedure to be carried out.	What procedure is and how it is carried out.
Describe what is to be done in general terms.	Reason for doing procedure and how it is
Describe why the procedure is important to his well-being.	expected to affect patient, both now and in longer term.
Give step-by-step description of procedure.	Identity and role of caregivers to be involved.
Name and describe the role of the caregivers who will be involved in his care during the procedure.	Expectations of medical team regarding cooperative behavior.
Describe what he needs to do to cooperate during the procedure.	
Actively choose to cooperate with care before and during procedure.	
General Goal: Maintenance	
Describe measures that will be taken to maintain normal physiological functioning (I.V., ventilation) during and after procedure.	How the integrity of body functions will be maintained.
Demonstrate deep breathing exercises.	Instruction/coaching in breathing exercises.
Ask questions about care.	Encouragement of active involvement in
Respond positively to supportive behavior of family members.	learning and preparation to maintain sense of control and self-esteem.
	Involvement of family in learning and preparation.
General Goal: Primary Prevention	
Describe how his well-being is to be safeguarded by use of special equipment, techniques, or materials.	Reasons for use of sterile technique or special equipment or materials.
Demonstrate correct/safe use of protective equipment or materials.	Instruction/coaching in use of protective measures.
General Goal: Developmental Prevention	
Describe basic principles of anatomy and physiology as they apply to present condition and anticipated procedure.	Basic anatomy and physiology to serve as basis of understanding own body's functioning and reasons behind procedure.
Describe expected progress of recovery after procedure.	Expected steps and timing of progress toward recovery.
Demonstrate through nonverbal behavior or describe lessened levels of stress.	Stress reduction as a result of knowing what to expect.

important to his recovery, but it is also reassuring to plan ahead for the success of the procedure.

Current nursing journals can provide the nurse with up-to-date details of many medical procedures. The nurse will also want to enlist the aid of colleagues and the patient's doctor in determining just what information should be included in preparatory teaching. The listing of learning objectives and teaching content shown in Table A–2 is necessarily general.

Relevant objectives vary from patient to patient and from situation to situation. Preparation for a minor procedure may have limited objectives and take only a few minutes, while preparation for major surgery may extend over several hours or even days and involve a multidisciplinary effort. In order for specific learning objectives to aid the nurse in focusing teaching and evaluating progress, they would need to include both details of the learning to take place and criteria for assessing the extent to which they had been met (see Section 4.3).

Teaching Strategies and Materials

The period of time during which surgery or a major treatment procedure is anticipated is one of high anxiety for most people. Adding to their psychological distress are the physical processes, often painful ones, that make the procedure necessary. In this less than ideal teaching environment, lengthy *explanations* of complex procedures will not be well comprehended. The key to the patient's understanding of information offered by the nurse is his active participation in learning. This is most easily achieved through *discussion* and other interactive teaching strategies. Interaction between nurse and learner accomplishes two other important goals of preoperative and pretreatment teaching: it helps to establish and further a *relationship of trust*, which will be even more important during the patient's recovery, and it inspires confidence in the patient that his needs will be individually considered and competently met.

Because of the complexity of material and of desired levels of learning associated with preparatory teaching, several teaching strategies may be used. These might include *small-group learning, experiential methods*, such as going to see the intensive care unit, or *self-paced* learning for topics such as anatomy and physiology in addition to discussion. Useful learning materials that will help the nurse emphasize important points and stimulate the learner's interest include *written material, pictures and diagrams, and videotapes or films*. It is essential, however, that such materials be used within the context of interactive strategies. Owing to the similarity of learning objectives which exist among preoperative or pretreatment patients on a particular unit, it is tempting for the nurse to treat materials as though they are able to teach by themselves, without her individual input. If teaching materials are presented in this way, the patient's confidence may actually be reduced and he may feel as though he is on some sort of depersonalized conveyor belt.

Some portions of preoperative or pretreatment teaching lend themselves well to a *small group* approach. In addition to the supportive aspects of a group, such subjects as basic anatomy and physiology, demonstration and practice of postprocedure exercises and deep breathing, the step-by-step sequence of expected events, or other areas of knowledge can be covered efficiently and effectively in a group setting (see Chapter 8).

Notes on Evaluating Preoperative and Pretreatment Teaching

As with other teaching situations in which learning needs are complicated by powerful feelings such as fear, confusion, a sense of helplessness, or panic and by physical conditions that cause pain or decreased mental alertness, continuing *feedback* from the learner during teaching is essential. If the learner is unable to comprehend the meaning of what the nurse is trying to present, she would do better just to comfort rather than try to teach him. Discussion strategies are ideally suited to continuing feedback from the learner and allow the nurse to tailor her input to his concerns and mental state as well as his individual learning needs.

Preoperative and pretreatment teaching can often be divided into segments and evaluated separately. Background information might be evaluated through having the learner label an appropriate diagram or his comprehension of the principles of sterility checked by using a multiple-choice test. *Pretests and posttests* can be used effectively to help both learner and teacher become aware of progress made. These written methods would, of course, depend on the physical and mental capabilities of the learner. Having the learner *"teach" a family member* what he has learned is effective because it allows him to "use" his new knowledge, share positive attitudes, practice skills, and identify gaps in his understanding. It is also unlike a formal "test" and therefore not as anxiety producing as a pen-and-paper evaluation. The point of evaluation is, after all, to help the learner become aware of what he has accomplished and what still needs to be done, not to give him a grade or rating.

As with admission teaching, the nurse can learn a great deal about common patient needs and the general effectiveness of the teaching strategies used by questioning patients after their surgery or treatment about what they learned beforehand that was helpful and why, what they would like to have known about and did not, and how they might have been better helped to prepare for the procedure. This kind of data can help the individual nurse evaluate her own teaching effectiveness and form the basis for organizing unitwide approaches and the development of teaching materials.

In summary, this section has offered guidance for the nurse on preoperative and pretreatment teaching. The general goal of this kind of teaching is to help the patient and his support group learn what to expect and why the procedure is to be carried out. With this understanding the patient is able to cooperate with caregivers, have an increased level of confidence in them, and anticipate an improvement in his well-being. Because of the major barriers to learning that often complicate teaching during the preoperative and pretreatment period, interactive strategies that encourage feedback and support materials that stimulate interest and motivation to learn are especially effective. The positive longer-term benefits of thorough preoperative and pretreatment teaching are an improved nurse-patient relationship of trust and accelerated postprocedure recovery.

App 3. TEACHING PATIENT CARE PROCEDURES

With hospital stays becoming shorter and patients being discharged still in need of care and treatment, the role of the nurse in preparing the patient and his family members to continue care at home has greatly increased. This is an area of teaching in which the nurse's knowledge and ability are unique and her ability to influence the well-being of the patient enormous. The patient care procedures that occupy this category of teaching may include a range of subjects from safe ambulation to care of the dying and a range of complexity from how to take a child's temperature to how to use a home dialysis machine.

In teaching patient care procedures, there are two major principles that ensure success: begin the teaching as early as possible and always include at least two learners.

There are at least three good reasons for beginning the teaching-learning process early. One of these is that the learning of skills requires time not only for understanding the procedure, but also for practicing and perfecting the manual skills required. A second reason, related to the first, is that patient care procedures must often be learned at high levels of complexity: not only must a person be able to perform the procedure, but he must also learn how to vary the procedure according to circumstances, and how to recover from an error. A third reason for starting early is that the time available to both learner and nurse teacher will often not coincide, making it necessary to delay teaching and practice sessions. A few such delays can destroy the most well-intentioned teaching plan unless additional time is available to restructure the plan.

There are also several reasons for including more than one learner in sessions devoted to the teaching of patient care procedures. One reason is the obvious backup that the learners provide for each other in the home setting. Another reason is especially important when complex procedures with exacting steps are involved: two learners can coach each other and watch for breaks in procedure that might endanger the patient. The learners thus provide quality control for each other.

Some of the major factors to be considered by the nurse as she plans and implements the teaching of patient care procedures are outlined in the following paragraphs.

Background Information

Because patient care procedures will ultimately be carried out in the home, information about that environment is important in all cases and essential in some. In some instances it may be necessary or advisable to have a public health nurse or social worker carry out a home assessment before beginning the teaching program. In other instances the information that can be supplied to the nurse by the learners in answer to carefully structured questions will be enough to allow her to plan adequately.

The performance of patient care procedures demands a high level of commitment and motivation, since they usually must be performed in the absence of health professionals who would be able to encourage, remind, and reinforce learning. It is therefore important that the nurse teacher be aware of the mental attitudes of the learner in terms of acceptance of the diagnosis, understanding of the need for continuing help, and a realistic view of the impact that continuing care will have on the patient.

Answers to the following questions, in addition to the usual assessment data, may be especially helpful to the nurse when planning to teach patient care procedures.

- What impact will limitations of sight, hearing, mobility, or comprehension have on learning or carrying out the procedure?
- What are the established patterns of relationships and responsibilities within the patient's home and how will these affect patient care?
- What experience has the patient previously had of being cared for by others at home? What previous experiences will help or hinder learning patient care procedures now?
- What are the perceptions of the patient and his family members about the need for continuing care and its implications for the patient's future well-being?
- What are the attitudes of the patient and other learners toward giving and receiving care such as that proposed? What cultural values may affect patient care?
- What environmental factors in the home will affect how patient care procedures are carried out? Is appropriate equipment available to the patient?
- What resources are available for follow-up and emergency consultation?

Although this list is far from comprehensive, it is included to help stimulate the nurse's thinking as she plans the teaching of patient care procedures.

Learning Goals and Objectives for Patient Care Procedures

A beginning point for the nurse in determining relevant learning goals and objectives are those objectives she already has formulated for her own care of the patient. She must then ask herself:

- Which of the care procedures now being done for the patient will need to continue after his discharge?
- Which of these have highest priority and which are the most complex, requiring the longest to teach?
- What equipment or materials will be necessary to carry out procedures at home and how can these be obtained?
- Who should learn these procedures?
- How can learning be organized to take advantage of the major principles of learning? (See Section 2.1.)

With answers to these kinds of questions as a basis, the nurse can begin to focus on what kinds of learning will be required (knowledge, attitudes, and skills) and at what level of complexity. The more complex the learning that is needed and the less previous experience the learner has to apply to this new situation, the more time will be required of the nurse teacher and the more carefully she must plan learning experiences. If it is possible to teach principles or portions of procedures that apply to several aspects of patient care, these should be separated out and taught first. Their application should then be clearly shown. Otherwise, only one procedure should be taught and practiced at a time to reduce confusion by both teacher and learner. When more than one teacher is involved, it is best to have one person teach a single procedure from beginning to end.

It is important that reality be duplicated in the learning situation as nearly as possible. If equipment is to be used at home, use the same equipment in teaching. If the learner is to take responsibility for assessing need and initiating care, plan to have him practice doing this with the nurse's guidance in the clinical setting as well.

The learning objectives and teaching content shown in Table A–3 are necessarily general. They are included in order to stimulate the nurse to think through major aspects of teaching patient care procedures. Effective teaching at high levels of complexity take considerable time and careful planning.

Strategies and Materials for Teaching Patient Care

The teaching of patient care procedures presents the nurse with a major organizational challenge. She must plan the presentation of material in an orderly, logical, and comprehensive way, steering a reasonable path between helping the person learn to do what is necessary and preparing him for all possible eventualities. At the same time she must minimize teaching time while motivating, but not frightening, learners. To be able to do all of these things well requires developed skills and considerable practice. For the nurse just beginning to develop such skills, it is suggested that she seek the consultation of more practiced colleagues in the initial organizational and planning stages.

A major factor in the effective teaching of patient care procedures is the development of *positive attitudes* toward helping and receiving help in learners. Just as the nurse herself must learn to offer assistance without sabotaging a patient's independence and self-esteem, so, too, must the caregiver at home. And just as the nurse herself sometimes must make a special effort to help a patient accept having things done for him and having his personal privacy invaded, so, too, must she help both caregivers and patient accept needed but unaccustomed care and breaches in privacy at home. To not resolve these kinds of attitudinal problems while the care procedures are being taught is to seriously reduce the chance of procedures being carried out regularly and correctly.

The nurse teacher's most important ally in resolving attitudinal issues is an open and trusting interpersonal relationship with learners. Such a relationship allows for the honest discussion of anticipated problems and mutual problem solving. Whenever major procedures will be the responsibility of family members, the nurse must plan time to sit down with them and the patient to realistically discuss these issues. (See Chapter 3 for guidance on the conduct and modeling of effective listening and use of "open" questions.)

Another important consideration for the nurse in planning teaching strategies is the potential sources of stress that may affect learning ability. Because the teaching of patient care procedures must start early, the patient is often still in an acute stage of illness. This makes it difficult for him to think clearly and realistically about future care. Once the acute phase has passed, he may begin to eagerly anticipate going home. While this may add to his motivation to learn self-care

TABLE A–3. Sample Objectives and Content for Teaching Patient Care

Learning Objectives—For the patient to:	Teaching Content
General Goal: Treatment	
Describe the patient care procedure in general terms, including its specific objective.	Introduction to patient care procedure.
Describe criteria for initiating procedure.	Background information and concepts on which procedure is based.
Demonstrate major/basic skills necessary for procedure.	Initial demonstration of complete procedure.
Describe each step in procedure in detail and correct sequence.	Demonstration, return demonstration, and coaching of:
Perform each step in procedure in correct sequence.	major/basic skills, each procedure step, correct sequence,
Perform assessment of need for procedure.	assessment procedure,
Perform initiation of procedure correctly, using assessment data.	initiation of procedure, variations in procedure.
Describe criteria used to vary procedure.	Coaching, encouragement, and positive feedback during practice.
Demonstrate variations in standard procedure.	
General Goal: Maintenance	
Describe abilities and limits that affect procedure.	Limitations and abilities affecting patient's well-being generally and care procedures specifically.
Demonstrate methods of maintaining and protecting:	Demonstration, return demonstration, and coaching of methods for maintaining body systems and functions.
cardiovascular function, respiratory function, gastrointestinal function, excretory functions, motion and mobility, etc.	Discuss need for and help plan maintenance of independence, mental stimulation, and social contacts.
Describe division of responsibility for care, including maintenance of independence and mental health.	Help caregivers decide on realistic division of patient care responsibilities.
Describe plan for maintaining social interaction with family and friends.	
General Goal: Primary Prevention	
Describe principles of safety and protection as they apply to care procedure.	Introduction to principles of safety and patient protection.
Demonstrate safe acquisition, use, storage, and disposal of equipment and materials necessary to patient care procedure.	Demonstration, return demonstration, and coaching of safe equipment and materials handling and of correct techniques for cleanliness or asepsis.
Demonstrate correct use of handwashing, asepsis, or other protective techniques.	
General Goal: Developmental Prevention	
Describe, rehearse/demonstrate steps in contacting resources to report/resolve:	Introduction to possible variations in expected procedure outcome.
unexpected procedure outcome, side effects, equipment failures, errors.	Demonstration, behavior rehearsal, and coaching of assessment, reporting, and resolution of problem.
Describe realistic expectations for positive impact of procedure on well-being and overall improvement in condition.	Realistic expectations for patient improvement. Availability of community resources.
Describe plan for use of appropriate community resources.	Help make plan for appropriate use of resources.

procedures, he may have difficulty seeing the importance of having other family members learn how to give him care. In his relief at having a crisis past and eagerness to be well again, he may not be realistic about his continuing needs. At the same time it is anxiety producing to have unpracticed hands carrying out nursing care procedures, especially when professional care is available. *Practicing procedures* within range of coaching is, however, essential to a home care program.

Because of the complexity of learning that often must take place, it is appropriate to use a variety of teaching strategies and materials to help learners acquire patient care skills. *Explanation and discussion* are useful for knowledge areas, while *demonstration and coaching* are the strategies of choice when manual skills are involved. *Behavior rehearsal* is an especially effective strategy for helping caregivers learn to deal with "What if..." scenarios.

Teaching materials come in many forms; it is difficult to think of any that could not sometimes be usefully adapted to the teaching of patient care procedures. Written materials, pictures, and diagrams are invaluable aids to discussions of concepts and principles. Videotapes and films can effectively show required skills and the resolution of problems. Self-paced instructional materials can be helpful for covering background information, such as anatomy and physiology, as well as the sequence of procedure steps and the protocol for identifying and handling problems. Hands-on learning involving the manipulation of actual equipment and materials as well as practicing procedures are, of course, essential. The creative nurse teacher will *vary approaches* in order to stimulate interest and motivation as well as technical skill learning.

Group approaches are often useful for the teaching of patient care procedures. The mutual support and quality control that group members offer to one another are especially valuable. Both theory and practice can be handled effectively in a group setting. The nurse can then focus her one-to-one teaching on individual problem solving and personal variations in standard procedures.

When follow-up care after discharge will include the involvement of a public health or visiting nurse or a representative of a community group, the nurse teacher may find it possible to involve this person in the teaching of patient care procedures. Community professionals are familiar with techniques of realistically "translating" procedures into terms easily understood by patients and their family members. It is well worth the time and effort it takes the nurse teacher to coordinate efforts with her community colleagues in order to facilitate continuing care and the reinforcement of her own teaching. The visiting nurse, for example, if introduced to the patient while he is still in the hospital, can begin to understand his needs and form a relationship of trust with him. These beginnings will then allow her to smooth the transition to home care and be immediately effective in providing consultation, backup, and continuing assessment to the patient and his family.

Notes on Evaluating the Teaching of Patient Care Procedures

If there is any area of patient education that requires thorough evaluation of learning, the teaching of patient care procedures is it. The limitation of evaluation in the clinical setting is that only the ability of the learner to carry out procedures correctly can be assessed. One has no direct way of knowing in advance that he actually will do this at home. However, to not *check out understanding and skill* before the patient is discharged is to come dangerously close to professional irresponsibility and negligence. Detected early, a lack of understanding and skill might be resolved through further teaching or the use of other care resources, such as home care agencies, public health nurses, or institutional convalescent care.

Initiating and inviting continuing *feedback* during the teaching-learning process is one way to avert the disaster of finding out belatedly that skills are inadequate for safe care. The quality of feedback is greatly improved by the setting of realistic learning objectives and clear standards for the demonstration of skills at staged intervals.

If the nurse teacher has done a good job of helping learners appreciate the benefits of carefully performed care procedures, they will expect, and consequently not feel threatened by, evaluation sessions. Knowledge areas of learning can be tested by *verbal* means, either oral or written. The nurse must be careful in preparing such evaluation materials to be sure that they adequately test the specific learning objectives appropriate to the learner involved. *Return demonstrations and behavior rehearsal* are the methods of choice for evaluating skill learning. *Checklists or rating scales* may assist both teacher and learner in identifying strengths and weaknesses in skill performance.

The use of *patient contracts* offers a means of making the learner an active participant in the identification of learning needs and the setting of realistic objectives. Because learner-kept records are often part of the contract, the learner is helped to develop skills and establish habits of complete record keeping. Such records verify that procedures have been carried out as planned, even in the absence of a supervising health professional. When a care procedure is initiated or modified according to need, the records also function as a valuable tool for the medical team to continue monitoring the patient's progress.

In summary, the teaching of patient care procedures is one of the more complex areas of patient education and presents a sizable challenge to the nurse teacher in terms of identification of learning needs, prioritizing objectives, organizing learning opportunities, and evaluating progress. At the same time the nurse is in a position to make a unique contribution to the patient's future well-being, independence, and self-responsibility through helping him and his family learn care procedures. The content of this teaching area is so well known to nurses, that they are able to concentrate their effort on effective teaching. For this reason it offers the nurse the opportunity to develop and perfect her teaching skills to a degree seldom available in other teaching areas. In order to realize the rewards of effective teaching and learning, the nurse is urged to help the learner begin early in his experience as a patient to prepare for the transition to home care and to accept and support his family members in their effort to learn how to help him effectively.

App 4. DISCHARGE TEACHING

Discharge teaching is oriented specifically to patient preparation for the transition from the clinical to the home setting. Like admission teaching, the learning that occurs just before discharge is usually complicated by high levels of anxiety and is focused largely on knowledge and attitudes rather than on skills. As discussed earlier, when care must be continued at home, the teaching of care procedures needs to begin well in advance of discharge in order to help learners develop complex skills.

> Discharge teaching appropriately focuses on what the patient can expect the course of his recovery to be and how to manage the medical resources available to him for follow-up care and consultation.

Once again, the inclusion of other people significant to the patient in the teaching-learning process helps to ensure correct recall and reinforcement of learning as well as provide emotional support to the patient during the transitional period.

A major source of stress just before discharge is the patient's uncertainty about the degree to which he will be physically able and expected by others to play his normal "well" role with its full share of responsibilities and tasks. Alternatively, he will be facing the frustration of still being "sick" and unable to function normally. It is important that the nurse include clarification about the patient's *role and limitations* in her teaching both with him and with his support group.

A second source of stress is a form of "separation anxiety" experienced by most hospitalized patients who have been acutely ill as they face the possibility of not having care available if they should again need it. For this reason discharge teaching will, at least in part, be directed toward helping the patient learn how and in what circumstances to seek professional help or consultation. He should leave well aware of what to look for and how to handle medication side effects and complications during recovery as well as with a plan for regularly scheduled medical follow-up.

Discharge teaching is one of the most common areas of teaching in which the nurse is involved. Sometimes nurses are not even aware that they are assuming a teaching role when they "tell" the patient what the doctor has written as discharge orders. This is unfortunate because effective discharge teaching that has as its general goal preparing the patient to make the transition to home care is sufficiently complex that just "telling" is not adequate. Some of the major factors to be considered by the nurse as she plans and implements an effective approach to discharge teaching are outlined in the following paragraphs.

Background Information

Discharge teaching has the advantage of readily available background information to guide the nurse as she plans her teaching intervention. Ideally, the nurse brings with her a personal knowledge of the patient's attitudes and values as well as his medical history and can offer help with learning within the context of already established communication patterns and a well-developed trusting relationship. In addition to an assessment of the patient's present health balance, answers to the following questions may be especially helpful to the nurse as she plans discharge teaching.

- To what degree is the patient currently limited in his ability to hear, see, or think clearly?
- How has the patient and his support group responded to his medical care? Has he been anxious to take self-responsibility, or relatively passive in accepting care? How involved have significant other people been in providing emotional and other forms of support?
- What clues has the patient given caregivers about his perception of what it will be like for him to be home?
- What is of most concern to the patient and his family about the transition to home care? What is his stress level and is that likely to increase or decrease before actual discharge? Have financial arrangements been clarified with the medical facility?
- To what degree has the patient and caregiving family members had the opportunity to develop patient care skills for use at home?
- What resources are realistically available to the patient for follow-up care and emergency consultation? To what degree is he already aware of these and know how and when to use them?
- What are the attending physician's instructions regarding limitations, the likely consequences of not following orders, and planned follow-up care? To what degree has he or she been actively involved in patient instruction?

The answers to these kinds of questions give the nurse a basis for planning discharge teaching and alert her to special learning needs that should best be approached well before actual discharge.

Learning Goals and Objectives for Discharge Teaching

In order for discharge teaching to effectively help patients learn how to take over responsibility for their care, planning and implementation must begin early. Although the nurse might not know the specifics of the doctor's orders until hours or even minutes before discharge, this must not operate as an excuse to put off beginning to help the patient make the transition to home care. Some predictable learning needs that will be experienced by all patients on a particular medical care unit are as follows:

- *Medications*: How and when to take medications, what side effects may occur, and how these are to be reported.
- *Activity*: What limitations apply to patient activities and the consequences of exceeding them. What activities are encouraged and how can the patient expect abilities to increase.

TABLE A–4. Sample Plan for Discharge Teaching

Learning Objectives—For the learner to:	Teaching Content
General Goal: Treatment Identify medications by name. Describe how and why medication is to be taken. Describe precautions to be taken and side effects to be noted. Describe in detail planned follow-up medical care, including dates and times of appointments. Describe in detail plan for continued care at home, including division of responsibilities. Demonstrate relevant self-care procedures.	Medications: instructions and reasons for use, potential side effects. Medical follow-up: plan for doctor or other appointments. Continued care at home: procedures, routines, and responsibilities.
General Goal: Maintenance Demonstrate willingness to limit activities to those advised. Describe anticipated schedule of activity limitations and changes. Describe consequences of exceeding activity limitations. Verbalize positive attitude toward continuing care at home. Describe in detail nutritional limitations or special diets. Describe realistic plan for nutritional control.	Activities: limitations, consequences of exceeding, preferred activities, and schedule of changes in activity levels. Self-care: understanding and skills needed for self-care, motivation to continue care and take self-responsibility. Nutrition: reasons for and details of special diets or food limitations.
General Goal: Primary Prevention Describe reasons for and details of safety precautions to be taken. Demonstrate ability to transfer from bed to chair or ambulate safely. Describe plan for infection control in detail. Demonstrate cleanliness techniques. Confirm modifications to home environment or acquisition of equipment for increased safety.	Safety: general principles, good body mechanics, transfer and ambulation techniques, use of special equipment, and plan for household modifications to improve safety. Infection protection: general principles, handwashing, asepsis, and use of special materials.
General Goal: Developmental Prevention Describe events and observations that are to be reported. Demonstrate knowledge of how to contact medical help. Describe anticipated changes in his condition in realistic terms. Name community resources available. Describe how and why these resources can be contacted.	Follow-up care: side effects of treatment or medication that require medical attention, how to obtain emergency care and medical consultation. Expectations for changes in condition/improvement during recovery. Community resources: what resources available, services offered, how to contact.

- *Nutrition*: What special diets are to be followed and why. What foods are encouraged and how can the patient get help with nutritional questions or problems.
- *Minor patient care procedures*: What special information or skills does the patient need to take care of himself at home. What precautions must be taken during baths or showers or other activities of daily living.
- *Follow-up medical care*: What plan should be followed for doctor visits,

telephone calls to report progress or problems, or the use of other community resources for care or information.

Although these content areas for teaching are predictable, the specific needs of individual patients must be carefully considered by the nurse before she initiates teaching intervention. Some general learning objectives are shown in Table A–4. In order to function as a useful teaching plan, these objectives and content areas would need to be made more specific and individualized to reflect the learning needs of a particular patient. The scope of knowledge, attitudes, and skills that are needed by the patient and his family members before discharge demand careful planning and early initiation of teaching interventions by nurses.

Strategies and Materials for Discharge Teaching

Just as in admission teaching, the nurse is tempted to limit her teaching strategy for discharge teaching to explanation, owing to the pressure of time. Although in this instance explanation is less likely to fail because of communication difficulties, it is not, by itself, adequate for preparing a patient to make the transition to home care. At the very least an explanation should be accompanied by *discussion* of how an instruction is to be implemented at home and what difficulties are anticipated by the patient or his family. *Written reminders* of essential information are a valuable adjunct to interactive teaching strategies. *Behavior rehearsal* is a useful strategy for helping learners with assessment and action in "What if..." scenarios. Being provided with specific guidance for how to behave if an unexpected event should occur reduces the stress of wondering whether learners will be able to handle an emergency situation.

Because of the general nature of the information they contain, films, videotapes, and self-paced learning programs are much less useful approaches to discharge teaching than to other areas of instruction. *Small learning groups* can, however, be valuable to patients anticipating discharge. They are especially appropriate and efficient when a number of patients share concerns about self-care, for example, on a postpartum unit.

Notes on Evaluating Discharge Teaching

The only valid and complete evaluation of discharge teaching occurs in the patient's home setting, when he discovers whether his preparation was adequate to allow him to manage his self-care and handle any unexpected events that have arisen. Without the ability to follow the patient home, the nurse's evaluation of the effectiveness of teaching is limited to *feedback* from learners during the teaching sessions and descriptions of anticipated behavior. The nurse will particularly want to encourage realistic discussions of how plans for self-care are to be implemented as evidence that explanations have been understood and some motivation for action exists. *Oral or written tests* of knowledge can be used to reinforce essential information. In this way nurses can become aware of gaps in understanding or uncertainty about instructions and take measures to repeat or extend teaching.

In summary, the major goal of discharge teaching is to help the patient assume self-responsibility for continued care. If the patient and his family members are encouraged to participate actively in his acute care, this transition will be less difficult. As in any of the transitional periods discussed in this appendix, discharge from acute care is accompanied by a number of anxieties and stresses. Careful planning by the nurse and early teaching intervention will alleviate the intensity of these anxieties and give the patient the best chance for uncomplicated recovery of his health.

SUMMARY

In this appendix four transitional events commonly experienced by patients in acute care have been discussed. For each transition we have outlined background information that is useful to the nurse in planning teaching intervention, specific goals and objectives of learning, strategies and materials that are especially applicable, and some notes on evaluating learning. Although this material is not intended to be used as it is to formalize teaching approaches, it is hoped that nurses will be stimulated by it to consider the broad scope of learning needs related to each of these transitions and plan their intervention accordingly. Other transitional events may be added to this list for certain clinical areas. For example, nurses on an oncology unit may want to plan teaching interventions for post-chemotherapy or care of the terminally ill patient at home. In all cases the nurse will want to individualize her approach so as to meet patient learning needs as fully as possible.

Appendix B

SOURCES OF EDUCATIONAL MATERIALS INFORMATION*

PATIENT EDUCATION MATERIALS

Ash, Joan, and Michael Stevenson. *Health: A Multimedia Source Guide*. New York: R. R. Bowker, 1976. 185 pp. $16.50

An annotated guide to 700 organizations that deal with health-related matters—publishers, audiovisual producers and distributors, libraries, government agencies, and professional and voluntary societies. For each organization listed, the availability of publications and other media is indicated. Three indexes are provided: an alphabetical listing; an index to sources that provide free or inexpensive pamphlet material to the layman; and an index to sources by subject. This publication is useful to those desiring to develop health information collections either within the hospital or in public library settings.

Bibliography of Patient and Community Health Education. Chicago: American Society for Health Manpower Education and Training, 1980.

A comprehensive bibliography of patient and community health education resources.

Commercially Produced Patient and Community Health Education Audiovisuals Used by 224 Hospitals. Chicago: American Hospital Association, Center for Health Promotion, 1979. 209 pp.

Listing was compiled under the American Hospital Association—Bureau of Health Education contract by the Mental Health Materials Center. Six hundred audiovisuals are listed, which are used by 224 hospitals in their patient and community health education programs. No evaluation has been attempted. Audiovisuals are grouped by subject such as arthritis, mastectomy, prenatal care, and so forth. In each instance, brief information is supplied with respect to source, cost, format, running time, primary audience, and context. Particularly helpful is the indication of the number of hospitals that report the use of each audiovisual. An appendix lists the names and addresses of distributors.

Critiques. (Wisconsin Clearinghouse, 1954 E. Washington Ave., Madison, Wisc., 53704) Bimonthly. $15 individuals; $25 libraries/institutions.

Excellent resource for evaluative reviews of materials on preventive and alternative health care, alcohol and drug abuse, mental health, youth development, and wellness. Items are divided by format: audiovisuals, pamphlets, books, curricula, posters, and multimedia packages. Each review includes information on subject area, date of publication, distributor, and cost, along with a synopsis of content; comments on what reviewers liked or did not like about each item; an overall rating (not recommended, poor, average, good, excellent); intended audience; notation of reading level, if appropriate; and recommendation for use. Highly recommended.

---

*Sources: Alan M. Rees and Blanche A. Young, *The Consumer Health Information Source Book*. New York: R. R. Bowker, 1981, pp. 44–49, and Alan M. Rees and Jodith Janes, *The Consumer Health Information Source Book*, 2nd Ed. New York: R. R. Bowker, 1984, pp. 18–29. Selections reprinted with permission.)

Duke, Phyllis, comp. "Audiovisuals: Patient Education." In *Journal of Biocommunication* 5 (March 1978): 18–23.

A list of some 80 producers of patient education materials. Most of the major suppliers are noted with a brief description of the principal health topics covered by each source. Types of media available, such as films, audiocassettes, charts, models and videocassettes are indicated. Addresses are provided for the ordering of 21 university catalogs of rental films for general public education.

Gotsick, Priscilla, Janice Branham, and Bruce Conley. *Sources of Patient Education Materials*. Detroit: Kentucky-Ohio-Michigan Regional Medical Library Network, Health Information Library Program, 1979. 17 pp.

Contains 121 health-related organizations, professional associations, and companies that produce and/or distribute patient education materials. Each entry indicates available formats (slides, filmstrips, videocassettes, films, audiocassettes, and so forth) and the major subject areas covered, such as muscular dystrophy, nutrition, and family planning. A good selection of the many sources currently available.

Martin, Rebecca, and Sen Yee. *Patient Education Audiovisuals: A Core List*. San Francisco: Veterans Administration Hospital, n.d. 5 pp.

A core list of highly recommended programs from the collection of the Patient Education Resource Center, Veterans Administration Hospital, San Francisco. The composition of the list reflects the common medical problems of a veterans population, as encountered in a general hospital. The programs cover alcoholism, arthritis, colostomy, diabetes, diet and nutrition, eye, gastrointestinal tract, heart disease, hip replacement, lung disease, medication, surgery and general health. The total cost of the programs listed is approximately $8,000. Purchase of the basic items, indicated by an asterisk, would amount to $2,200.

Martin, Rebecca, and Sen Yee. *Sources for Patient Education Materials*. San Francisco: Veterans Administration Hospital, August 1977. 14 pp.

A good summary of 140 voluntary health organizations, professional associations, media producers, publishers, government agencies, pharmaceutical companies, and universities that supply audiovisuals, books, and pamphlet materials relating to patient education.

Martyn, Dorian, Dorothy Spencer, and Phyllis Duke. *Source List for Patient Education Materials*. Milledgeville, Ga.: Health Services Communications Association (HESCA), Education Committee, 1978. 47 pp. $3.

The most comprehensive listing to date of organizations that supply books, pamphlets, or audiovisual materials. The 530 entries were derived from an extensive survey of health organizations designed to identify available materials. Each entry contains the name and address of the organization, types of materials available, availability of catalogs, and the source from which the entry was obtained for inclusion. The list is not selective and includes all organizations that reported the availability of educational materials. A subject index is provided utilizing subject headings modified from MeSH (Medical subject headings used by the National Library of Medicine). Apart from the subject indexing of each source there is no listing of specific materials available. The objective of the publication is, however, to serve as a list of sources rather than as a compilation of materials. Highly recommended.

Rees, Alan M. (Ed.). *Consumer Health & Nutrition Index*. Phoenix, Ariz.: Oryx Press. Quarterly. $79.50/yr.

Provides indexed information on health-related articles and book reviews appearing in 73 popular consumer magazines and newsletters. Topics such as exercise, alcoholism and drug abuse, cancer, pregnancy, Alzheimer's disease, vegetarianism, and osteoporosis are included.

Rees, Alan M. (Ed.). *CHIS 86: The Consumer Health Information Service*. Ann Arbor, Mich.: University Microfilms International, 1987. $390

A microfiche file of the full text of some 2,000 health-related pamphlets, booklets, and leaflets published by the federal government, voluntary health associations, pharmaceutical companies, etc., together with selected articles from *The New York Times*. An Index and Subject Guide are included. Material is updated regularly.

Some Sources for Patient Education Videotape Programs: Some Commercial Suppliers of Patient Education

Materials. Chicago: American Hospital Association, February 1977. 4 pp. (Distributed by the Centers for Disease Control, Bureau of Health Education, Atlanta, Ga.)

Lists the names, addresses and phone numbers of the principal suppliers of audiovisual materials.

The Videolog: Programs for the Health Sciences, 1979. New York: Esselte Video, 1979. 399 pp. $35.

Contains descriptions of over 7,000 videotape and videocassette programs and series for both professional and patient health education. An annotated description is provided for each entry. A subject index lists titles of programs. Reference to the alphabetical listings then provides a short description of each item together with price and ordering information. Patient health education programs, over 800 in number, are listed by title under the heading "Patient Education." This section is further divided into topics such as alcoholism and drug abuse, cardiology and cardiovascular system, dental health, nutrition, obstetrics, and so forth.

SPANISH-LANGUAGE MATERIALS

Aqui Se Habla Español: A Guide to Spanish-Language Health and Patient Information. Rockville, MD: Office of Communications and Public Affairs, 1980. 78 pp. DHHS Pubn. No. (HSA) 81-7006.

Describes over 450 publications and audiovisuals available in Spanish from more than 100 distributors, including government agencies, professional and voluntary health associations, pharmaceutical companies and commercial publishers. Materials are arranged in 51 subject categories, including accidents and first aid, cancer, epilepsy, family planning, health-care costs, hemophilia, infant and child care, orthopedics, sickle cell anemia, and venereal disease. In each category, entries are divided into print and nonprint materials. Information incorporates a short nonevaluative description of each item: its format— booklet, poster, miniguide, 16-mm film, video-cassette—and whether the item is free, for sale or for rent. No publication dates are given. A valuable resource for Spanish-language materials for librarians, patient educators, and consumers.

Guide to Audiovisual Aids for Spanish-Speaking Americans: Health-Related Films, Filmstrips and Slides, Descriptions and Sources. Health Services Administration, 1974. DHEW Pubn. No. (HSA) 74-30. 37 pp.

Materials, mainly films, are grouped by topics such as aging, cancer, diabetes, heart disease, multiple sclerosis, venereal disease, mental health, and prenatal and infant care. Short nonevaluative descriptions are provided. Also contains names and addresses of 44 distributors of materials. The dates of the materials are from 1940 to 1973.

Korzdorfer, Kamala, and Irene Yeh, comps. *Spanish Language Health Materials: A Selected Bibliography*. Hayward, Calif.: California Ethnic Services Task Force, 1978. 41 pp.

This bibliography is designed for use by medium-sized public libraries in either initiating or expanding a Spanish-language materials collection in health. The materials listed (books, pamphlets, and texts) are either in Spanish or bilingual Spanish-English form and represent a wide range of reading levels and interests. Most of the annotations include a critical description of contents and an evaluation in terms of language and reading level. The major topics covered are alcohol and drugs, consumer health information, diseases, human physiology, medical care, medicinal plants and herbs, mental health, nutrition, pediatrics and child care, physical fitness, pregnancy and childbirth, sex education, and women's health. Also included is a list of titles only of materials that were unavailable for examination and names and addresses of sources. An excellent guide —evaluative and informative.

Spanish-language Health Communication Teaching Aids: A List of Printed Materials and Their Sources. Health Services and Mental Health Administration, 1973. 55 pp. DHEW Pubn. No. (HSM) 73-19.

A compilation of pamphlets, books, posters, and other information materials available from state health agencies, pharmaceutical companies, publishers, and community health organizations. Although many of the teaching aids may now be unavailable because of the age of the listing, this is still a useful guide to some 90 sources of such materials. Annotations are nonevaluative.

GOVERNMENT PUBLICATIONS

Consumer Information Catalog: A Catalog of Selected Federal Publications of Consumer Interest. Pueblo, Colo.: Consumer Information Center. Qtrly. Free.

Each issue lists and briefly describes over 200 selected federal publications on a variety of popular topics, including an extensive assortment of free or low-cost publications on general health; diseases and common ailments; children's health and prenatal care; drugs and medicines; and food, diet and nutrition. A limit of 20 free publications is imposed on each order. There is a $1 user fee for processing an order of two or more free titles. Orders are filled by the Consumer Information Center.

MEDOC: A Computerized Index to U.S. Government Documents in the Medical and Health Sciences. Salt Lake City, Utah: Eccles Health Sciences Library, University of Utah. Qtrly. $35/yr.

MEDOC lists health-related government documents received at Eccles Health Sciences Library. The coverage is broad and includes a large number of health-related topics. Four indexes are provided: Superintendent of Documents Number Index; Title Index; Subject Index; and Series Number Index. Consumer health and patient education publications are indicated as such by the use of "G" for general. MEDOC contains many omissions; some lay health publications fail to receive the "G" designation; and the materials listed are in many instances not current. Nevertheless, MEDOC is a useful guide to health-related government publications and is worth the price.

Monthly Catalog of United States Government Publications. Washington, D.C.:Superintendent of Documents, Government Printing Office. Monthly. $25/yr.; $50/yr. microfiche.

Each issue contains between 1,500 and 3,000 entries of new items for sale. Entries are arranged by the Superintendent of Documents classification number and contain four indexes: author, title, subject, and series report. Complete bibliographic data are provided for each document. A rich source for health-related documents.

NIH Publications List. Bethesda, MD: National Institutes of Health, Division of Public Information, January 1983. NIH Pubn. No. 83-7. 91pp.

Many of the publications listed are oriented toward the general public. Nineteen component divisions of the National Institutes of Health are detailed, including the National Cancer Institute; National Heart, Lung, and Blood Institute; National Institute of Arthritis, Diabetes, and Digestive and Kidney Diseases; and the National Institute on Aging. In most cases, one copy of each publication listed is available free from the Public Inquiries Office of the appropriate NIH component (Institute, Division, or Center) at Bethesda, Maryland 20205. Some are for sale from the Superintendent of Documents, although Government Printing Office numbers are not given. Lists several hundred publications and includes a title index.

Subject Bibliography Index. Washington, D. C.: Superintendent of Documents, United States Government Printing Office, SB-888, March 1, 1983. 8 pp.

A listing of over 250 subject bibliographies available without charge, which provides access to the more than 16,000 different books, pamphlets, posters, periodicals, subscription services, and other government publications available for purchase from the Superintendent of Documents. To keep up with the 3,000 or so new titles entering the GPO's inventory each year, as well as the many titles that are superseded by revised editions, the subject bibliographies are periodically updated. Currently, there are some 24 subject bibliographies of interest for consumer health and patient education.

> *Alcoholism.* SB-175, July 1, 1983. 8 pp.
> *Care and Disorders of the Eyes.* SB-028, April 15, 1983. 4 pp.
> *Children and Youth.* SB-035, October 22, 1983. 38 pp.
> *Consumer Information.* SB-002, September 8, 1982. 20 pp.
> *Dentistry. SB-022, March 3, 1983. 4 pp.*
> *Diseases in Humans.* SB-008, November 18, 1982. 20 pp.
> *Drug Education.* SB-163, July 1983, 13 pp.
> *Family Planning.* SB-292, March, 1983. 5 pp.
> *Food, Diet, and Nutrition.* SB-291, June 1982. 19 pp.
> *The Handicapped.* SB-037, March 15, 1983. 12 pp.
> *Hearing and Hearing Disability.* SB-023. March 4, 1983. 3 pp.
> *Heart and Circulatory System.* SB-104, October 29, 1982. 4 pp.

Hospitals. SB-119, April 1, 1983. 6 pp.
Medicine and Medical Science. SB-154, November 24, 1982. 29 pp.
Mental Health. SB-167, February 9, 1983. 16 pp.
Nurses and Nursing Care. SB-019, August 1, 1983. 5 pp.
Physical Fitness. SB-239, April 25, 1983. 3 pp.
Public Health. SB-122, June 23, 1983. 8 pp.
Rehabilitation. SB-081, June 1, 1983. 5 pp.
Retirement. SB-285, December 2, 1982. 6 pp.
Smoking. SB-015, June 22, 1983. 3 pp.
Social Security. SB-165, May 26, 1983. 5 pp.
Vital and Health Statistics. SB-121, May 12, 1983. 9 pp.
Women. SB-111, November 5, 1982. 17 pp.

REFERENCES AND BIBLIOGRAPHY

American Journal of Nursing, "Patients Are Now Products at Some Hospitals." In "News," *American Journal of Nursing* 86:476, April 1986.

American Hospital Association. *A Patient's Bill of Rights*. Chicago: American Hospital Association, 1972.

American Nurses' Association. *Model Nurse Practice Act*. Kansas City, Mo.: American Nurses' Association, 1976.

American Nurses' Association. *The Professional Nurse and Health Education*. Kansas City, Mo.: American Nurses' Association, 1975.

Ausubel, D. P., and F. G. Robinson. *School Learning: An Introduction to Educational Psychology*. New York: Holt, Rinehart and Winston, 1969.

Bailey, Ronald F. *The Role of the Brain*. Netherlands: Time-Life International, 1976.

Barrett, J., B. A. Gessner, and C. Phelps. *The Head Nurse*. 3rd ed., Norwalk, Conn.: Appleton-Century-Crofts, 1975.

Beach, Dale S., ed. *Managing People at Work*. New York: Macmillan, 1975.

Becker, M. H. "The Health Belief Model and Sick Role Behavior." *Health Education Monograph* 2:409–419, 1974.

Becker, M. H., and L. Maiman. "Sociobehavioral Determinants of Compliance with Health and Medical Care Recommendations." *Medical Care* 13:10–24, 1975.

Becker, M. H., and L. Maiman. "Strategies for Enhancing Patient Compliance." *Journal of Community Health* 6:113–135, 1980.

Benne, K. D. "The Process of Re-education: An Assessment of Kurt Lewin's Views." In W. Bennis, K. Benne, R. Chin, and K. Corey. *The Planning of Change*, 3rd ed. New York: Holt, Rinehart & Winston, 1976.

Bennis, W., K. Benne, R. Chin, and K. Corey. *The Planning of Change*, 3rd ed. New York: Holt, Rinehart & Winston, 1976.

Berne, Eric. *The Structure and Dynamics of Organizations and Groups*. New York: Ballantine Books, 1974.

Black, Kathleen. *Short-term Counseling*. Menlo Park, Calif.: Addison-Wesley, 1983.

Bloom, Benjamin. *Taxonomy of Educational Objectives: The Classification of Educational Goals*. New York: David McKay Co., 1956.

Bradway, K. "Jung's Psychological Types." *Journal of Analytical Psychology* 9:129–135, 1964.

Brammer, L. *The Helping Relationship: Process and Skills*. Englewood Cliffs, N.J.: Prentice-Hall, 1973.

Bramson, R. S. *Coping with Difficult People*. New York: Ballantine Books, 1981.

Breckon, D. J., J. Harvey, and R. B. Lancaster. *Community Health Education*. Rockville, Md.: Aspen Publishers, 1985.

Brown, E. L. *Nursing for the Future*. New York: Russell Sage Foundation, 1948.

Bruner, J. S. "The Act of Discovery." *Harvard Educational Review* 31:21–32, 1961(a).

Bruner, J. S. *The Process of Education*. Cambridge, Mass.: Harvard University Press, 1961(b).

Burnside, Irene. *Working with the Elderly: Group Process and Techniques*, 2nd ed. Monterey, Calif.: Wadsworth, 1984.

Caplan, G. *Principles of Preventive Psychiatry*. New York: Basic Books, 1964.

Carkhuff, R. *The Art of Helping*. Amherst, Mass.: Human Resources Development Press, 1973.

Carkhuff, R. *The Art of Helping IV*. Amherst, Mass.: Human Resources Development Press, 1980.

Carkhuff, R., and B. Berenson. *Teaching As Treatment: An Introduction to Counseling and Psychotherapy*. Amherst, Mass.: Human Resources Development Press, 1976.

Clark, C. C., and C. A. Shea. *Management in Nursing*. New York: McGraw-Hill, 1979.

Cohen, I. B. "Florence Nightingale." *Scientific American* 250: 3, March 1984.

Cunningham, M. A., and D. Baker. "How to Teach Patients Better and Faster." *RN* 86:50–52, Sept. 1986.

Darkenwald, G. G., and S. B. Merriam. *Adult Education: Foundations of Practice.* New York: Harper & Row, 1982.

Davis, A. Jann. *Listening and Responding.* St.Louis: C. V. Mosby Co., 1984.

Davis, Anne. "Informed Consent: How Much Information Is Enough?" *Nursing Outlook* 33:40–42, 1985.

Davis, Anne, and M. Aroskar. *Ethical Dilemmas and Nursing Practice.* Norwalk, Conn.: Appleton-Century-Crofts, 1978.

Doak, C. C., L. Doak, and L. Root. *Teaching Patients with Low Literacy Skills.* Philadelphia: J. B. Lippincott, 1985.

Douglas, T. *Group Processes in Social Work.* New York: John Wiley & Sons, 1979.

Dyche, June. *Educational Program Development for Employees in Health Care Agencies.* Tri-Oak Educational Division, 1982.

Egan, Gerard. *The Skilled Helper.* Monterey, Calif.: Brooks/Cole Publishing, 1975.

Elgin, S. H. *More on the Gentle Art of Verbal Self Defense.* Englewood Cliffs, N.J.: Prentice-Hall, 1983.

Elms, R. R., and R. C. Leonard. "Effects of Nursing Approaches During Admission." *Nursing Research* 15:39–48, Winter 1966.

Erikson, E. *Childhood and Society.* New York: W. W. Norton, 1950.

Falvo, Donna R. *Effective Patient Education: A Guide to Increased Compliance.* Rockville, Md.: Aspen Publishers, 1985.

Faulkner, A. *Recent Advances in Nursing 7: Communication.* New York: Churchill Livingstone Inc., 1984.

Furth, H. G. *Piaget for Teachers.* Englewood Cliffs, N.J.: Prentice-Hall, 1970.

Garvin, C. *Contemporary Group Work.* Englewood Cliffs, N.J.: Prentice-Hall, 1981.

Gayles, A. R. "Lecture vs. Discussion." *Improving College and University Teaching* 14:95–99, 1966.

Gelman, D., et al. "The Social Fallout from an Epidemic." *Newsweek,* August 12, 1985, pp. 28–29.

Glaser, P., R. Sarri, and R. Vinter, eds. *Individual Change Through Small Groups.* New York: Free Press, 1974.

Goffman, E. *Presentation of Self in Everyday Life.* Harmondsworth: Penguin, 1971.

Gordon, D. *Health, Sickness and Society.* St. Lucia, Queensland: University of Queensland Press, 1976.

Green, L. W., M. W. Kreuter, S. G. Deeds, and K. B. Partridge. *Health Education Planning: A Diagnostic Approach.* Palo Alto, Calif.: Mayfield Publ. Co., 1980.

Haimann, T., and W. G. Scott. *Management in the Modern Organization,* 2nd ed. Boston: Houghton Mifflin, 1974.

Hallal, J. C. "The Relationship of Health Beliefs, Health Locus of Control and Self-Concept to the Practice of Breast Self-examination in Adult Women." *Nursing Research* 31:137–142, 1982.

Harron, J., and J. Schaeffer. "DRGs and the Intensity of Skilled Nursing." *Geriatric Nursing* 7:24–25, 1986.

Herje, P. A. "Hows and Whys of Patient Contracting." *Nurse Educator* 5:30–34, 1980.

Hobson, W. *The Theory and Practise of Public Health,* 4th ed. London: Oxford University Press, 1975.

Holmes, T., and R. Rahe. "Social Readjustment Rating Scale." *Journal of Psychosomatic Research* 11:213–218, 1967.

Honey, Peter. *Solving People Problems.* London: McGraw-Hill, 1980.

Houston, B. K. "Control Over Stress, Locus of Control and Response to Stress." *Journal of Personality and Social Psychology* 21:249–255, 1972.

Inhelder, B., and J. Piaget. *The Growth of Logical Thinking from Childhood to Adolescence.* New York: Basic Books, 1958.

Ivey, A. E. *Microcounseling: Innovations in Interviewing Training.* Springfield, Ill.: Charles C. Thomas, 1971.

Janis, I. L., and J. Rodin. "Attribution, Control and Decision-Making: Social Psychology and Health Care." In G. C. Stone, F. Cohen, and N. E. Adler, eds., *Health Psychology: A Handbook.* San Francisco: Jossey-Bass, 1979.

Johnson, J. E., and H. Leventhal. "Effects of Accurate Expectations and Behavioral Instructions on Reactions During a Noxious Medical Examination." *Journal of Personality and Social Psychology* 29:710–718, May 1974.

Johnson, R. B., and S. R. Johnson. *Toward Individualized Learning.* Menlo Park, Calif.: Addison-Wesley, 1975.

Joint Commission on Accreditation of Hospitals. *Accreditation Manual for Hospitals.* Chicago: American Hospital Association, 1980.

Jung, Carl. *Psychological Types.* New York: Harcourt Brace Jovanovich, 1923.

Keirsey, D., and M. Bates, *Please Understand Me.* Del Mar, Calif.: Prometheus Nemesis Books, 1978.

Kirscht, J. P. and I. M. Rosenstock. "Patients' Problems in Following Recommendations of Health Experts." In G. Stone, F. Cohen, and N. Adler, eds. *Health Psychology: A Handbook.* San Francisco: Jossy-Bass Publ., 1980.

Klein, Donald. "Some Notes on the Dynamics of Resistance to Change: The Defender Role." In W. Bennis, K. Benne, R. Chin, and K. Corey. *The Planning of Change*, 3rd ed. New York: Holt, Rinehart & Winston, 1976.

Klevins, C., ed. *Materials and Methods in Adult Education*. New York: Klevins Publ. Inc., 1972.

Knowles, M. *The Modern Practice of Adult Education*. New York: Association Press, 1975.

Knowles, M. *The Modern Practice of Adult Education: From Pedagogy to Andragogy*. Chicago: Follett Publ. Co., 1984.

Knowles, M., et al. *Andragogy in Action*. San Francisco: Jossey-Bass, 1984.

Kübler-Ross, E. *On Death and Dying*. London: Tavistock, 1970.

Kübler-Ross, E. *Death—The Final Stage of Growth*. Englewood Cliffs, N.J.: Prentice-Hall, 1975.

Lau, R. "Origins of Health Locus of Control Beliefs." *Journal of Personality and Social Psychology* 42:322–334, 1982.

Lazarus, R. S. *Patterns of Adjustment*, 3rd ed., New York: McGraw-Hill, 1976.

Leahy, K., M. M. Cobb, and M. Jones. *Community Health Nursing*, 3rd ed., New York: McGraw-Hill, 1977.

Lefcourt, H. *Locus of Control: Current Trends in Theory and Research*. Hillsdale, N.J.: Lawrence Erlbaum Assoc., 1982.

Lefrancois, G. *Psychology for Teaching*. Belmont, Calif.: Wadsworth Publishing Co., 1975.

Lenz, Elinor. *The Art of Teaching Adults*. New York: Holt, Rinehart & Winston, 1982.

Lewin, K. "Group Decision and Social Change." In T. M. Newcomb, and E. L. Hartley, eds. *Readings in Social Psychology*. New York: Holt, Rinehart and Winston, 1947(a).

Lewin, K. "Frontiers in Group Dynamics." *Human Relations* 1:5–41, 1947(b).

Lewin, K., and P. Grabbe. "Principles of Re-education." In W. Bennis, K. Benne, and R. Chin. *The Planning of Change*. New York: Holt, Rinehart & Winston, 1966.

Longest, B. B. "Job Satisfaction for Registered Nurses in the Hospital Setting." *Journal of Hospital Administration* 4:46, May-June, 1974.

McGovern, W. N., and J. A. Rodgers. "Change Theory." *American Journal of Nursing* 86:566–568, 1986.

McKibbin, R., et al. "Nursing Costs and D.R.G. Payments." *American Journal of Nursing* 85:1353–1357, 1985.

Mager, Robert. *Preparing Instructional Objectives*, 2nd ed. Palo Alto, Calif.: Fearon Publ., 1975.

Maslow, A. H. "A Theory of Human Motivation." *Psychological Review*, July 1943, 370–396.

Maslow, A. H. *Toward a Psychology of Being*. Princeton, N.J.: D. Van Nostrand, 1962.

Maslow, A. H. *Motivation and Personality*, 2nd ed. New York: Harper & Row, 1970.

Mattoon, Mary Ann. *Jungian Psychology in Perspective*. New York: Free Press, 1981.

Merton, R. K. *Social Theory and Social Structure*. New York: Free Press of Glencoe, 1957.

Muldary, T. W. *Interpersonal Relations for Health Professionals: A Social Skills Approach*. New York: Macmillan, 1983.

Mumford, E., and J. K. Skipper. *Sociology in Hospital Care*. New York: Harper & Row, 1967.

Murray, R., and J. Zentner. *Nursing Assessment and Health Promotion Through the Life Span*. Englewood Cliffs, N.J.: Prentice-Hall, 1975.

Myers, I. *Manual: The Myers-Briggs Type Indicator*. Palo Alto, Calif.: Consulting Psychologists Press, 1962.

Narrow, B. *Patient Teaching in Nursing Practice*. New York: John Wiley & Sons, 1979.

National League of Nursing Education. *Standard Curriculum for Schools of Nursing*. Baltimore: Waverly Press, 1918.

Nightingale, F. *Notes on Nursing, What It Is and What It Is Not* (facsimile of 1859 edition). Philadelphia: J. B. Lippincott, 1946.

Northen, H. *Social Work with Groups*. New York: Columbia University Press, 1969.

Northen, H. "Psychosocial Practice in Small Groups." In R. W. Roberts, and H. Northen. *Theories of Social Work with Groups*, 2nd ed. New York: Columbia University Press, 1976.

Orlando, I. J. *The Dynamic Nurse-Patient Relationship*. New York: Putnam, 1961.

Peplau, H. E. *Interpersonal Relations in Nursing*. New York: Putnam, 1952.

Perls, Fritz. *The Gestalt Approach and Eye Witness to Therapy*. Palo Alto, Calif.: Science and Behavior Books, 1973.

Phares, E. J. *Locus of Control in Personality*. Morristown, N.J.: General Learning Press, 1976.

Polit, D. F., and B. P. Hungler. *Nursing Research: Principles and Methods*, 2nd ed. Philadelphia: J.B. Lippincott, 1983.

Pressey, S. L. "A Third and Fourth Contribution Toward the Coming Industrial Revolution in Education." *School and Society* 36:668–672, 1932.

Quelch, J. A. "Marketing Principles and the Future of Preventive Health Care." *Health and Society* 58:310–347, 1980.

Rakich, J. S., B. Longest, and T. O'Donovan. *Managing Health Care Organizations*. Philadelphia: W. B. Saunders, 1977.

Rankin, S. H., and K. Duffy. *Patient Education: Issues, Principles and Guidelines*. Philadelphia: J. B. Lippincott, 1983.

Redman, B. K. *The Process of Patient Education*, 5th ed. St. Louis: C. V. Mosby, 1984.

Ridgeway, V., and A. Mathews. "Psychological Preparation for Surgery: A Comparison of Methods." *British Journal of Clinical Psychology* 21:271–280, 1982.

Riehl, J. P., and C. Roy, eds. *Conceptual Models for Nursing Practice*, 2nd ed., Norwalk, Conn.:Appleton-Century-Crofts, 1980.

Robinson, Lisa. *Psychological Aspects of the Care of Hospitalized Patients*, 4th ed., Philadelphia: F. A. Davis Co., 1984.

Rogers, Carl. *On Becoming A Person*. Boston: Houghton Mifflin, 1961.

Rogers, Carl. *Encounter Groups*. Harmondsworth: Penguin, 1975.

Rogers, Martha. *An Introduction to the Theoretical Basis of Nursing*. Philadelphia: F. A. Davis, 1970.

Rosenstock, I. M. "The Health Belief Model." *Milbank Memorial Fund Quarterly* 44:94, 1966.

Rosenstock, I.M. "The Health Belief Model and Preventative Health Behavior." *Health Education Monograph* 2:354–386, 1974.

Rosenstock, I. M., and J. Kirscht. "Why People Seek Health Care." In G. Stone, F. Cohen, and N. Adler, eds. *Health Psychology: A Handbook*. San Francisco: Jossey-Bass, 1980.

Rosenthal, C., V. Marshall, A. Macpherson, and S. French. *Nurses, Patients and Families*. New York: Springer Publishing Co., 1980.

Rosenthal, R., and L. Jacobson. *Pygmalion in the Classroom*. New York: Holt, Rinehart & Winston, 1968.

Rothman, E., and N. Lloyd. *The Professional Nurse and the Law*. Boston: Little, Brown, 1977.

Rotter, J. "Generalized Expectancies for Internal Versus External Control of Reinforcement." *Psychological Monographs: General and Applied*. 80, 1966.

Saranson, S. *Caring and Compassion in Clinical Practice*. San Francisco: Jossey-Bass Inc., 1985.

Satir, Virginia. *Conjoint Family Therapy*. Palo Alto, Calif.: Science and Behavior Books, 1971.

Schein, E. H. "Interpersonal Communication, Group Solidarity and Social Influence." *Sociometry* 23:148–161, June 1960.

Schultz, Duane. *Growth Psychology: Models of the Healthy Personality*. New York: D. Van Nostrand, 1977.

Seligman, M. *Helplessness*. San Francisco: Freeman Press, 1975.

Selye, Hans. *Stress Without Distress*. New York: Lippincott & Crowell, 1974.

Sime, A. M. "Relationship of Preoperative Fear, Type of Coping, and Information Received About Surgery to Recovery from Surgery." *Journal of Personality and Social Psychology* 34:716–724, 1976.

Skinner, B. F. *The Behavior of Organisms*. Norwalk, Conn.:Appleton-Century-Crofts, 1938.

Skinner, B. F. *The Technology of Teaching*. Norwalk, Conn.: Appleton-Century-Crofts, 1968.

Smolensky, J. *Principles of Community Health*, 4th ed., Philadelphia: W.B. Saunders, 1977.

Sorensen, K. C., and J. Luckmann. *Basic Nursing: A Psychophysiologic Approach*. Philadelphia: W.B. Saunders, 1986.

Squyres, W. D., et al. *Patient Education and Health Promotion in Medical Care*. Palo Alto, Calif.: Mayfield Publ. Co., 1985.

Thorndike, E. L. *The Psychology of Wants, Interests and Attitudes*. Norwalk, Conn.:Appleton-Century-Crofts, 1935.

Travelbee, J. *Interpersonal Aspects of Nursing*. Philadelphia: F. A. Davis, 1966.

Tuckman, B. "Developmental Sequence in Small Groups." *Psychological Bulletin* 63:384–399, 1965.

Tulving, Endel. *Elements of Episodic Memory*. Oxford: Oxford University Press, 1983.

Wallston, B. S., K. A. Wallston, G. D. Kaplan, and S. A. Maides. "Development and Validation of the Health Locus of Control (HLC) Scale." *Journal of Consulting and Clinical Psychology* 44:580–585, 1976.

Waring, Judith, and James McLennan. *Community Health Nursing: Helping with Health*. Sydney: McGraw-Hill, 1979.

White, R., and K. Mitchell. "Goal Attainment: An Alternative Method of Treatment and Programme Evaluation." *Journal of the Australian and New Zealand Student Services Association*. Counselling Monograph 4, 1975.

Wiedenbach, E. *Clinical Nursing, A Helping Art*. New York: Springer, 1964.

Wingfield, A., and D. Byrnes. *The Psychology of Human Memory*. New York: Academic Press, 1981.

Wittig, Arno. *Psychology of Learning*. New York: McGraw-Hill, 1981.

Woldum, K.M., et al. *Patient Education: Foundations of Practice*. Rockville, Md.: Aspen Publishers, 1985.

Yura, H., and M. Walsh. *The Nursing Process*, 4th ed., Norwalk, Conn.: Appleton-Century-Crofts, 1983.

INDEX

Page numbers in italics indicate figures. Page numbers followed by t indicate tables. Page numbers followed by e indicate case examples.

Abdominal pain, 178e
Acceptance of help, 67
Accountability, 104, 256–257, 264
Accuracy of teaching materials, 148–149
Acquired Immune Deficiency Syndrome (AIDS), 45e
Activity group, in community, 205e
Adaptation, 91. See also *Stress.*
Administration of care facilities, costs affecting, 15–18
  gaining support for patient teaching in, 16–18, 17t
Admission teaching, 267–272
  background information for, 268
  evaluation of, 270–271
  goals and objectives of, 268, 269
  strategies and materials for, 270
Advice, consequences of giving, 173–176, 174–175e, 180
  handling requests for, 171–176
  ineffectiveness of, 124–125, 200, 220
Affective domain, 26. See also *Attitudes, complexity levels of; Learning process.*
AIDS, 45e
Alert, 55. See also *Stress response.*
Alzheimer's disease, 75–77e
American Hospital Association, 12. See also *Informed consent.*
American Nurses' Association (ANA), 11
Analyzer, 82–84. See also *Personality, dimensions of.*
Anxiety. See *Stress.*
  separation, 199, 284
Appointment cards, 146–147e. See also *Teaching materials, written.*
Arthritis, symptoms of, 177e
Assessment, patient, 8, *8*, 48, 53, 90–97, 96t. See also *Communication skill(s); Health balance; Nursing process, phases of; Social system.*
  CONE interview for, 97–100
  interpretation of, 95
  of complex problems, 181–182
  of mental alertness, 152–153
  of patient's beliefs, 43–46, 44t
  of problem-solving stage, 172–173
  of visual acuity, 152–153

Assessment data, collection of, 94–101
  for program development, 242–243, 258–259
  kinds and sources of, 95–97, 96t
  methods for, 75, 96t, 97–100
  objectivity in, 95
  "traps" in, 94–97
Attending, 71–74. See also *Communication, nonverbal.*
Attention, gaining learner's, 120, 144–145. See also *Lesson sequence.*
Attention span, 144, 161, 210
Attitudes, changes in, 53–54e, 158, 202
  complexity levels of, 26, 37t, 109t
  evaluation of, 232
  nurses', 69, 70t
  values expressed as, 42–43
Attribution. See *Locus of control.*
Audiovisual programs, 160–164
  preparation of, 160–162, 163–164e. See also *Programmed learning.*
  sources of, 162, 289–290
Authority and responsibility, 249, 254, 260, 264
Awareness, 172. See also *Problem solving, personal.*

Balance, dynamic, 90. See also *Health balance.*
Barriers to learning, 144–145, 152–153, 162
  environmental, 118
  in groups, 207
Behavior(s), 78, 235–236. See also *Trial and error learning.*
  analysis of, 133, 225, 226t, 234
  as part of learning objective, 105, 108, 120
  attending, 71–74. See also *Communication skill(s).*
  evaluation of, 228–231
  indicating stress, 53, 53–54e, 60–61, 79
  interpretation of, 5e, 6, 6e. See also *Teaching approaches, indirect.*
  nurse's, 72, 99, 131
  sociocultural support for, 47, 50–52, 109, 197
  trying out, 34, 210
  unmet needs and, 38–42, 45–46
  values and beliefs as basis for, 42–43

Behavior change, 21, 27, 125. See also *Change process; Learning process.*
  in group, 193, 210, 213
  observation of, 226–231
  sociocultural factors in, 50–51, 50e
Behavior modification, 224–226, 226t
Behavior rehearsal, 133, 138–139, 231
Beliefs, 42–46
  about control over health, 44t
  nurse's, 68, 70t, 95
Beta-blocking medication, 120–121e
Bloom, Benjamin, 26, 36–37, 37t, 109t
Brammer, L. M., 67
Breast self-examination, 152–153, *154–155*
Brown, Ester Lucille, 20

Caplan, Gerald, 56, 104, 104t
Cardiac catheterization, preparation for, 117e
Cardiopulmonary resuscitation (CPR), evaluating learning of, 228e, 229t, 230t
CARE, attending behaviors of, 71–74
  after open questions, 75
  Centered attention, 71
  Appropriate responsiveness, 71–72
  Relaxed posture, 72
  Eye contact, 72–73
  goals of. See *Goal(s) of care.*
Care facilities, administration of, 15–18
Carkhuff, Robert, 172–173, *172*, 196, 199
Challenge, 55–56. See also *Stress response.*
Change process, 21, 43–46, 103. See also *Behavior modification; Learning process.*
  in learning group, 203. See also *Group process.*
  in policies on patient teaching, 17–18, 243
  influenced by stress, 59–61, 107
  sociocultural influence on, 47, 50–51, 50e
  teaching as part of, 21, 103, 224, 234
Checklist(s), for developing education program, 257–265
  for evaluating behavior, 228e, 229, 229t
Children, communication with, 35–36
  cognitive development of, 35–36, 36t
  perception of needs by, 39
Children's Bureau, 19
Chronic disease, in elderly, 23
Closed circuit television, 143–144e. See also *Audiovisual programs.*
Closure, 80–81. See also *Personality, dimensions of.*
Coaching. See *Demonstration-coaching strategy; Teaching strategies.*
Color, 158. See also *Teaching materials, pictures and diagrams as.*
Committee, advisory, 246–247
  planning, 245–246
Communicable disease, beliefs about AIDS as, 45e
Communication, 3, 5–6, 117–118
  barriers to, 14, 14e
  congruence in, 69–70, 222–223

Communication (*Continued*)
  during discussion, 128
  in "expressive" role of nurse, 65
  learning skills in, 84, 135–139
  modeled by nurse, 208
  nonverbal, 70–74, 145, 171, 229, 232
  of CARE, 71–74
  of empathy, 69
  of genuineness, 69–70
  of openness, 68, 71
  of respect, 68–69
  of warmth, 68
  one-way, 160, 127
  qualities of interpersonal, 68–70, 117–118
  sociocultural determinants of, 72–73, 153
  teaching skills of, 178–179
  with children, 35–36
Communication skill(s)
  active listening, 67, 70–74, 73e, 127, 130. See also *CARE.*
  "minimal encouragement" in, 71, 76e
  closed questions in, 75
  collecting subjective data, 96, 97
  feedback in, 124, 222–223
  "following," 77, 77e
  group leadership in, 195
  handling complaints, 179–181
  helping with personal problem solving, 175. See also *Problem solving, personal.*
  open questions in, 75–77, 75–77e, 128
  program coordination, 255
Community care, coordination of, 278, 282–283
  for Alzheimer's patient, 75–77e
  goals of, 101–102
Community services, 92. See also *Health balance model, resources for; Group(s), community.*
Competition for patients, 22
Complaints, handling of, 179–181
Compliance, 34, 51, 56, 175
Computer-assisted instruction, 164–166
Computers in medical care, 22. See also *Technology.*
Conceptual development, in children, 36t
Confidentiality, of information, 67, 98, 268
Conflict, avoidance of, 253, 254, 257
  in groups, 198, 210. See also *Group process.*
  of values and beliefs, 43, 49–50
  skills in resolution of, 257
Confrontation. See *Nurse-patient interaction, confrontation in.*
Congruence, 69–70, 222–223. See also *Communication.*
Consensus, in learning group, 211. See also *Group process.*
  in planning committee, 246
Consent. See *Informed consent.*
Continuing education, for program manager, 257
  referral to, 215–216. See also *Group(s), community; Group(s), learning.*
Contracts, patient, 106, 234

Coordination, of education program, 254–255, 263–264
of patient teaching, 117, 117e. See also *Nursing intervention, coordination.*
Cost-effectiveness. See *Administration of care facilities.*
Counseling intervention, open questions in, 75–77, 116. See also *Nursing intervention, counseling.*
referral to, 182
CPR. See *Cardiopulmonary resuscitation.*
Creative thinking, 128, 198–199, 198–199e
Credibility, establishing, 122, 123, 246
Crisis, teaching during, 40–41e, 60–61, 174. See also *Stress response.*
Crisis intervention, 21, 57–59, 57–58e, 181. See also *Stress.*
listening behavior and, 74
Criteria, as component of objective, 105–106
Curriculum plan, for program, 247

Data collection, 75. See also *Communication skill(s); Assessment data.*
health balance and, 90–94. See also *Interview, CONE.*
"traps" in, 94–97
Decision making, based on informed consent, 13. See also *Patient participation.*
behavior rehearsal for evaluation of, 231
by trial and error, 33–34
in program planning, 247–249
personality influences on, 77–84
Defense mechanisms, 79
Defensiveness, in asking for help, 170, 170e
in nurse, 71
Deficits in health balance, 91. See also *Health balance.*
Delegation, of teaching, 117, 117e
Demonstration-coaching strategy, 131–134. See also *Teaching strategies.*
advantages of, 132
equipment for, 132, 158–159
evaluation of learning using, 228–231
failure of, 134
guidelines for, 133–134
levels of teaching by, 131
Dependence, 43
Depression, personality and, 82
Developmental prevention, 103–104. See also *Goal(s) of care.*
group goal of, 203
Diagnosis, nursing, 90, 100–101
requests for, responding to, 176–179
Diagnosis related groups (DRGs), 22
Diagrams, use of in teaching, 157–160. See also *Pictures and diagrams.*
Dimensions of personality. See *Personality, dimensions of.*
Discharge, early, 2, 22, 60, 193, 277

Discharge teaching, background information for, 284–285
evaluation of, 287
goals and objectives for, 285–287, 286t
remembering, 147, 147e
scope of, 284
strategies and materials for, 287
Discovery learning, 128. See also *Discussion strategy.*
Discussion strategy, 127–131. See also *Teaching strategies.*
advantages of, 128
audiovisual programs and, 161
experiential learning and, 136
goals and objectives for, 129
guidelines for, 129–130
in admission teaching, 270
in learning group, 211, 214t
preparing for, 128–129
recovering from failure of, 130
Disease prevention, history of, 18–19
Distress. See *Stress; Stress response.*
Domains of learning. See *Objectives, learning.*
DRGs, 22

Early discharge from hospital, 2, 22, 60, 193, 277
Education, nursing, 19
Education programs. See also *Program development.*
assessment phase of, 241–245
checklist for development of, 257–265
implementation phase of, 253–257
organizational phase of, 249–253
patient, 240, 240t
planning phase of, 245–249
Egan, Gerard, 66, 74
Emotion(s), expression of, 79. See also *Verbalization, of feelings.*
interference of, 67
Emotional disturbance, referral of person with, 182, 213–217
Emotional involvement, in learning, 125, 135, 146, 157
Emotional support, 82, 103, 135, 194, 201
by group members, 207
Empathy, 69. See also *Communication.*
Environmental factors, in learning, 67, 71, 79, 91, 103, 118, 144, 206. See also *Barriers to learning; Health balance.*
Erikson, Eric, 20
Ethical issues, 13, 13t, 21–22
Ethnic patterns, 47t, 48–50. See also *Social system.*
"Eustress," 55. See also *Stress response.*
Evaluation of learning, 219–238
errors in, 234–237
expectations of teacher in, 235–236
feedback in, 122, 221–226

Evaluation of learning (*Continued*)
  in admission teaching, 271–272
  in patient education program, 252
  objectivity in, 228–234
  observation of behavior in, 226–231
  of group process, 213
  verbal methods of, 231–234
Example, learning by, 33. See also *Role model;*
    Teaching approaches.
Exercises, experiential, examples of, 139–140
  guidelines for use of, 139. See also *Experiential*
    strategies; Teaching strategies and examples at
    the end of each chapter.
Experience, as factor in learning, *28*, 29, 32–38,
    35–36e. See also *Learning, principles.*
  beliefs and values based on, 42
  interpretation of need based on, 171
Experiential strategies, 134–141. See also
    Behavior rehearsal; Exercises, experiential;
    Teaching strategies.
  advantages of, 135
  microteaching and, 142
  preparation for, 135–136, 136e
Explanation strategy, 123–127. See also *Teaching*
    strategies.
  advantages of, 123
  guidelines for, 124–125
  lack of feedback in, 126–127, 126–127e
  length of, 126
  preparation for, 124
Exploration, preceding problem solving, 172,
    172, 176–177
Expression, facial, when listening, 72. See also
    Communication, nonverbal.
"Expressive" role of nurse, 65–66. See also
    Role(s) of nurse.
"External" locus of control, 43–44, 44t
Extrovert, 78–80
Eye contact. See *CARE; Communication, nonverbal.*

Facial expression, when listening, 72. See also
    Communication, nonverbal.
Family. See also *Social system.*
  educational program for, 203, 243–244e
  emotional support by, 103
  participation in learning by, 51, 105, 109–110,
    134
  primary relationship of, 48–50, 68
Feedback, 7, 221. See also *Communication;*
    Communication skill(s).
  correction and coaching using, 133, 223–224
  during teaching, 70, 121, 126, 194, 221–226,
    235, 271–272
  in Nursing Process system, 7, *8*
  in self-paced learning programs, 164
  interpreting, 222–223
  lack of, 126–127e
  motivation and reinforcement using, 224–226
  nurse to patient, 71

Feedback (*Continued*)
  sources of, 221–222, 221t
  to complainer, 180
  to program sponsor, 255–256
Feeling, verbalization of. See *Communication;*
    Verbalization, of feeling(s).
Films. See *Audiovisual programs.*
Financial issues, 15–18
Flip charts, 156. See also *Teaching materials.*
Frame of reference, patient's, 74. See also
    Communication skill(s).

"Games," computer, 165
  used in teaching, 139–140. See also *Exercises,*
    experiential.
"Yes, but...", 175
Genuineness, communication of, 69–70
Goal attainment, 227–231. See also *Evaluation of*
    learning; Objectives, learning.
Goal(s) of care, 102–104, 104t, 107, 107t. See
    also *Objectives, learning.*
  developmental prevention as, 103–104
  in patient education programs, 240
  maintenance as, 102–103
  patient objectives reflecting, 106
  primary prevention as, 103
  treatment as, 102
Governmental publications, sources of, 291–293
Group(s), community, 213–217
  health service, 217
  human relations and therapy, 216
  learning programs and continuing
    education, 215–216
  preparation of learner for, 215
  self-help and rehabilitation, 51, 216
  sources of information about, 213, 215
  learning, 193–196. See also *Group leadership;*
    Group process.
    advantages of, 194
    as preparation for teachers, 251
    communication skills in, 84
    conducting patient education program with,
      255
    for families of patients, 40–41e
    functions within, 195–196
    goals and objectives in, 195–196, 201–203
    planning and organizing, 200–208
    problem solving in, 198–199e
    selection of members for, 80, 83t, 203–206
    size limitation of, 206
    teaching patient care in, 278, 282
  multidisciplinary, 244e, 251
Group leadership, 208–213. See also *Group(s),*
    learning; Group process.
  in assessment and testing stage, 210–212
  in group formation stage, 209–210
  in problem solving stage, 212–213
  in termination stage, 213
  meeting organization and, 206–208

Group leadership (*Continued*)
  positive behaviors for, 208t
  teaching strategies for use in, 214t
Group process, 196–208. See also *Group leadership; Group(s), learning.*
  behaviors that promote, 208t
  evaluation of, 213
  interaction patterns during, 198
  preparation of members for, 204–206, 205e
  special approaches to, 200
  stage of, assessment and testing of, 197–198
    group formation, 186–197
    problem solving, 198–199
    termination, 199

Health, definitions of, 90
Health balance, 8
  assessment of, 90–94, 181–182
  CONE interview using, 99–100
  factors that influence, 90–92
  goals of care determined by, 102–104
  restoration of, 60, 178, 178e
  spontaneous teaching and, 169
Health balance model, *91*
  advantages of, 92–93, 95, 101
  application of, 92–94, 92–93e
    to planning learning groups, 201–203
  resources for, 92, 93e, 101t
  strengths in, 92, 93e, 101t
  stressors in, 91, 93e, 101t
  unmet needs in, 91, 93e, 101t
Health belief model, 45–46
  elements of, 45t
Health education pamphlets, 152, *154–155*. See also *Teaching materials, written.*
Health locus of control, 43–44, 44t
Health promotion, 2, 8. See also *Wellness.*
Health service groups, 217. See also *Groups, community.*
Help, acceptance of, 67
Helplessness, 43–44
  learned, 43
  perception of, 56–57, 179, 203, 276
  personality and feelings of, 81–82
Historical perspective, on patient teaching, 18–23
History, patient's. See *Assessment data, collection of.*
Holmes, T., 53
Home care, 194. See also *Community care; Patient care procedures.*
Homeostasis, 52. See also *Health balance; Stress response.*
Hospital care, changes in, 2, 16. See also *Discharge, early; Medical care.*
Hypertension, learning to manage, 35–36e

Iatrogenesis, 102
Identification, with patient, 69
Illustrations. See *Pictures and diagrams; Teaching materials.*

Immunization, introduction of, 21
Indirect teaching. See *Teaching approaches, indirect.*
Individuality of patient, in stress response, 60–61
Industrial Revolution, 19
Infantile paralysis (polio), 21
Influence, nurse's, 57, 60–61. See also *Stress response.*
Informal teaching. See *Spontaneous teaching.*
Information, requests for, handling, 171–176
  social acceptability of, 170, 170e
Informed consent, 11–13, 13t
Instructions, giving, 186, 186e
  writing, 156–157. See also *Teaching materials, written.*
"Instrumental" role of nurse, 65–66. See also *Role(s) of nurse.*
Insurance, third party reimbursement and, 250t, 261
Interaction, nurse-patient. See *Communication; Communication skill(s); Nurse-patient interaction*
Intervention, nursing. See *Nursing intervention, Nursing Process.*
Interview, assessment, 97–100. See also *Assessment, patient; Assessment data, collection of.*
  comparison with discussion, 129
  CONE, 97–100, 116
    health balance as basis of, 99–100
    introducing patient to, 98
    preparation for, 97–98
    steps in, 98–99
Introvert, 78–80
Issues, economic, in program development, 243, 250

Jargon, inappropriate use of, 68, 125, 205
Job satisfaction, 40. See also *Need(s), perception of.*
Joint Commission on Accreditation of Hospitals (JCAH), statement on informed consent by, 11
Jung, Carl, 78

Knowledge, as basis of teaching, 116–117
  evaluation of, 232. See also *Evaluation of learning.*
  levels of complexity in, 37t, 109t. See also *Objectives, learning.*
Knowles, Malcolm, 32, 60
Kubler-Ross, Elisabeth, 57

Language barrier, 153. See also *Teaching materials, written.*
Leadership, group, 208–213. See also *Group leadership.*
  styles of, 254–255

Learned helplessness, 43–44

Learning, principles of, 31–32, 31t, 34–38, 47, 52, 66
  styles of, 80

Learning complexity, levels of, 26, 37t, 108–109, 109t, 232. See also *Objectives, learning.*

Learning goals, identifying, 101–108. See also *Goals of care; Learning process.*

Learning needs, determining, 89, 96. See also *Assessment, patient; Objectives, learning.*

Learning process, 27–31. See also *Group process.*
  factors that influence, *28,* 28–31, 224
  identifying goals and stating objectives, 101–108
  in children, 35–36
  Lewin's model of, 27–28
  modelling or example in, 32–34, 131
  motivation and, 38–42
  perception of need in, 38–42, 42t
  phases of, 27
  progression from simple to complex in, 34–38
  reinforcement and practice in, 131, 161
  role of experience in, 135
  trial and error in, 33–34
  sociocultural context of, 30–31, 46–52, 92–93, 109, 125
  stress and, 55–57, 59–61

Learning sequence and style, 81. See also *Personality, dimensions of; Lesson sequence.*

Lecture, 123. See also *Explanation strategy; Teaching strategies.*

Legal issues in patient teaching, 10–13, 227. See also *Informed consent; Patient's rights.*

Lesson plan, 111, 112t. See also *Nursing intervention, teaching.*

Lesson sequence, steps in, 119–123

Lewin, Kurt, 27–28

Life-style, changes in, 203, 211. See also *Stress.*

Life-support systems, ethical issues and, 21–22

Listening skills, active. See *CARE; Communication skill(s), active listening.*

Locus of control, 43–44, 44t

Mager, Robert, 105

Maintenance, goal of, 201–202. See also *Goal(s) of care.*

Management, nursing, 22

Management, program, 256–257. See also *Program development.*

Manipulation, 69, 184, 225

Marketing, of educational programs, 250–251, 250t, 261

Maslow, Abraham, 20, 27–28, 38–42, *39,* 55–56

Media, use of, 251. See also *Marketing, of educational programs.*

Medical care, coordination of, 14, 14e, 15
  learning how to seek, 178–179
  technology and specialization in, 13–15, 22
  use of computers in, 22

Medicare, 22

Medication, teaching about, 120–121e

Memory, stimulation of, 145–146, 151, 157

Mental alertness, 152–153. See also *Assessment, patient.*

Micro-social world, 48. See also *Social system.*

Microteaching, 142. See also *Experiential strategies.*

Mind-body connections, 177–178, 177e

"Minimal encourage to talk," 71. See also *Communication skill(s).*

Modeling or example, 32–33. See also *Experience; Role model.*

Motivation, assessment of, 119. See also *Assessment, patient.*
  to learn, 38–42. See also *Need(s), perception of; Readiness to learn.*
    concern as expression of, 183, *183*
    effect of beliefs on, 43–46, 45e
    in adults, 39–40
    in group setting, 194, 203–206
    Maslow's hierarchy of needs, *39*
    role of stress on, 56–61
    through reading, 153

Multiple sclerosis, 73e

Multiple-session teaching, 111. See also *Nursing intervention, teaching; Program development.*

Narrow, Barbara, 8, 237

National League for Nursing, 19

Need(s), affect motivation, 38–42
  health beliefs and, 45–46
  learning, identification of, 8, 20, 95
    perception of, 38–46, 169
  nurse's influence on, 29–31, *29,* 42t
  referral based on, 214
  sociocultural aspects of, 47–50
  stress and, 40–41e, 56–57, 59
  teaching priorities based on, 44, 106, 119, 124, 171

Negotiation, in problem management, 257. See also *Program development.*

Nightingale, Florence, 19

Nonclosure, 80–81. See also *Personality, dimensions of.*

Non-compliance, 34, 51, 56, 175

Nonverbal communication, 70–74. See also *CARE; Communication skill(s).*

Northen, Helen, 196

Nurse(s), roles of. See *Role(s) of Nurse.*

Nurse-patient interaction, 68–70. See also *Communication; Communication skill(s); Trust relationship.*
  confrontation in, 127, 130, 184, 223
  developing trust and rapport in, 117–118, 222
  in assessment, 46, 95
  in preparation for learning group, 205
  in problem solving, 178, 178e

Nurse-patient interaction (*Continued*)
  in teaching, 3–6, 75, 97, 128, 158, 194, 210
    by experiential strategies, 135–141
  personality affecting, 83
  planned to meet needs, 40–41e, 41, 42t
  questions used in, 75–77, 75–77e
  readiness to learn and, 29–31, *28, 29*
Nurse Practice Acts, 11
Nurse teachers, specialized, 110
Nursing Care Plan, 105, 107, 107t
Nursing diagnosis, 90, 100–101
Nursing education, 19
Nursing intervention, 9, 67. See also *Nursing Process.*
  coordination, 14, 15
  counseling, 9, 65–66
  factors influencing, 3, *3*, 59–61, 101
  referral, 182–183, 182–183e
  teaching, 7–10, 65–66, 107, 108–112
    at patient admission, 267–272
    at patient discharge, 284–288
    patient care procedures, 277–283
    preoperative or pretreatment, 272–277
Nursing management, 22
Nursing practice, principles of, 20
Nursing Process, 6–10. See also *Nursing intervention.*
  combination of roles in, 65–66, *66*
  feedback in "system" of, 221, *221*
  phases of, 7–8, *8*
    assessment, 94–95, 97–100
    evaluation, 220
    planning, 106–107
  relationship of teaching to, 89, 185
Nursing roles. See *Role(s) of nurse.*
Nursing theory, development of, 20–22

Objectives, learning, 8, 44, 104–108, 120–121, 220
  complexity of goal in, 26, 37, 37t, 107t
  components of, 105
  for education program, 244e, 248
  importance to evaluation of, 122, 235
  of teaching materials, 150
  patient responsibilities reflected in, 105–106
Objectives of patient care, 9–10e, 106–107. See also *Goal(s) of care.*
Objectivity in evaluation, 228–234
"Organizer," definition of, 120
  use of, 120–121, 120–121e, 151, 161

Pamphlets. See *Teaching materials, written.*
Pasteur, Louis, 19
Patient care planning, goals of care in, 102–107
  guided by patient responsibilities, 108
  using health balance model, 92–94

Patient care procedures, teaching, 277–283
  background information for, 278–279
  evaluating, 282–283
  goals and objectives for, 279–280, 281t
  strategies and materials for, 282–283
Patient contracts, 106, 234
Patient education materials, sources of, 289–290
Patient education programs. See *Education programs; Program development.*
Patient participation, in behavior analysis, 225. See also *Contracts, patient.*
  in decision making, 2, 60, 89. See also *Self-care.*
  in learning, 115–116, 119, 121–122, 140, 203–206
Patient rights, 2, 12. See also *Informed consent.*
Patient self-responsibility, as goal of teaching, 89, 130, 132, 133
Patient teaching, issues influencing, 10–18
  administrative, 15–18
  ethical, 13, 13t, 21–22
  legal, 10–13, 227
  medical care, 13–15
Performance standards, of skills, 132, 133. See also *Objectives, learning.*
"Personal space," invasion of, 72
Personality, dimensions of, 77–84, 83t, 95, 130
  analyzer-personalizer, 78, 82–84, 83t, 223
  closure-nonclosure, 78, 80–81, 83t
  extrovert-introvert, 78–80, 83t
  sensate-intuitive, 78, 81–82, 83t
Personalizer, characteristics of, 82–84, 223
Philosophy, of patient education programs, 247–249, 248e
  nursing and, 21
Piaget, Jean, 35–36, 36t
Pictures and diagrams, guidelines for, 158–159, *159*
  sources of, 159–160
  use of, 157–160
Planned or prepared teaching, 4
Policies, organizational, changes in, 17–18, 17t
  on patient teaching, 16–18
Polio, 21
"Positive regard, unconditional," 68. See also *Communication.*
Postpartum patient, health balance of, 92–93e
  nursing diagnosis for, 101
  patient care objectives for, 106
Posture, while listening, 72. See also *Communication, nonverbal.*
Power and control, personal, 43–44, 69, 75, 81–82, 115, 127, 132
Power struggles, avoiding, 249, 259
PRECEDE model, 241–242, *242*
Prenatal patient, uncommunicative, 126–127e
Preparation for surgery, on videotape, 163–164e
Pretest, use of, 120
Prevention, 2, 103–104. See also *Goal(s) of care.*
  beliefs about, 45–46, 45e
  primary, 103, 202

Primary social relationships, 48–50, 68
Principles of learning, 31–32, 31t, 34–38, 47, 52, 66
Privacy, physical, 67–68, 81. See also *Confidentiality*.
Problem(s), sharing of, 66–67. See also *Verbalization, of feelings*.
Problem solving, based on informed consent, 13
  effect of stress on, 55–56
  in learning groups, 196, 211–113
  influence of personality on, 77–84
  learning through, 7–8, 34, 101, 135
  of complex problems, 181–183
  personal, 172–173, *172*, 180–181
Procedures, in patient education program, 252–253, 252–253e
Program development, 239–266, 240t
  assessment phase of, 241–245
    checklist for, 258–259
    identifying resources for, 242–243
    PRECEDE model for, 241–242, *242*
  implementation phase of, 253–257
    checklist for, 263–265
    coordination of, 254–255, 263–264
    problem management in, 257–259, 264–265
    quality control and accountability of, 255–256, 264
  organizational phase of, 249–253
    checklist for, 261–263
    deciding on procedures in, 252–253, 262–263
    marketing in, 250–251, 250t, 261
    preparation of staff in, 250–252, 261–262
  planning phase of, 245–249
    checklist for, 259–260
    committee for, 245–247, 259–260
    decisions to be made during, 247–249, 260
Program Evaluation and Review Technique (PERT), 243–244, 259
Programmed learning, 165–166, *165*. See also *Audiovisual programs*.
Projectors, overhead, 156. See also *Teaching materials*.
Psychological "safety," while learning, 135, 212, 237
Psychology, contribution of, 20
Public health, history of 19–21
Public relations, effect of on patient teaching, 17–18, 248–249, 254
Publications, government, sources of, 291–292
"Pygmalion effect." See *Self-fulfilling prophecy*.

Quality control, in education program, 256–257, 264
Quality of life, patient's, 241, 248, 258
Question(s), answered by evaluation, 220
  asked of nurse, 171
  for understanding complex problem, 181
  in patient assessment, 97–100, 102–104

Question(s) (*Continued*)
  ineffective, 126
  to evaluate learning, 231–234
  to explore problems, 176–177
  use of "open," 75–77, 76e, 124, 129. See also *Communication skill(s)*.
Questionnaires, 100, 120, 232–233, 272
  statistical analysis of, 233

Rahe, R., 53
Rapport, establishing. See *Communication skill(s)*; *Trust relationship*.
Rating scales, 229–231, 230t. See also *Evaluation of learning*.
Readiness to learn, assessment of, 117–118
  factors in, 28–31
  influences on, 42–46, 50–51, 59–61, 96
  nurse's impact on, 28–31, *28, 29*
  perception of need in, 38, 169, 173
  "unfreezing" and, 27
Reading ability, assessment of, 153
Record keeping, 94, 96, 104–105
Records, patient-kept, 231, 234
Red Cross, American, 19
Referral, of complex problems, 182
  to community groups, 213–217
"Refreezing." See *Change process*.
Rehabilitation unit, patient teaching in, 139–140
Reinforcement of learning, 74, 121–122, 146. See also *Learning process*.
  in behavior modification, 225, 226t
Relationship(s), primary. See *Social system*.
  "therapeutic," 21
  trust. See *Trust relationship*.
Relationship skills. See *Communication skill(s)*: *Nurse-patient interaction*.
Research, 233, 248–249, 260. See also *Evaluation of learning*.
Resistance to learning, 59–61. See also *Learning process*.
Risk-taking, during learning, 135, 140
Rogers, Carl, 68
Role model, nurse as, 5–6, 33, 49, 131–134, 208
Role(s) of nurse, 21–23, 65–66, *66*, 75–77, 80, 129, 168, 177, 179, 222–226, 265
  as advocate of patient teaching, 16–17, 17t
  as "expert," 125, 127
  as group leader, 198, 204, 209–210, 212
  during role play, 136, 136–137e
  teaching, 3, *3*
Role play, 136–138. See also *Experiential strategies*.

Self-care, preparation for, 2, 21, 67, 131–134, 207
Self-concept and self-esteem, 47, 60
Self-fulfilling prophecy, 235, 236e. See also *Evaluation of learning*.

Self-paced learning programs, 164–166
Self-responsibility, patient, 89, 130, 132, 133
Seligman, Martin, 43
Selye, Hans, 52–53, 56
Separation anxiety, 199, 284
Skills, levels of. See *Learning complexity, levels of.*
Skinner, B. F., 225
Slides, as a teaching material, 164. See also
    Audiovisual programs.
Social relationships, primary, 48–50, 68
Social system, components of, 47t, 48–50
    ethnic patterns and cultural values in, 48–50
    medical and health care as a, 47t, 49
    primary relationships in, 48–50, 68
    secondary influences in, 48
Spanish language materials, sources of, 290–291
Specialization, 13–15, 22
Spiral, learning, 34–35. See also *Learning process.*
Sponsorship, of educational program, 248–249,
    254, 256, 260. See also *Program development.*
Spontaneous teaching, 4–5, 170–171, 184–189
    about seeking medical help, 178–179
    when advice or information requested, 171–
        176, 268
    when complaints involved, 179–181
    when complex problems involved, 181–184
    when diagnosis requested, 176–179
Staff development units, as resource for nurse-
    teacher, 157, 162, 251–252, 261–262
Statistical analysis of tests and questionnaires,
    233
Stereotypes and prejudices, 69, 83, 235–236. See
    also *Beliefs; Values.*
Stimulus-response learning, 33. See also *Learning
    process.*
Stress, definition of, 52–53
    effect of on learning, 6, 30–31, 52–61, 70,
        107, 144
    influence of on attitudes, 53–54e, 79, 179–181
    management of hypertension and, 35–36e
    reduction of, 53–54e, 56, 60–62, 119
Stress gauge, four levels of, 54–57, 55
    causing crisis, 57
    causing threat, 56, 284
    environmental, 79
    learning as, 59–60, 197, 199
Stress response, levels of, 55–59, 55
    to learning and change, 59–61, 136, 141
    variability of, 54–59, 91
Stressor(s), definition of, 52–53
Styles of leadership, 254–255
Styles of learning, 80
Surgery, exploratory, and nonverbal behavior,
    73e

Taxonomy, of learning complexity, 37t, 108–
    109, 109t
Teaching, preoperative or pretreatment, 272–
    277

Teaching (*Continued*)
    preoperative or pretreatment, background
        information for, 273–274
    evaluating, 276–277
    goals and objectives for, 274–276, 275t
    strategies and materials for, 276
Teaching approaches, indirect, 5–6, 49
    prepared or planned, 4, 88
    spontaneous, 4–5, 117
Teaching materials. See also specific teaching
        materials designated by *
    accuracy of, 148–149
    *audiovisual programs as, 160–164
    choosing appropriate, 145–150, 270, 276, 280,
        282, 287
    content and organization of, 149–150, 152,
        154–155
    for use in learning groups, 210, 211, 214t,
        252, 262–263
    individualizing, 147–148, 150
    *pictures and diagrams as, 157–160
    review of, 148–150
    *self-paced learning programs, 164–165
    sources of, 289–293
    written, 120–121e, 150–157
        advantages of, 151–152
        guidelines for reviewing and choosing, 152–
            156, *154–155*, 223
        preparation of, 156–157
        presentation of, 40–41e, 156, 161, 205, 252
Teaching plan, 112t. See also *Lesson plan.*
Teaching strategies. See also specific teaching
        strategies designated by *.
    choosing appropriate, 55, 60–61, 116–123,
        270, 276, 280, 282, 287
    combining, 119, 146–147
    for learning groups, 210, 211, 214t
    using *demonstration-coaching, 131–134, 224
    using *discussion, 127–131
    using *explanation, 79, 83t
Teaching styles, formality and structure in, 115–
    116
Technology, effect of on patient teaching, 14–
    15, 14e, 20–23
Television, closed circuit, 163–164e
Tests, statistical analysis of, 233
    to evaluate learning, 232–233, 277. See also
        Evaluation of learning.
Time, limitations in teaching, 118–119
    required for group teaching, 197, 198, 202,
        207
    required for individual teaching, 110, 124,
        130, 132, 136
"Total patient care," 7, 30
Trial and error learning, 33–34. See also
    Learning process.
Treatment, goal, 201. See also *Goals of care.*
Trust relationship, advantages of, 122, 135,
    140–141, 177
    encouraging development of, 66–70, 86, 93,
        99, 117–118, 270

"Unconditional positive regard," 68. See also
Communication.
Unplanned teaching. See Spontaneous teaching.
Unmet needs. See Need(s), perception of.

Validity, of evaluation measurement, 229
Values, conflict of, 38, 42–48, 68, 210. See also
Beliefs.
Verbalization, of feelings, 73–74, 75, 75–77e,
82–83, 95–96, 146. See also Communication
skill(s); Nurse-patient interaction.
  as feedback during learning, 129, 130, 136,
  136–137e, 140, 213
  in personal problem solving, 172, 179–181,
  198

Videotapes, 228–231. See also Audiovisual
programs.
Visual acuity, 152–153, 233. See also Assessment,
patient.

Warmth, quality of, 68
Wellness, 2, 89, 90, 94, 201. See also
Developmental prevention; Health balance.
World Health Organization, definition of health,
90
World War II, influence on nursing, 19–20
Written teaching materials, 150–157, 252. See
also Teaching materials, written.